Career Development for Health Professionals

Career Development for Health Professionals

LEE HAROUN, MA, MBA

Formerly director of Maric College and
Regional Director of Education for Quest Education Corporation

W.B. SAUNDERS COMPANY
A Harcourt Health Sciences Company
Philadelphia London New York St. Louis Sydney Toronto

W.B. SAUNDERS COMPANY
A Harcourt Health Sciences Company
The Curtis Center
Independence Square West
Philadelphia, Pennsylvania 19106

Library of Congress Cataloging-in-Publication Data

Haroun, Lee.
Career development for health professionals / Lee Haroun.
p.; cm
ISBN 0-7216-8454-8
1. Medical personnel—Vocational guidance. I. Title.
[DNLM: 1. Health Personnel. 2. Career Choice. 3. Vocational Guidance. W 21 H292c 2001]
R690.H377 2001
610.69—dc21 00–067950

Publishing Director: Andrew Allen
Acquisitions Editor: Maureen Pfeifer
Editorial Assistant: Erin Nihill
Production Manager: Donna L. Morrissey

CAREER DEVELOPMENT FOR HEALTH PROFESSIONALS ISBN 0-7216-8454-8

Printed in the United States of America

Last digit is the print number: 9 8 7 6 5 4 3 2 1

To Dad, Bob, and David –

Thank you for your love, encouragement, and support.

Preface

This book was written as the result of the author's desire to assist health care students achieve four important goals that will improve the quality of their own lives and make meaningful contributions to the lives of others:

1. Complete their educational programs
2. Think like health care professionals
3. Find the right jobs
4. Attain long-term career success

Many students who begin health care studies with great enthusiasm drop out when they discover that they lack some of the study and organizational skills necessary for academic and career success. This book shows students that becoming a health care professional begins as soon as they start school and that many of the skills needed for academic success are the same as those needed on the job.

The need for competent, thinking health care professionals has never been greater. Health care is one of the fastest growing industries in the United States. Helping students succeed in their programs has the larger benefit of providing society with the competent, caring employees needed to fill the growing number of positions available.

Content

Career Development for Health Professionals is divided into two major sections. The first, consisting of Chapters 1–7, introduces students to the world of health care and teaches them the life-management and study skills essential for learning and working successfully in various health care occupations.

- Understanding what it takes to be a competent and caring health care professional
- Planning and preparing ahead for employment success
- Developing a positive attitude and effective personal organizational skills
- Taking effective notes
- Reading to learn
- Conducting research efficiently
- Improving writing skills
- Preparing to take tests successfully
- Overcoming math anxiety
- Getting the most from lab classes and clinical experience
- Communicating and working effectively with others
- Applying productive problem-solving techniques

The second section, consisting of Chapters 8–13, focuses on job search skills and how to achieve and maintain career success.

- Locating job leads
- Creating an appealing resume
- New trends, such as using the Internet and preparing a scannable resume
- Presenting oneself effectively and confidently at interviews
- Increasing the chances of being hired
- Becoming a valued employee
- Keeping career progress on course

All information is current and based on interviews with health care employment personnel and employers.

The book is written in a conversational, reader-friendly style. Much of the material is organized into list formats for efficient reading and later reference. Tables and charts are also used to summarize information to make it easier for students to study and review. Examples from a variety of health care occupations illustrate how concepts are applicable on the job.

Special Features

Each chapter contains a variety of features to help students benefit fully from the material.

- *Learning Objectives* that focus on the most important success skills and provide direction for both students and instructors
- *Key Terms* that include definitions to ensure understanding of important concepts and ideas
- *Quotes* to inspire, motivate, and promote thinking
- *Take a Moment to Think* questions to encourage students to explore their own ideas about important concepts
- *Prescription for Success* exercises to provide students with a wide variety of opportunities to apply the ideas presented, collect additional information, and develop their skills

How to Use This Book

This book is designed to be flexible and meet a variety of textbook needs. It can be used in a number of courses and learning contexts:

- Orientation and study skills classes for new students
- Introductory health care courses
- Professional development courses
- Job search courses
- Academic refresher and review classes for math, writing, and communication
- As a supplement to health care specialty courses to expand the coverage of oral and written communication skills; provide a math review; teach note-taking, research, and test-taking strategies; and enhance personal organization and problem-solving skills
- Independent study in which students are assigned to work on the development of specific skills

Instructor's Manual

The accompanying Instructor's Manual is designed to help busy instructors make the most of the text. It includes the following features:

- Suggestions for organizing courses
- Chapter lesson plans
- Ideas for class activities
- Transparency masters
- Forms to copy for student exercises
- Supplemental instructional resources
- Chapter quizzes

Message to Students

The author's professional career has been devoted to working in education and helping students achieve their goals. It is her sincere desire to help you succeed in school and in life. The purpose of this book is to provide you with the tools to become your best and realize your dreams.

One of life's most exciting discoveries is learning that you can achieve almost anything you are willing to work for. Accepting responsibility for your own choices and actions empowers you to create your own life. This book contains many of the tools that will help you make positive choices and achieve academic, personal, and career success.

To make the best use of these tools, the author suggests the following:

1. Trust yourself. You have the power and ability to succeed.
2. Be willing to try new ideas. If something in the book looks like "too much trouble" or even a little crazy, give it a try anyway.
3. Don't be overwhelmed by the number of ideas and suggestions in each chapter. They are intended to cover a wide range of learning styles, personal preferences, and student needs. You are not expected to do all of them, but to choose the ones that work best for you.
4. Put forth your best efforts when doing Prescription for Success exercises. Use them as opportunities to learn, not as "must-do's" necessary to complete an assignment and get a grade.
5. Apply the ideas to your own life. The material is meant to be practical, not simply topics to read about and discuss in class.

Start now to become a competent, caring health care professional who will enjoy a satisfying career while making a positive contribution to the lives of others.

Acknowledgments

The author wishes to express sincere thanks to those who provided the valuable suggestions necessary to ensure the completeness and accuracy of a project this size. They include the following professionals who have dedicated their careers to providing education or employment services for today's students and tomorrow's professionals: Sharon Ackroyd, Brenda Bracken, Victoria Courtney, Mary Ann Crone, Melva Duran, Sandra Madges, Sue Royce, Debbie Schroller, Carol Walters, and Sandi Watson.

Contents

1

Your Career Starts Now

OBJECTIVES

THE INFORMATION AND ACTIVITIES IN THIS CHAPTER CAN HELP YOU TO:

- ➢ Explain the meaning of the sentence "Study skills are job skills."
- ➢ Give five examples of study skills that can help you to succeed in school, obtain the job you want, and increase your worth as a health care professional.
- ➢ Identify and describe what you consider to be the benefits and responsibilities of a health care professional.
- ➢ Explain the purpose and content of the SCANS competencies and National Health Care Skill Standards.
- ➢ Identify skills and attitudes you believe you need to develop more fully.
- ➢ Describe what you believe patients expect from health care professionals.
- ➢ Use visualization techniques and affirmations to help you achieve your academic and professional goals.
- ➢ List ways that you can maximize your school experience.

KEY TERMS

Affirmation: A positive statement created to describe a characteristic or possession you want to have. A form of self-talk, affirmations are repeated out loud. The use of affirmations has been shown to help people become or have what they verbalize.

Attitude: Your mental approach to any situation. Attitudes are often referred to as being either positive or negative and affect the way you approach life. They are under your control and can be improved if you work to become aware of them and want to make changes.

Career ladders: The organization of occupations or positions that are in a related field and involve progressively higher levels of skill and responsibility. Additional education or training is usually needed in order to move up the ladder. In physical therapy, for example, the ladder starts with physical therapy aide and moves up to physical therapist assistant and physical therapist.

Certification: Documentation from a recognized professional organization that you have acquired the knowledge and demonstrated the skills necessary to perform satisfactorily in a specific occupation. Earning certification often requires taking written and/or hands-on tests.

Commitment: Dedication to something, such as an idea, a relationship, or an organization. It includes taking the action necessary to follow through with your beliefs. Fulfilling commitments requires focus and persistence.

Competency: A skill that is performed well enough to meet preestablished standards. This term often refers to job skills, such as "correctly perform a blood draw" and "accurately fill out an insurance claim form."

Confidentiality: Refers to keeping something absolutely private. For example, a patient's medical records are confidential. Patients' information cannot be shared with anyone who is not directly associated with their care unless the patients have given written permission for its release.

Consequence: The result of taking a certain action. Consequences can be either positive or negative.

Empathy: Understanding the experiences and feelings of another person by considering a situation from his or her point of view. This is often described as feeling *with* others and requires good listening skills and paying careful attention to what others say and do. The verb describing the action of acting with empathy is "to empathize."

Ethics: Concepts of right and wrong that guide ideal behavior. Ethics are developed and agreed upon by groups of people such as the citizens of a country or members of a religious organization. In health care, the principal ethical rule is that all patients are entitled to competent care. Professional health care organizations have developed codes of ethics that set **standards** of professional conduct for members.

Ethnic: Referring to the customs and behaviors practiced by a specific racial or national group of people as distinguished from other groups. The word is commonly used to describe groups that are not part of the majority group of a society. For example, "ethnic restaurants" in the United States refer to those serving nontraditional American cooking, such as Chinese or East Indian. On the other hand, in Japan, McDonalds is an ethnic restaurant!

Habits: Actions or ways of thinking that are developed over time and become automatic, without thought. With effort, negative habits can be recognized and changed, and positive habits can be formed.

Informational interview: A meeting with someone who works in the career field in which you are interested. The purpose is not to obtain a job, but to ask questions and learn as much as possible about the nature of work in a specific area, such as nursing. The information gathered is used to make informed career decisions and prepare for employment success.

Integrity: Behavior that is based on honesty, sincerity, and good intentions. We refer to people who strive to always do the right thing as "having integrity."

License: Legal approval given to professionals to ensure that only those who are properly trained can perform duties that might cause harm to others. Licenses are granted by governmental bodies and require that applicants meet specific educational requirements and pass tests to demonstrate their competence.

Prioritize: To determine which is the most important of a group of items. For example, if you have a number of tasks that must be completed in a limited amount of time, you prioritize by listing the tasks in order from most to least important.

Reason: To organize facts so that they make sense and help you to draw correct conclusions. In math, this means to use the facts given in a problem correctly to arrive at the answer. On the job, reasoning is used to review a situation, collect facts, and choose the best course of action.

Self-esteem: The way people see themselves and the opinions they have about their appearance, competence, intelligence, and other characteristics.

Standard: A predetermined measure, such as a test score, of the quality of a performance or behavior. Some standards are stated as the minimum levels that meet safety requirements. Others are set at higher levels to serve as goals for achieving one's best.

Visualization: A technique in which you create detailed pictures in your mind of something you want to have or become. For example, if you are studying respiratory therapy, you create an image of yourself working as a successful respiratory therapist. Research has shown that people tend to become, in reality, what they first create in their imaginations.

First Step on the Road to Success

Today is the first day of the rest of your life.

Congratulations! Choosing to study for a career in health care is the first step toward achieving a productive and satisfying future. You have made a significant **commitment** to yourself and your community. By enrolling in an educational program, you have demonstrated that you have the ability to set your sights on the future, make important decisions, and follow through with action. You have proven that you have the strong personal foundation on which you can build the skills and habits that will help ensure your success in school and in your career.

The purpose of this book is to help you be successful in this building process by sharing the knowledge and techniques that have helped other students achieve their goals. It is written with the hope that you will apply what you learn here to maximize your investment in education, secure the job that you want after graduation, and find satisfaction in your career as a competent and caring health care professional.

Connecting School and Career

The process of becoming a health care professional began the day you started classes. Much more than learning technical skills, this process involves acquiring the attitudes, personal characteristics, and habits of a successful professional. What you think and do while in school will determine, to a great extent, the quality of the professional you will become. Your career has indeed started *now.*

The skills described in this book to help you succeed in school can also be applied to your professional and personal life. In fact, the term "study skills" is misleading, because skills are not isolated sets of activities that are restricted to school situations. They have many applications on the job. Let's look at four examples of skills that can be applied to your studies, the job search process, and your future work in health care.

1. *Time management.* For busy people, time is one of their most precious possessions (Table 1–1). Juggling class attendance and study time with family responsibilities, work, and time for yourself involves **prioritizing** and careful planning. Your success in school is heavily influenced by how well you organize your time.

An effective job search typically requires that you devote time each day to identifying leads, making appointments, attending interviews, and carrying out follow-up activities. You must allocate adequate amounts of time for these efforts and organize your time to avoid delays that could cost you employment opportunities.

The effective use of time is critical in health care work. Some professionals are responsible not only for their own time, but also for planning that of others. Medical assistants are often in charge of the physician's daily appointment scheduling, a task that can affect the profitability of the practice. Insurance coders and billers must submit claims on time to avoid rejections and financial losses. Nurses have patient care responsibilities during designated hours, and it is essential that they plan a schedule that permits them to see every patient on their shift.

2. *Oral communication.* Strong communication skills are essential to success (Table 1–2). Expressing yourself clearly is important for giving presentations in class, as well as for asking and answering questions in class. It also contributes to your ability to establish and maintain satisfactory relationships with your instructors and classmates.

A critical part of the job search process is the interview, in which you combine your abilities to think clearly and use verbal skills effectively. Feeling confident about your ability to express yourself will allow you to present your qualifications in a convincing way.

All jobs today demand good communication skills. This is particularly true in health care because you will constantly interact with others, including patients, coworkers, supervisors, and the general public. Physical and occupational therapy

TABLE 1–1 ***Applications of Time Management Skills***

School	Job Search	Career
Plan study schedule	Pursue leads without delay	Schedule and track patient appointments
Attend classes on time Meet deadlines for assignments Prepare for exams	Schedule interviews Arrive for appointments on time Keep track of interviews and other appointments	Balance work, family, and personal needs Allocate time for patient treatments Arrive for work on time
Balance school and job schedules	Send thank-you notes promptly	Follow facility schedules
Allocate time for family	Follow up in a timely way	Schedule time for continuing education activities

TABLE 1–2 ***Applications of Oral Communication Skills***

School	Job Search	Career
Ask questions in class Answer questions in class Present oral reports Share information with classmates	Make telephone inquiries about job openings Introduce yourself to potential employers Ask questions of potential employers Present your qualifications at interviews	Participate in staff meetings Give instructions to patients Relay information to coworkers Present reports to supervisor

assistants, for example, are among the many health professionals who do extensive patient education. The effectiveness of their explanations of exercises and self-care techniques influences the time it takes their patients to return to normal activity.

3. *Taking notes.* You may think of notetaking as being limited to use in lecture classes, but this skill is used extensively outside the classroom. During the job search, it will be important to record information about openings accurately, along with interview appointment dates and times and directions for locating facilities. After interviews, you may want to make notes about the job requirements, additional information you need to send the prospective employer, and other facts that are important to remember.

When you become employed, you will be expected to absorb a great deal of new information about your facility's rules and procedures, the location of supplies and equipment, people's names, and many other details. You can use your notetaking skills to create a personal reference notebook, a resource that will increase your efficiency on the job. Furthermore, notetaking is an important health care job skill. Many professionals are responsible for interviewing patients and taking notes on special forms called "patient histories." Another specialized form of medical notetaking is called "charting." This involves writing notes on patient medical records which include information about symptoms, treatments, and medications prescribed. Both procedures impact patient care and require total accuracy. Their quality depends on the professional's notetaking ability (Table 1–3).

4. *Taking tests.* You may think that you have escaped the dreaded test once you leave school, but tests are just one form of evaluation. The truth is that life is full of tests. Job interviews are a form of test designed to assess your ability to present yourself and your qualifications. Many health care fields, such as nursing, radiology, and physical therapy, require that you pass a professional exam before you can work at certain occupational levels.

Once on the job you are, in a sense, being tested every day. While you may not think of your everyday tasks as tests, they are applications of what you have learned, and your ability to perform them correctly will be noted by your patients, coworkers, and supervisor. The annual employee performance evaluation is the formal documentation of this continual assessment of your work. Learning to perform "when it counts" is a valuable skill and represents the ultimate ability to take and successfully pass a test (Table 1–4).

You can see that the skills traditionally labeled as "school skills" have valuable applications during the job search and on the job. Throughout this book we will continue to point out ways that school skills are in fact valuable job skills.

TABLE 1–3 ***Applications of Notetaking Skills***

School	Job Search	Career
Take notes during lectures Write instructions during lab demonstrations List important ideas when reading	Write down facts about job openings Note times, directions, and other information about interviews List facts learned during interviews	Fill out medical history forms Accurately record phone messages Make notes on patient charts

TABLE 1–4 ***Applications of Test-Taking Skills***

School	Job Search	Career
Take daily quizzes	Pass professional exam	Perform your daily work accurately and competently
Review and take final exams	Present self successfully at interviews	Participate in annual performance evaluations with supervisor
Demonstrate practical skills	Answer interviewer's questions	It's all a test!

Success Is More Than Grades

An important thing to keep in mind is that school success is much more than simply earning good grades. Many students believe that students with straight As will always get the best jobs. This is not necessarily true. Students who *only* have good grades, without developing other important success skills, are not likely to keep the jobs they do get. Long-term success is determined by many factors.

Students who have mastered the study habits and memory techniques needed to perform well on written exams may earn high grades, along with high hopes for landing and keeping a great job. But if they lack other key characteristics, such as consideration for others, effective time management, and the ability to problem-solve, they will be disappointed. Patients, it turns out, will not ask to see your grade transcript. Most employers don't either. But both of them *do* ask that you arrive on time, treat them with consideration, and communicate clearly. Mastery of facts is not enough for today's health care professional. More than test performance, you must demonstrate effective job performance.

The Nature of Work in Health Care

Health care is a complex, ever-changing field that offers both opportunities and challenges for those who choose to work in it. The more you know about the nature of modern health care delivery and what is expected of professionals, the better you can prepare for your future. As you read through the following sections, think about how the information presented corresponds with your own ideas and how it fits your expectations of the future.

SOURCES OF SATISFACTION IN HEALTH CARE WORK

1. *Meaningful work.* Good health is a basic need for both human survival and happiness. Working in a field that promotes health gives you the opportunity to make meaningful contributions to the well-being of others. Whether you provide direct patient care or perform supporting activities, your work has a direct impact on patients, and the quality of your work can truly make a difference in their lives. A career in health care has a valuable and meaningful purpose.

2. *Opportunity to serve.* People seek the services of health care professionals when they need help. They come with the hope that you can help them solve their problems, and they entrust themselves to your care. You have opportunities to enter both the physical and emotional space of others, sharing close personal contact. People who are ill or injured are often afraid and anxious. You are in a position to influence their recovery.

3. *Career stability.* The need for health care will always exist, even if job titles change over time. The reorganization that is taking place in today's health care delivery systems is causing continual shifts in the need for specific occupational positions. A decrease in the number of job openings for one position is usually balanced by an increase in another. While you may need to redefine your job in the future, you will always have a solid knowledge base on which you can add the experience or training needed to qualify for new positions.

4. *Interesting work environment.* The world of health care is changing at a rapid rate, both scientifically and organizationally. Advances in our understanding of how the body works, along with discoveries about the causes and treatments of diseases, are reported almost weekly. Computers have increased our capacity to collect and organize information, as well as providing us with a sophisticated tool that is itself

constantly being upgraded. You will witness advances in knowledge that will extend and improve the quality of human life. The health care environment is never boring. There will be a steady stream of interesting information to learn, apply, and use to stimulate your imagination.

5. *Opportunities for advancement.* The health care field offers many opportunities for upward mobility if you are willing to continue learning and adding to your skills. Many jobs offer opportunities for on-the-job learning that enable you to increase your value to your patients and employer, as well as your eligibility for promotion. In addition, many occupational specialties in health care present the chance for **career laddering.** This refers to the organization of job titles that move upward to progressively higher-level positions that require more knowledge and increasingly complex skills. The higher-level positions almost always require further education and additional **certifications** or **licenses.**

RESPONSIBILITIES OF WORK IN HEALTH CARE

1. *Take your work seriously.* The health care worker who has direct patient care responsibilities has the potential to affect the well-being of those patients, both positively and negatively. How well you perform your duties is of critical importance, and you must ensure that you master and conscientiously apply the knowledge and skills necessary for your job. Some tasks, such as the administration of medications, literally have life and death implications. Less dramatic perhaps, but very important, are the results of work carried out in the business section of a health facility. Medical and financial record keeping can seriously impact the efficiency and success of a health care delivery system.

2. *Serve as a positive role model.* Americans have traditionally relied heavily on the medical community to solve their health problems. We have now conquered many of the infectious diseases that used to be the primary causes of death. Today's top killers in the United States—cancer, heart disease, and stroke—are greatly influenced by lifestyle choices such as diet, exercise, smoking, and the use of drugs and alcohol. Society is realizing that individuals must take more responsibility for their own health and that health care workers must take an active role in promoting sound health habits. Many professional organizations formally recognize the importance of their members serving as role models and have prepared statements outlining these responsibilities.

Excerpts from "Role Model Statement for Respiratory Care Practitioners"*

As health care professionals engaged in the performance of cardiopulmonary care, the practitioners of this profession must strive to maintain the highest personal and professional standards. A most important standard in the profession is for that practitioner to serve as a role model in matters concerning health.

The respiratory care practitioner shall support research in all areas where efforts could promote improved health and could prevent disease.

The respiratory care practitioner shall serve as a physical example of cardiopulmonary health by abstaining from tobacco use and shall make a special personal effort to eliminate smoking and the use of other tobacco products from the home and work environment.

3. *Be dependable.* Patients depend on health care professionals to deliver the services they need in a timely way. They cannot wait for care, and it is critical that you can be relied on to be present and punctual. High-quality care requires consistency, and your work habits significantly impact the effectiveness of the health care team.

4. *Keep current.* The changes that make work in health care interesting also demand that you continually keep up with advances in your field. Some developments, such as the increased use of computers, have made it necessary for professionals to learn new skills. In addition to new discoveries and technologies, recent

* Prepared by the American Association of Respiratory Care

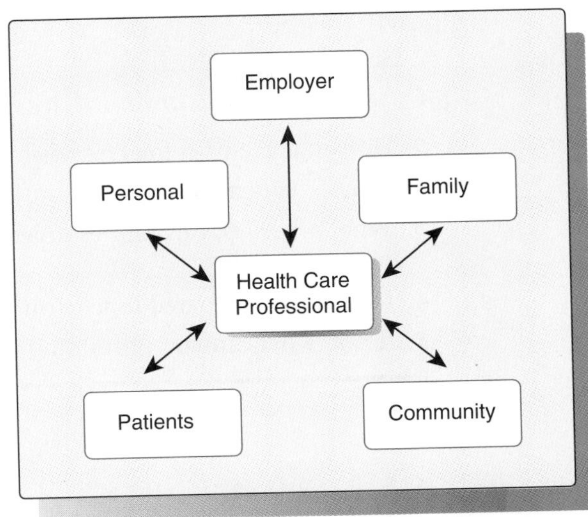

FIGURE 1–1 Health care professionals must meet a variety of needs.

reorganization of the health care industry has expanded many job titles to include duties not previously assigned to them. For example, medical assistants are now expected to master the intricacies of medical insurance coding and billing. And the extended duties of respiratory therapists include performing electrocardiograms (EKGs), drawing blood, stress testing, and keeping records of charges to patients. All health care professionals must keep up with increasing numbers of government regulations. You can count on changes occurring in your future job requirements, and you must be willing to adapt and learn new skills.

5. *Act professionally.* The term "professionalism" is used to describe the appearance and behavior expected of someone in a work situation. Professionals guide their actions by the responsibilities demanded by their positions. In health care, this means that you apply all your efforts to performing your duties in a competent and caring manner. It means that you put the needs of patients above your own and always act in their best interest, even under difficult and stressful circumstances. It means that you work cooperatively with your coworkers and contribute willingly to team efforts (Fig. 1–1).

The practices of health care professionals can have significant human and legal consequences, so an important component of professionalism is to always think about what you are doing on the job. Nothing is routine, and you can never take your duties for granted. You must give your work constant attention, carefully apply your knowledge and skills, and know when to ask for help from your supervisor or coworkers.

PRESCRIPTION FOR SUCCESS 1–1

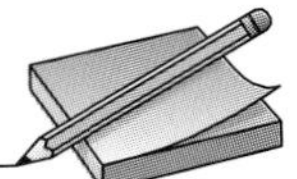

Let's Hear from You

1. Why did you choose a career in health care?
2. What do you hope to contribute?
3. What do you hope to accomplish?
4. What do you know about the requirements of health care occupations in general? Your occupational area?
5. What do you know about current trends in health care?
6. How do you think these trends might affect your future work?

PRESCRIPTION FOR SUCCESS 1–2

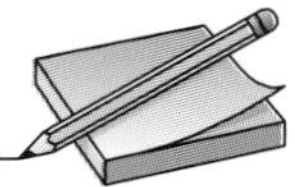

Consider the Responsibilities

1. Do you agree with the responsibilities listed?
2. Why or why not?
3. What other responsibilities do you believe are required of health care professionals?
4. Do you feel prepared to take on these responsibilities?
5. If not, what can you start doing now to become prepared?

PRESCRIPTION FOR SUCCESS 1–3

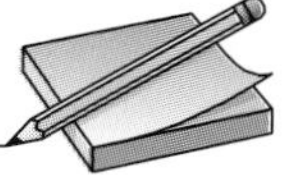

Knowing Ahead Gives You the Edge

Research your targeted career to see how it has changed over the last twenty years. To gather information, interview someone who has worked in the field for several years, contact the appropriate professional organization, and speak with the instructors at your school.

1. Does it require more training than it did in the past?
2. Have new duties and responsibilities been added? Deleted?
3. Have licensing or certification requirements been added or changed?
4. What changes are anticipated for the future?
5. How can you start preparing now to be ready for these changes?

What Do Employers Want?

In recent years, employers in all industries have expressed concerns that entry-level workers are not adequately prepared for the modern workplace. They seek job candidates who are not only qualified technically, but who bring essential supporting skills such as the ability to communicate effectively, work cooperatively with others, accept responsibility, and problem-solve. These skills are especially critical in the health care industry, because it is service-based and depends heavily on the quality of its personnel. This is even more true today as health care facilities strive to provide higher-quality care at lower costs.

BOX 1–1. SCANS REPORT HIGHLIGHTS

Employers want workers who can:

Think creatively
Make decisions
Solve problems
Continue to learn
Reason
Identify, organize, plan, and allocate resources
Work with others
Acquire and use information
Understand complex interrelationships
Work with a variety of technologies
Be responsible
Believe in self-worth
Demonstrate **empathy**
Manage themselves
Demonstrate **integrity** and honesty

SCANS REPORT

In the late 1980s, a commission appointed by the U.S. Secretary of Labor conducted a nationwide employer survey to determine the **competencies** needed by all entry-level workers. The resulting report compiled and organized these needs into a format known as the SCANS Competencies (SCANS stands for "Secretary's Commission for Achieving Necessary Skills") (Box 1–1).

Earlier in this chapter, we discussed how the sets of skills commonly referred to as study skills can be applied to all areas of your life. Look at the SCANS Competencies and you will see that the same is true for them. For example, acting with integrity means that you set high standards for yourself as a student and do your own work to complete assignments and take exams; that you present yourself honestly in job interviews and apply for only those positions for which you are competent; and that you never cut corners when working with patients and fellow workers.

PRESCRIPTION FOR SUCCESS 1–4

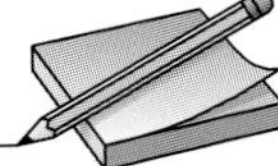

Self-Assessment

How would you rate yourself on each of the SCANS Competencies? Fill out the following self-assessment guide as a first step in creating an action plan to fully develop the competencies most needed in the modern workplace. Check the column that best describes you.

	Often	*Sometimes*	*Not Often*
1. Creative thinking: I generate new ideas and come up with original approaches to everyday problems and situations.	___	___	___
2. Decision making: I gather lots of information, identify alternatives, consider **consequences,** select an alternative, and evaluate the effectiveness of the results.	___	___	___
3. Problem solving: I recognize problems that need attention, identify possible solutions, create a plan, and carry out the plan.	___	___	___
4. Continuous learning: I am interested in knowing everything I can that will help me succeed in my work and life, and I try to keep up with advances that will help me to do so.	___	___	___
5. Reasoning: I understand relationships between ideas and am able to apply them when learning and solving problems.	___	___	___
6. Responsibility: I am dependable and complete any tasks that I am given or for which I volunteer.	___	___	___
7. Self-worth: I believe in myself and my ability to succeed.	___	___	___
8. Empathy: I try to understand the experiences and feelings of others and see situations from their point of view.	___	___	___
9. Self-management: I set personal goals, monitor my progress, and use self-discipline to ensure that I achieve them.	___	___	___

continued

PRESCRIPTION FOR SUCCESS 1–4 (*continued*)

	Often	*Sometimes*	*Not Often*
10. Integrity: I guide my actions by a set of principles that defines right and wrong.	___	___	___
11. Honesty: I tell the truth to myself and to others.	___	___	___

PRESCRIPTION FOR SUCCESS 1–5

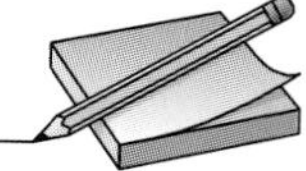

How Did You Rate Yourself?

Review the ratings you gave yourself in the previous exercise.

1. Do any areas need further development?
2. Which ones?
3. What can you do now to work on these areas?

Review the completed assessment periodically to monitor your self-development as you complete your educational program. Prescription for Success exercises later in the book will build on your answers to Prescription for Success exercises 1–4 and 1–5.

NATIONAL HEALTH CARE SKILL STANDARDS

A project of special interest to future health care professionals is the creation of the National Health Care Skill Standards, a list of entry-level worker competencies (Box 1–2). Like the SCANS Competencies, they include many personal habits and behaviors that can be applied to a wide variety of occupations. And they are not limited to purely technical expertise but include the ability to communicate, maintain good attendance, and demonstrate responsibility.

BOX 1–2. EXAMPLES OF THE NATIONAL HEALTH CARE SKILL STANDARDS

Health care workers will:

- Exhibit personal skills such as good attendance, time management, and individual responsibility.
- Maintain professional conduct and appearance.
- Understand accepted **ethical** practices with respect to cultural, social, and **ethnic** differences within the health care environment.
- Encourage the practice of preventive health behaviors among their clients.
- Communicate effectively, both orally and in writing.
  - Know the various methods of giving and obtaining information.
  - Understand how to explain planned procedures and goals to clients.
  - Understand how to communicate client information within a team.
  - Understand the need for precise, accurate, and timely reporting.
  - Interact effectively and sensitively with all members of the health care team.

BOX 1-3. WHAT'S NEEDED? A WORD FROM HEALTH CARE PROFESSIONAL ORGANIZATIONS

American Association of Respiratory Care

"If you want to join this field, you must be sensitive to the needs of patients who have serious physical impairments. You must work well as a member of a team. You need superior communication skills to deal with other members of the health care team, your patients, and their families. The ability to pay close attention to detail and to follow instructions are prerequisites for practitioners. Since much of your work will center on the equipment you use, you should have an interest in learning the mechanics of medical technology."

American Academy of Physician Assistants

The types of people who should consider becoming a physician's assistant should:

"Enjoy helping people
Want to learn and grow
Want a challenging and rewarding career
Want responsibility
Want to make a difference."

American Society of Podiatric Medical Assistants

"Enjoy contact with people and a willingness to help them . . . the ability to do neat and precise work . . . good manual dexterity . . . along with cooperativeness, good judgment, and a pleasant personality are valuable and necessary assets for a successful podiatric assistant."

American Pharmaceutical Association

"Qualifications:

Professional demeanor
Ability to respect **confidentiality** of patient data
Strong communication skills
Courteous **attitude**"

Did you notice how many standards mention the ability to communicate well? The lack of effective communication skills among health care workers is reportedly the leading contributor to patient dissatisfaction and personnel problems in health care facilities. Your future success can be greatly enhanced by your ability to listen and convey information effectively.

PROFESSIONAL ORGANIZATIONS

Most professional organizations for specific health care occupations have prepared statements outlining the characteristics needed to work in their fields (Box 1-3). Notice how certain requirements appear again and again.

INFORMATIONAL INTERVIEWS

Conducting **informational interviews** gives you opportunities to learn more about the specific needs of employers in your career area, the skill requirements, and the everyday duties performed by professionals. Supervisors, as well as working professionals, are excellent sources of information. The goal of this type of interview is *not* to seek employment; it is only to seek information. You may already know someone who you would like to interview. If not, ask your instructor or the career services department (sometimes called "job placement") at your school for suggestions. If you are a student member of a health care professional organization, this can be a good source of leads.

Once you have a contact, call and make an appointment. Explain that you are a student and want to learn more about your career area. Be considerate of the person's time, and if he or she is very busy, ask if you can schedule fifteen or twenty minutes. Arrive a few minutes early and dress professionally. Take along a list of prepared questions and a small notebook and pen. Here are some suggestions of questions for a supervisor:

1. What skills are most important to be successful as a ______?
2. What personal characteristics do you look for in a candidate seeking work as a ______?
3. What type of work is performed by a ______ in your facility?
4. What type of orientation or on-the-job training is given to new employees?
5. What is your best advice for someone who is interested in becoming a ______?
6. What learning and promotional opportunities are available for professionals who work as ______?

Examples of questions to ask a working professional include:

1. What are the typical duties of a ______?
2. What percentage of the day is usually spent on each duty?
3. Describe a typical day. (Is there a typical day? If not, describe a typical week.)
4. How many patients do you see in a day? How many tests do you perform? How many reports do you transcribe?
5. How much independent decision making is required?
6. What is most challenging about your work?
7. What is most satisfying about your work?

To keep a record of what you hear, take brief notes during the interview or summarize the information as soon as possible afterward. What did you learn? Did you gain any new insights? What else do you need to find out? What do you need to concentrate on while you are in school? Be *sure* to send a thank-you note to the person you interviewed.

PRESCRIPTION FOR SUCCESS 1–6

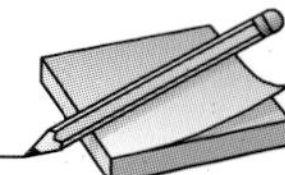

Conduct an Informational Interview

1. Make an appointment with a health professional or supervisor.
2. Prepare at least ten questions.
3. Conduct the interview.
4. Write a summary report of your findings.
5. Send a thank-you note.

PRESCRIPTION FOR SUCCESS 1–7

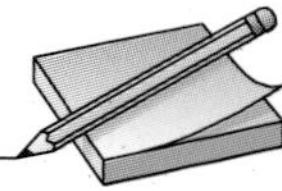

The Ideal Candidate

1. Imagine yourself as a busy pediatrician who runs a clinic in a low-income neighborhood. You need to hire a medical assistant. You have found a candidate who appears to have the necessary technical skills and experience. List other characteristics you think would be important. Explain why you chose them.
2. Explain how understanding the needs of employers can help you to better prepare for your future career.
3. Which of your own personal qualities do you believe will be of most value to future employers?

BOX 1-4. WHAT DO PATIENTS WANT?

Clear communication
Competent care
Courtesy
Empathy
Understanding

What Do Patients Want?

Patients want to receive competent care delivered with consideration and respect. When seeking health care, people are often at their most vulnerable. They fear what might be discovered during a diagnostic test or that they will experience pain during a necessary treatment. The **self-esteem** of patients can be threatened by the feeling of powerlessness that usually accompanies illness and injury.

Many patients want to participate in decision making regarding their care. They have the right, both ethically and legally, to be fully informed about their conditions, treatment options, and possible outcomes. Health care professionals must give clear explanations in everyday language and offer patients the opportunity to ask questions and receive honest answers. At the same time, they want and have the legal right to confidentiality, and you must be willing to guard the privacy of your patients. Nothing can be discussed with anyone other than the health care team members directly involved with a patient's care, and all files and paperwork must be securely stored.

Changes in American society and the development of managed care organizations, designed to control medical costs, have brought special challenges for patients as well as for health care professionals. In the past, many people had the same physician throughout their lives. Doctor and patient belonged to the same community, and a sense of trust developed over the years. Patients today may see a different physician each time they visit their health care facility. They may face a serious illness or life-threatening situation in the care of a stranger, adding to the stress of an already difficult situation. Studies have shown that patients who belong to a caring, supportive community recover more successfully than patients who don't. Providing a supportive health care community can improve patient outcomes. As a health care professional, you can demonstrate a caring attitude and help develop a bond of trust with patients by being attentive, listening carefully, and practicing empathy.

Health care professionals today face the challenge of working with patients from many different ethnic backgrounds, some of whom have beliefs about health care practices that differ from those of traditional Western medicine. Patients also come from many different economic and social groups, races, and religions. They may have lifestyles or personal beliefs with which you disagree. Regardless of your opinions about individual patients, they all have the right to be respected and receive appropriate, high-level care. Every patient deserves your best efforts.

Patients seek help in solving their health problems, but your responsibilities in meeting their needs go beyond performing a painless blood draw, giving effective breathing treatments, or sending out accurate bills for payment. You must be willing to combine caring with technical competence, treating each patient as worthy of your full attention (Box 1-4).

PATIENT'S BILL OF RIGHTS

Health care organizations have formally recognized the rights of patients to receive proper care. The American Hospital Association has written a "Patient's Bill of Rights" which many health care facilities nationwide have adopted. These include, among others, affirmation of patients' rights to:

- be treated with consideration and respect

- receive clear and complete information on which to base decisions regarding treatment
- be assured privacy and confidentiality
- participate in making decisions regarding their care, including the right to refuse treatment
- receive continuity of care

PRESCRIPTION FOR SUCCESS 1–8

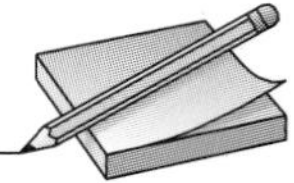

And the Patient Is . . . YOU

Imagine that you have arrived at an urgent care facility with a suspected broken arm. You were out for an enjoyable Sunday afternoon, skating with friends, when you hit a hole in the pavement and fell. Your arm is very painful, and you are worried about your ability to work if you end up in a cast.

1. Describe how you would feel if you found yourself in this situation.
2. How would you hope to be treated by the health care professionals at the urgent care center?
3. What would be most important to you?
4. What would be least important to you?
5. Did you learn anything from this exercise that might affect your approach to working with future patients?

PRESCRIPTION FOR SUCCESS 1–9

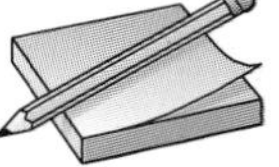

Create an Occupational Portrait

Use the information from your informational interview, the National Health Care Skill Standards, and the appropriate professional organization (see Appendix 1) to prepare a summary report about your future career. Include the following:

1. Major responsibilities.
2. Typical duties performed.
3. Skills and personal characteristics required.
4. Job outlook and salary information.
5. Sources of continuing education.
6. Promotional opportunities.

Creating a Successful Future

You have to take life as it happens, but you should try to make it happen the way you want to take it.—Old German saying

Human beings have the unique ability to create their own lives. They can generate ideas, form mental images, and plan ways to achieve what they imagine. You have generated the idea of becoming a health care professional and have completed the first step toward achieving that goal by enrolling in school. Whether you graduate and find satisfactory employment will depend on your belief in your ability to succeed and your willingness to take the necessary actions to achieve your goals.

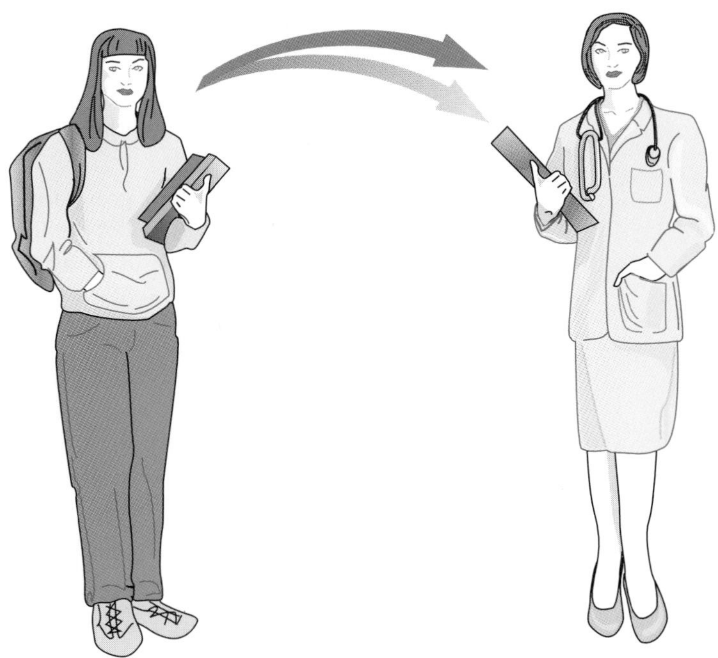

FIGURE 1–2 You create your future.

Henry Ford, who not only created fame and riches for himself but changed the history of transportation, is quoted as saying, "Whether you think that you can, or you can't, you are right." The tendency for people to get what they expect is known as the "self-fulfilling prophecy." In a classic test of the power of expectations, a group of first-grade teachers were given two lists of students at the beginning of the school year. They were told that the first list contained the names of children who had been identified as "high achievers," while the second contained the names of "low achievers." The final grades of the children's progress at the end of the school year closely reflected their reported abilities: most "high achievers" earned As, and most "low achievers" earned Ds. In reality, these students were not necessarily either but had been randomly selected for the experiment. Perceptions were proven to shape reality. This applies to what we believe about ourselves.

You can use this principle as you begin your career journey. All achievements begin as ideas, and what you picture mentally can become your reality. Positive images of you succeeding as a student act as powerful motivators. In addition to visual suggestions, your self-talk influences your success—or lack of it. We are continually holding internal conversations that either provide encouragement ("I know I can pass this test" or put ourselves down ("I'll never be able to get this report finished"). By taking control of the pictures and words in your mind, you can apply their power to help you create the life that you want.

Visualization is one popular technique for harnessing this power. If your goal is to become a medical assistant, create a detailed mental picture of yourself working as a professional (Fig. 1–2). See yourself preparing instrument trays, working with the physician, and talking with patients. Try the technique for yourself by following these steps:

I. Find a quiet, private place where you won't be disturbed.

II. Close your eyes.

III. Imagine yourself as a ______ (occupation of your choice).

  A. Create the details. Attempt to make the image as real as possible.

    1. What are you wearing?
    2. Who are your coworkers?
    3. What is the setting? Hospital? Physician's office? Business office?

4. What are you doing? Interacting with a patient? Performing a procedure? Working on a computer?

B. Create positive thoughts and feelings for yourself in the scene. You are competent. You work well with patients and coworkers. You like what you are doing.

IV. Try to keep your scene going for a few minutes. Make it as specific as possible and keep filling in the details. The idea is to have a clear, firm image of yourself carrying out the duties of your chosen profession.

V. Repeat this exercise regularly. Think of it as your own television series, with you as the star. Give your program a name.

A second technique for creating the future you want involves filling your self-talk with positive statements. These statements are called **affirmations,** and, like visualizations, they are based on the principle that we become what we first create in our minds (Box 1–5).

To create and use affirmations effectively:

1. State them in the present tense.
2. Include your name.
3. Keep them positive.
4. Say them aloud several times each day.

Write your affirmations on cards to carry with you or post them in an area where you will see them every day. The important thing is that you remember to repeat them regularly over a period of time.

PRESCRIPTION FOR SUCCESS 1–10

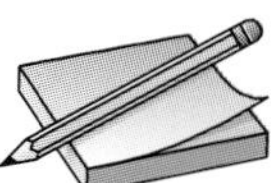

Give It a Try

1. Do a visualization exercise. It may feel strange at first, but this technique has helped many people achieve their goals. Concentrate on seeing yourself as clearly as possible. Fill in the details such as how you get to work, what you are wearing, your interactions with others, and the duties you are performing.
2. Write three affirmations and repeat them each day for the next week.

In addition to visualization and affirmations, there is a third technique based on the idea that you can realize your goals by conducting yourself as if you've already achieved them (Fig. 1–3). In other words, you increase your chances of becoming a successful health care professional if you start approaching life as if you were already that person. Develop **habits** that you know will be expected on the job. For example, because accuracy and efficiency are important characteristics for the health care professional, complete all class assignments as if the well-being of others depended on their accuracy. Working effectively with others as part of a team will be required in your work, so start using every opportunity to develop your teamwork

BOX 1–5. EXAMPLES OF EFFECTIVE AFFIRMATIONS

I, Rosa Maria, am a highly skilled dental assistant.

I, Kenisha, perform my radiology duties with confidence.

I, Jaime, conduct accurate laboratory tests.

I, Andrea, am a competent, caring nurse.

I, Pham, help patients with my therapeutic skills.

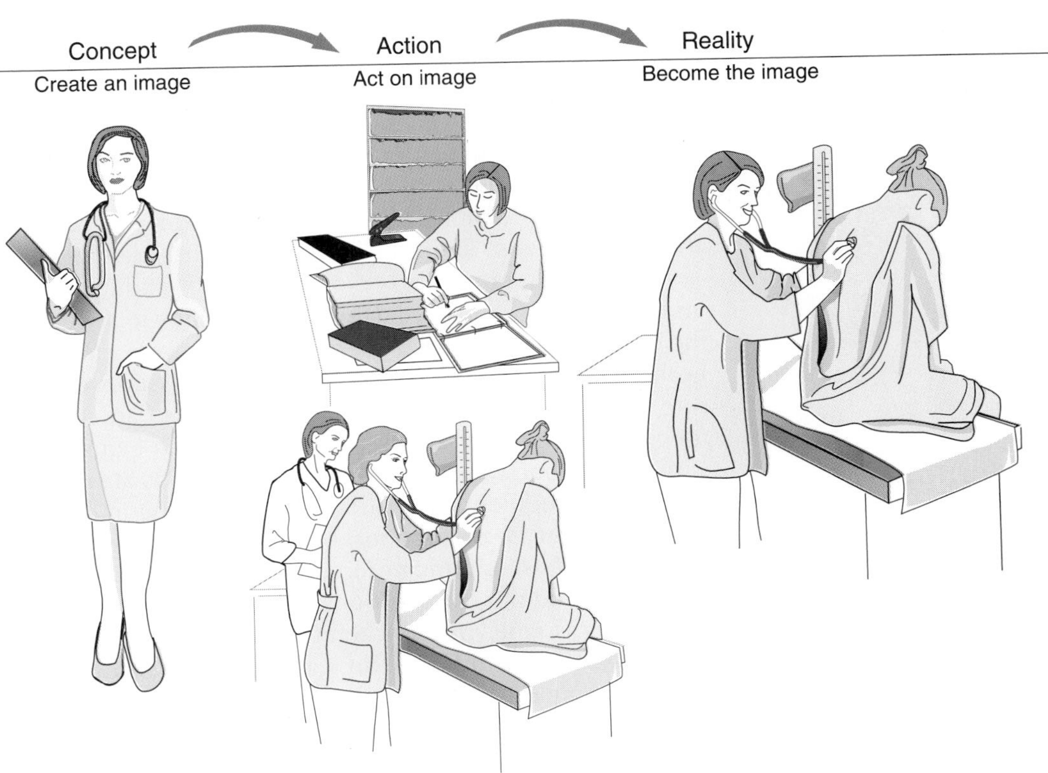

FIGURE 1–3 Achieve your goals through actions. Develop habits that you know will be expected of you on the job.

skills. Strive to cooperate with your classmates and instructors. If you see yourself as a person who works well on a team and practice being an effective team member, you will indeed become a team member who makes positive contributions. By the time you graduate, you will have truly become the health care professional you aspire to be.

Maximizing Your Education

You are making a significant investment of time, effort, and money in your education. You can simply get by, doing only what is required to pass your classes, or you can fully benefit from this investment. A worthy goal is to do everything possible to become the best health care professional possible. Both you and your school have responsibilities to ensure that this happens.

YOUR RIGHTS AS A STUDENT

Making mistakes is inevitable. Not learning from them is inexcusable.

1. *Make mistakes.* This may sound a little strange. After all, aren't you supposed to do the best you can, earning the highest grades possible? Yes, but many students see grades as ends in themselves, rather than as the signs of having mastered the skills they will need in the future. Good grades do not guarantee mastery, nor do you receive grades for all the skills that will determine your future success. To place too much emphasis on grades is to miss the real purpose of school, which is to master a wide range of skills such as those we saw in the SCANS Competencies and National Health Skill Standards.

Compare your educational experience with learning to ride a bike. First, you use training wheels, go slowly, and tip over once in a while. Eventually you become a proficient cyclist, ready for the big race. School offers you a rehearsal for professional life, providing you with opportunities to learn from mistakes that would be unacceptable if made on the job. If you do not score 100% on an exam, it has still served you by allowing you to make mistakes, learn from them, and avoid making them on the job when the consequences are more serious.

2. *Ask questions.* You are attending school to benefit from the knowledge and experience of your instructors. Take advantage of this opportunity by being an active participant in your classes. Don't be an invisible student. Even if the textbooks and lectures are excellent, you may still need to ask for explanations, examples, and additional resources. If there is anything that you don't understand, ask questions. Students aren't expected to understand everything the first time they hear it. Maybe not even the second. Think about it—there would be no need for you to attend school at all if you already knew the information presented in your program!

Many adults are afraid of "looking stupid" and hesitate to admit that they don't understand or are confused. However, the failure to ask questions not only decreases the chances of maximizing your education, it prevents you from learning a critical health care skill. Consider the serious consequences of professionals who are not sure of drug dosages or steps in a procedure but are afraid to ask their supervisors for direction. In these situations, risking the well-being of patients is indeed stupid, while asking questions demonstrates intelligence. Start learning now to be comfortable asking questions. If it is too difficult for you to speak up in class the first few times that you have questions, start out by speaking with your instructor during break, after class, or during office hours.

You should not use questions, however, to substitute for reading your textbook or studying assigned material before each class meeting. This results in class time being misused and is unfair to those students who are prepared for class. A related on-the-job example involves employees who arrive late and unprepared for meetings, thus wasting their coworkers' time. Develop habits now that show consideration for others and contribute to the efficiency of the classroom and the workplace.

3. *Take advantage of school resources.* Every school wants every student who enrolls to graduate, and considerable resources are allocated to services to support this effort. Find out now what services are available to you, the hours they can be accessed, and whether appointments are necessary. Two of the most important services that all students should become familiar with are the library (or resource center) and career services (sometimes called "job placement").

If you are having personal problems or academic difficulties, ask whether the school provides counseling and/or tutoring. Some schools will refer you to outside agencies that offer assistance to students for such difficulties as dealing with domestic abuse and finding reliable child care. Asking for help when you need it can make the difference between dropping out or graduating and becoming successfully employed.

The school catalog is an often overlooked source of information that can help you succeed in school. Many students never take the time to read it and, as a result, are unaware of the resources available for them. Even worse, they risk unknowingly breaking rules or missing important deadlines. Spend a few minutes reading and become an informed student.

Find out if your school gives awards and honors for which you might qualify. While some are based on grades, many are given for nonacademic achievements such as perfect attendance, citizenship, and most improvement. If these are available, build them into your goals as incentives to reward your performance.

PRESCRIPTION FOR SUCCESS 1–11

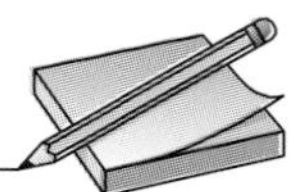

Treasure Hunt

When you need help, school services can seem like treasures. But in order to take advantage of everything your school has to offer, you must know about it. Ask questions and read your school's literature to collect the information needed to fill in the following chart. Not every school will offer all of these services. If not, find out if they are available elsewhere in the community.

PRESCRIPTION FOR SUCCESS 1–11 (*continued*)

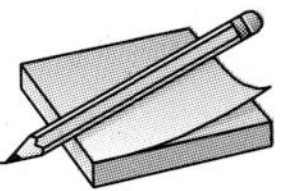

Service Availability Chart

Resource	Services Provided	How to Access/Qualify
Library Books Journals Internet access Reference assistance Other		
Advising Academic Personal		
Tutoring Instructors Other students Study groups		
Career Services Job placement Job fairs Networking Part-time jobs Resumes Employer contacts Classes/workshops		
Professional Organizations (student chapters)		
Volunteer Opportunities		
Refresher and Basic Skills Classes		
School Organizations Special interest groups Social clubs		
Information Sources and Referrals Child care Transportation Financial assistance Other		
Special Needs and Referrals Alcohol abuse Drug dependency Family planning Domestic abuse Other		
Honors and Awards		

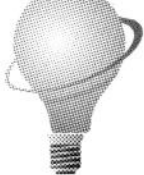

Take a Moment to Think

In what ways can students take responsibility for their own learning?

YOUR RESPONSIBILITIES AS A STUDENT

1. *Attend all scheduled learning activities.* Health care educational programs feature a variety of learning opportunities including lectures, lab sessions, guest speakers, field trips, and hands-on experiences in health care facilities. Your instructor

may also recommend additional activities outside of those organized by the school, such as watching a television documentary or visiting a medical supply company. These activities are designed to ensure that you understand and master all the knowledge and skills necessary for your future work, and you cannot afford to miss them. They are opportunities to develop the competencies essential for work in health care. Learning to perform essential tasks, such as the administration of injections, requires that you spend time and put forth effort under the guidance of your instructors. *Now* is the time for learning and making mistakes, not when you are faced with your first patient. Your future ability to carry out the duties that affect the well-being of others makes it essential that you fully participate in every learning activity offered in your program.

Employers routinely request information about a student's attendance record. Good attendance is considered a valuable job skill because health care services are driven by time requirements. The success of a private physician's practice depends heavily on efficient patient scheduling. Hospitals have daily responsibilities for performing hundreds of treatments, procedures, and surgeries which must be completed in a timely way. In both settings, effective care can be provided only if the staff is available to perform their work. Start now to develop the habit of consistent and punctual attendance.

2. *Apply your best efforts to learning.* As a student, you have the right to ask questions and make mistakes. At the same time, learning requires hard work, and it is your responsibility to complete all reading, written, and lab assignments and to participate actively in class. Understanding and applying new information can be challenging, and the techniques and suggestions presented in the following chapters were selected to help you learn more effectively.

In performing your work as a health care professional, you will need to assess situations, consider alternatives, and make sound decisions on which to base your actions. To master this essential competency, you must now focus on your studies, work hard, and be persistent. In an earlier section, we discussed how techniques such as visualization can help you achieve your goal of becoming a health care professional. Mental images and words can motivate you and help shape your behavior, but they do not take the place of effort, study, and application. The willingness to do the "shoulds" when you would rather be doing the "wants" is a major determinant of success. You will not always feel like studying after a day that includes classes, a few hours on the job, and family responsibilities. Being an adult student is not easy. Keeping your long-term career goals clearly in mind will help you to find the necessary self-discipline.

3. *Ask for help when you need it.* Instructors and administrators want to help their students succeed. They have chosen to work in education because they are interested in helping students complete their programs and graduate. However, you must take responsibility for requesting assistance. Ignoring problems will not solve them; they usually only get worse. Don't wait until you are hopelessly lost in a class and cannot possibly be ready for the final exam the following week before finally asking for help. Take charge of your learning and at the first sign of trouble, ask about tutoring, study groups, computer labs, and any other learning resources the school might have available.

If you experience problems of a personal or financial nature, refer to the list of school resources that you prepared in the last exercise. Asking for help when you need it is a sign of strength, not weakness, and is one of the main characteristics that distinguishes a graduate from a dropout.

The flip side of asking for help is being willing to give it. Offer your assistance to others in the school community. Volunteer to hand out papers for the instructor. Give a student who lives in your area a ride to school. Tutor a classmate who is struggling with a subject that you find easy. You have chosen a profession that is based on giving service, and this is a habit you can start practicing now in all areas of your life. Students who give of themselves are the type of people who become indispensable employees.

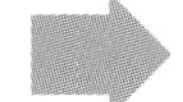

SUMMARY OF KEY IDEAS

1. Your career as a health care professional starts *now.*
2. What you do in school you will do on the job.
3. Being a good health care provider involves much more than mastering technical skills.
4. Visualization and affirmations are powerful tools for achieving goals.
6. As a student, you have both rights and responsibilities.
7. Keep your focus on your future.

BIBLIOGRAPHY

Occupational Outlook Handbook. Indianapolis: JIST Works, Inc., 1998.

Gawain, Shakti. *Creative Visualization.* Mill Valley, CA: Whatever Publishing, Inc., 1978.

Maltz, Maxwell. *Psycho-Cybernetics: Creative Living for Today.* New York: Pocket Books, Simon and Schuster, 1974.

McCutcheon, Maureen. *Exploring Health Careers,* 2nd ed. Albany, NY: Delmar Publishers, 1998.

Swanson, Barbara. *Careers in Health Care.* Lincolnwood, IL: VGM Career Horizons, Division of NTC Publishing Group, 1994.

2

Planning for Career Success

OBJECTIVES

THE INFORMATION AND ACTIVITIES IN THIS CHAPTER CAN HELP YOU TO:

- ➢ Describe how the principles of marketing can be applied to career preparation and the job search.
- ➢ Develop a personal philosophy of work.
- ➢ Identify and describe your job preferences.
- ➢ Understand the importance of aligning your preferences with the realities of the workplace.
- ➢ Identify skills you have now that you can apply to your health care career.
- ➢ Recognize the value of the resume as a planning tool for managing personal and professional development. Begin now to use it to your advantage.
- ➢ Begin professional networking activities.
- ➢ Start to identify potential references.

KEY TERMS

Civic organizations: Groups that are devoted to community projects. Lions Clubs, for example, raise funds and provide free eye care for people who cannot otherwise afford it.

Clinical experience: The term used in this book to describe supervised, unpaid work experiences performed by students in health facilities or offices to gain hands-on, practical experience. Depending on your school, occupational program, and type of experience, this may be called "clinical," "externship," "fieldwork," "internship," "practicum," or "preceptorship."

Documentation: Any type of material that serves as evidence of skills mastered, courses completed, and achievements and recognition earned. Examples include grade reports, nursing license, and the cardiopulmonary resuscitation (CPR) card.

Hygiene: All practices that contribute to good health and the prevention of disease. An example is proper handwashing techniques.

Networking: Meeting new people for the purpose of personal and professional development. It can take place at professional meetings and seminars or through personal encounters.

Per diem: Work performed on an on-call basis. Some health care professionals are employed by special organizations, called "registries," that send them to a variety of facilities for short-term assignments.

Philosophy: The system of beliefs that forms the foundation of a person's view of the world and ideas about the meaning of life. A person's philosophy influences all aspects of life, including profession, personal relationships, religion, and politics.

Portfolio: An organized collection of items that provide evidence of your job-related skills and capabilities. Portfolios are becoming common additions to the resume for presentation to a potential employer.

Proactive: Taking action before it is necessary or required. Proactive students learn all they can about employer requirements before they complete their education. On the job, proactive medical assistants anticipate the needs of physicians before being told.

Reference: Person who agrees to vouch for your professional skills and capabilities, such as a former supervisor. This may be done by letter or telephone.

Resume: A written document, prepared in one of several standard formats, that summarizes your professional skills and capabilities. It is sometimes called a "curriculum vitae."

Standard precautions: Practices that prevent the transmission of disease through the microorganisms present in blood and other body fluids. For example, used needles are disposed of in special containers that are removed by medical waste services.

Sterile technique: Special procedures used to create an environment that is free of all living microorganisms (germs). For example, surgical instruments are treated at high temperatures and placed in specially sealed packages until they are used.

Syllabi: Handouts prepared by instructors that give information about a course. They include course objectives, textbooks, lecture topics, reading assignments, and dates of quizzes and tests. (The singular form of the term is "syllabus.")

Transferrable skills: Skills that can be applied to different types of occupations, such as organizing and tracking supplies.

Work ethic: A positive approach to work, including the demonstration of responsibility, honesty, loyalty, and dedication to the needs of those served.

And the Product Is . . . You!

Give yourself a running start.

Marketing is a multistep process that begins with an idea for a new product and ends with the sale of that product. Mastering this process is a critical factor for the survival of any business. Successful marketing is similar to starting a new career successfully. *You*—the composite of your skills, characteristics, and talents—are the product. To ensure that you have the skills and qualities needed by employers, you must prepare appropriately for the workplace and learn to present yourself effectively during the job search.

The marketing process can be organized into a five-part plan called the "Five Ps of Marketing":

1. Planning
2. Production
3. Packaging
4. Presentation
5. Promotion

In this chapter, we discuss each of the Ps in detail and see how developing your own personal marketing plan now, as you begin your health care studies, can help ensure your future career success.

Planning

In Chapter 1, we discussed the expectations of potential employers and future patients, your future "customers." Studying the needs of customers is called "market research," and its purpose is to determine what customers want. Waiting until the end of your program to think about getting a job is like creating a product without doing market research. Designing and manufacturing a product that no one wants or needs doesn't make sense. Just like a business, you are investing time, effort, and money in the development of your product. The exercises in Chapter 1 gave you an opportunity to begin your own market research and learn as much as possible about the type of product needed by health care employers. You can apply your findings to start planning now for career success (Fig. 2–1).

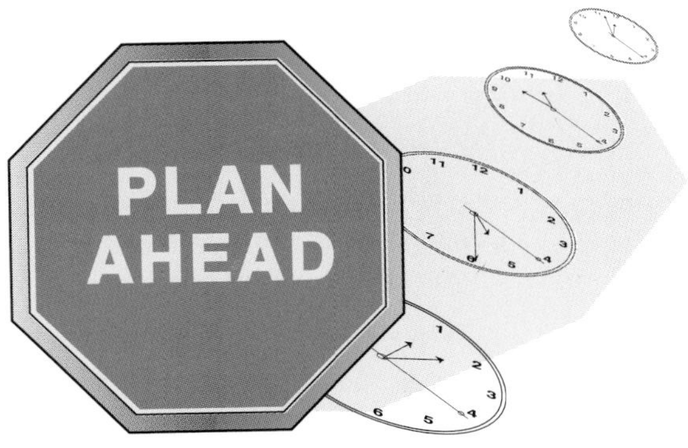

FIGURE 2–1 Success starts with a good plan.

WHAT DO YOU WANT?

If you don't know where you're going, chances are you'll end up somewhere else.

In addition to exploring the needs of your customers, an important aspect of planning is to identify what *you* want. You must consider your own needs and desires as you create your professional self. The clearer you are about your career goals and expectations, the greater the chance you have of achieving them.

Beginning now to think now about your specific career goals and workplace priorities will keep you alert to appropriate employment possibilities. Take every opportunity during your studies to observe, ask questions, and read about your field. Then compare your findings with your own interests. Many fields in health care today feature newly created positions and expanded responsibilities for traditional jobs. A wide variety of choices is available today for new graduates. Being aware of these opportunities improves your chances of finding employment that matches your priorities.

DEVELOPING A PHILOSOPHY OF WORK

Most of us spend a significant number of our waking hours on the job. How we spend that time determines, to a great degree, the quality of our lives. It makes sense, then, to think about what work means to you. Exploring your personal beliefs will help you increase the amount of satisfaction you get from your career. The following list* contains a variety of reasons why people work:

- Survive financially
- Define self
- Gain self-respect
- Demonstrate competence
- Gain power
- Fill time
- Measure self-worth
- Learn
- Experience variety
- Contribute to the community
- Experience enjoyment

People are generally happiest and most productive when their work provides them with more than material rewards. Some people are motivated by continual challenges, others value consistency, and still others are content with either condition as long as their work allows them to help others. Take some time to identify the workplace factors that motivate you.

* Adapted from Bingham & Stryker, 1990.

PRESCRIPTION FOR SUCCESS 2–1

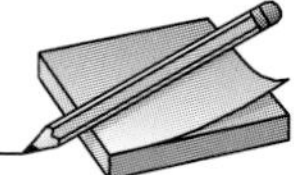

My Philosophy of Work

Use your answers from Prescription for Success 1-1 in Chapter 1, the previous list of suggestions, and your answers to the following questions to write a description of your **philosophy** of work.

1. What does work mean to you?
2. What needs do you want to be filled by your work?
3. Which of these needs were satisfied in previous jobs?
4. What is the overall purpose of the health care occupation you have chosen?
5. What significance does work in health care have for you?
6. How can you maximize your chances for satisfaction in health care work?

WORK PREFERENCES

It is also important to begin thinking about the kinds of tasks you like to do and the working conditions you prefer. There is a wide variety of work settings for health care professionals. Being clear about your own preferences will help you choose and prepare for the most appropriate types of positions in your career area.

PRESCRIPTION FOR SUCCESS 2–2

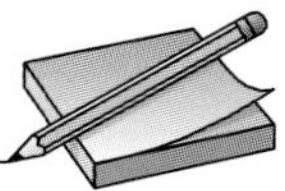

What Do I Want

1. Type of facility: large, small, urban, suburban, rural, in-patient, out-patient
2. Type of population served: economic status, age range, gender, ethnic groups
3. Work schedule: steady employment, **per diem** (daily, contracted), flexible hours, fixed hours, overtime, days only, evenings and weekends
4. Specialty area
5. Type of supervision
6. Work pace: fast, moderate
7. Interaction with others (*All* health care professionals are part of a team, although some work more independently than others.)
8. Range of duties: wide variety, concentration on a few

ALIGNMENT WITH EMPLOYERS

While it is important to try to meet your personal needs when seeking employment, you must also have realistic expectations. An essential activity in career planning is to compare your work preferences with the needs of potential employers to see how well they match. Students sometimes have unrealistic goals for the positions they hope to fill immediately following graduation. Recent graduates are qualified for *entry-level positions.* You can avoid frustration and disappointment if you understand the workplace and adjust your expectations. This way, you can maximize the benefits of your first work experiences in health care.

Formal training is only the beginning of your journey to developing competence as a health care professional. Your skills will continually grow and be refined as you accumulate hands-on practice and everyday experience in the field. When starting a new career, it may be wise—even necessary—to trade your "perfect-job" requirements for opportunities that lead to long-term career success. You will want to look for a first-time job that allows you to do the following:

1. Gain self-confidence
2. Work with a variety of people
3. Acquire additional knowledge
4. Increase your skill base
5. Explore specialties within your field of interest
6. Network with other professionals
7. Demonstrate your abilities

Your first employer is giving you the gift of confidence in your abilities. You will be entrusted with serious responsibilities that may include patient welfare, accuracy and confidentiality of important records, and other matters that influence the reputation and success of the facility. You will have a chance to prove your value by learning as much as possible, finding ways to help your employer and coworkers, and contributing to the overall success of the organization. Entry-level jobs, performed well, can be the first important step leading to positions that meet your hopes for a fulfilling career.

ALIGNMENT WITH YOUR PROFESSION

Health care professions vary in the type of work performed. You need to be aware of the daily tasks and working conditions of the occupation you have chosen. For example, respiratory therapy and radiology require the technical aptitude to work with complex equipment. Occupational therapy requires the ability to apply oral communication skills to teach patients and their families. Health information technology and insurance coding require accuracy and attention to detail when creating, filling out, and organizing medical records and forms.

You may need to consider trade-offs in order to obtain a balance that offers maximum career satisfaction. For example, a recent nursing graduate who wants the excitement of a hospital emergency room *and* the convenience of a 9:00 a.m. to 5:00 p.m. weekday schedule may have a conflict. To avoid a mismatch between your expectations and the real world, learn as much as possible about the specific requirements of your future profession so that, if necessary, you can rethink and reprioritize your requirements.

Adjusting your short-term expectations doesn't mean giving up your long-term goals. In fact, purposeful planning now can help you arrive at the place where you want to be in the future. If you discover that the specific type of job you want requires previous work experience, you can set short-term goals that will serve as stepping stones to acquire that experience. Find out now what skills are emphasized in your target position and look for opportunities to learn as many of them as possible during your studies, **clinical experience,** and first job. For example, Rosa wants to work as a back-office assistant with a plastic surgeon, assisting with out-patient procedures. Her research shows that there are only a few plastic surgeons in her area and that they prefer to hire assistants with previous work experience. Rosa decides to look for a job with a general practitioner or pediatrician who does minor surgery in the office. Her short-term goals are to gain experience with **sterile technique, standard precautions,** surgical assisting, and patient care. While in school, she asks her instructor to recommend reference works about plastic surgery and to allow her to spend extra practice time in the lab so that she can reach a high level of competence with sterile technique, surgical instruments, wound care, and related topics.

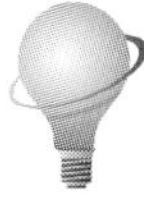

Take a Moment to Think

In addition to the preceding list of benefits, what else can you learn and gain from your first job?

PRESCRIPTION FOR SUCCESS 2–3

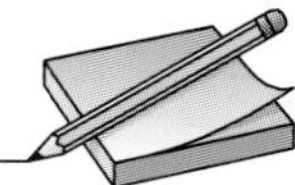

Are My Expectations Realistic?

Review your findings gathered in Prescriptions for Success 1-3, 1-6, and 1-9 in Chapter 1. Compare these findings with your responses to the last two exercises.

1. Do your preferences fit the occupation you have chosen?
2. In which areas might you have to adjust your expectations?
3. What short-term goals can you develop to serve as stepping stones to achieve your long-term goal?

Employees who are willing to meet the expectations of their employers are often rewarded with additional (and interesting!) responsibilities and promotions. Some employers even create new positions in order to use the talents of their employees. For new health care professionals who are well prepared and who contribute enthusiastically to the success of their employers, entry-level jobs can serve as launch pads for career success. You, too, may benefit by having new and interesting responsibilities added to your job description, receiving a promotion, or having a job created that brings you satisfaction. Serving the needs of others can provide you with opportunities to meet your own.

Production

The next step in the marketing process is to use the information gathered from market research to design and produce a product that meets the needs of the customer. Your school has developed an educational program that meets the technical specifications required for your chosen career. You and your school are partners in your development as a health care professional and each of you has responsibilities, as discussed in Chapter 1 (Fig. 2–2).

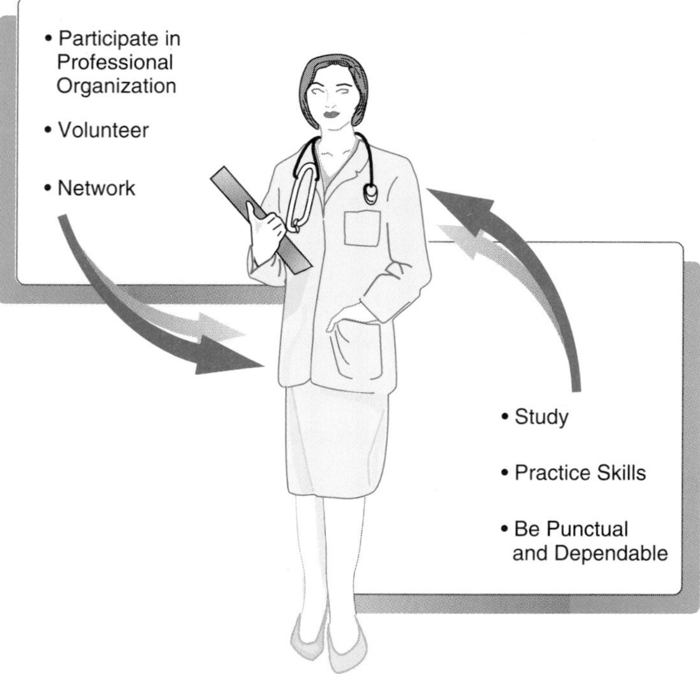

• Participate in Professional Organization
• Volunteer
• Network
• Study
• Practice Skills
• Be Punctual and Dependable

FIGURE 2–2 You are creating your professional self.

Accepting responsibility for creating your own life—your product—is empowering and satisfying. It can be one of the most exciting parts of starting a new career. Take an active role in creating a successful product. While in school, be **proactive** and look for opportunities to enhance your personal and professional growth. Turn mistakes into lessons and learn from them. Approach personal difficulties as strength-building exercises. Recognize your past achievements and take credit for new accomplishments. You already have many of the components for a successful "professional product," and these will serve as the foundation for acquiring new skills and habits.

Sometimes we don't recognize our own abilities or appreciate their value. We tend to overlook some of our greatest assets because they are not technical or job-specific. Here are just a few examples:

- Work Habits
  - Arrive on time for all required activities
  - Accept responsibility for all tasks assigned
  - Treat customers courteously
  - Work well in groups
- Personal Characteristics
  - Honesty
  - Kindness
  - Reliability
  - Good health

PRESCRIPTION FOR SUCCESS 2-4

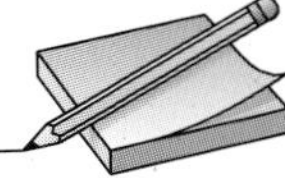

Personal Inventory

1. Make a list of your work habits that you believe will be valuable in your future employment in health care.
2. Do the same for your personal characteristics.

The purpose of the self-assessment you completed in Prescriptions for Success 1-4 and 1-5 in Chapter 1 was to help you identify areas that needed improvement or further development in order to increase your professional and personal effectiveness. Chapters 3 through 8 of this book can help you develop skills in areas such as problem solving, oral communication, and teamwork. Your program courses will also provide you with many opportunities to develop the skills outlined in SCANS and the National Health Care Skill Standards. The employment world has sent a loud, clear message that career success depends as much on your abilities in these areas as on your technical knowledge and performance. Do not underestimate their importance in creating a high-quality product that will be a winner in the marketplace.

Packaging

Even an excellent product may not sell if it is poorly packaged. Companies know this and invest a lot of time and money to ensure that products are visually appealing to customers. Appearance can make the difference between whether a product sells or collects dust on the shelf.

Most of us package ourselves to impress others or to fit into a specific social group. Americans spend billions of dollars annually on clothing, cosmetics, accessories, and hair in an effort to create a pleasing appearance. We realize that how we look often determines whether we will be given a chance to show who we are and what we can do.

Appearance is especially important in the health care field because it influences patients' opinions about the competence of the health care professional. Your

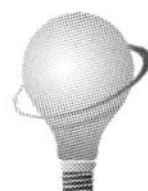

Take a Moment to Think

1. Are there any aspects of my appearance that might be inappropriate for the health care setting?
   a. Fashion trends
   b. Health habits
   c. Cleanliness and hygiene
   d. Safety issues
2. Am I willing to change these aspects, at least during working hours?
3. What can I start to do now to improve my professional appearance?

If you are not sure about aspects of your appearance or grooming, speak privately with your instructor or someone else you trust. Dealing with these issues now will give you time to take care of them before you begin your job search. Your ultimate goal as a health care professional is to provide for the needs of your patients, and as we have seen, packaging is an important factor in delivering effective patient care.

effectiveness in meeting patient needs can be impacted by your appearance, because patient satisfaction increases when health care professionals "look like they know what they are doing."

What is expected of the health care professional? How do you *look* competent? We will discuss four ways. The first is to be fairly conservative in dress and grooming. This means avoiding fashion trends that are outside the mainstream of society, such as brightly colored hair, tattoos, and body piercing. While these may simply represent a current style and a fun way to look, they may be interpreted as signs of rebellion, immaturity, and lack of common sense. Many patients are offended or even frightened by this type of appearance.

A second consideration is to strive for an appearance that radiates good health. As we discussed in Chapter 1, an important responsibility of the professional is to promote good health. This is partly achieved by example. Conditions such as teeth that need dental work, badly bitten fingernails, and dandruff indicate a lack of self-care, inappropriate in a profession that encourages the practice of good habits. Furthermore, the way you present yourself reflects your approach to life and your opinion of yourself. Failure to care for yourself projects a lack of self-confidence and undermines patient faith in your effectiveness.

Third, the issues of cleanliness and **hygiene** are vitally important for professionals whose work requires them to touch others. Patients literally put themselves in the hands of health care professionals and must feel assured that they will benefit from, and not be harmed by, any procedures performed. It is natural to want the professional to look clean and neat and be free from unpleasant odors. For example, while the hands of the dental assistant be may clean and gloved, a dirty uniform or shoes give an unfavorable impression to the patient who has the assistant's hands in his mouth. The patient may wonder if proper attention was given to sterilizing the equipment and cleaning the work area.

Finally, professionals must consider the safety and comfort of both patients and themselves. Perfumes and scented personal products cannot be tolerated by many patients. Long fingernails, flowing hair, and large hooped earrings may be attractive and appropriate for a social event. In a health care setting they can scratch patients, contaminate samples, get caught in equipment, or be grabbed by a small patient. Safety on the job cannot be compromised to accommodate fashion trends.

Presentation

Begin with the end in mind.—Stephen Covey

Your **resume** is a form of advertising. It tells potential employers what you can do for them: the features you offer and the benefits they will gain by hiring you. The main purpose of a resume is to convince them to give you an interview. In Chapter 9 you will learn how to write and organize an effective resume. The focus in this chapter is on learning about the content of the resume and how to use it as a guideline to create your professional self (Fig. 2–3). Starting to plan your resume now will help you to:

1. Recognize what you already have to offer an employer.
2. Build self-confidence.
3. Motivate yourself to learn the nontechnical skills that contribute to employment success.
4. Target areas for personal development.
5. Accumulate experiences that enhance your employability.

THE BUILDING BLOCKS OF YOUR RESUME

The following ten sections of your resume provide **documentation** of your professional qualifications.

Career Objective

A brief description, often only one sentence long, of the position or job title you are seeking. It can include the type of facility and environment you prefer. Examples of objectives are as follows:

- Obtain a position as an administrative and clinical medical assistant in a fast-paced office that offers challenging work and opportunities to acquire additional knowledge and learn new skills.
- Work as an occupational therapy assistant in a pediatric facility.

As we discussed earlier, it is wise to have reasonable expectations for your first employment positions. Set positive long-term goals, but be realistic when starting out. This is your chance to work with real people who have real problems. The more kinds of jobs you are willing to accept when first entering the field, the higher your chances of obtaining employment.

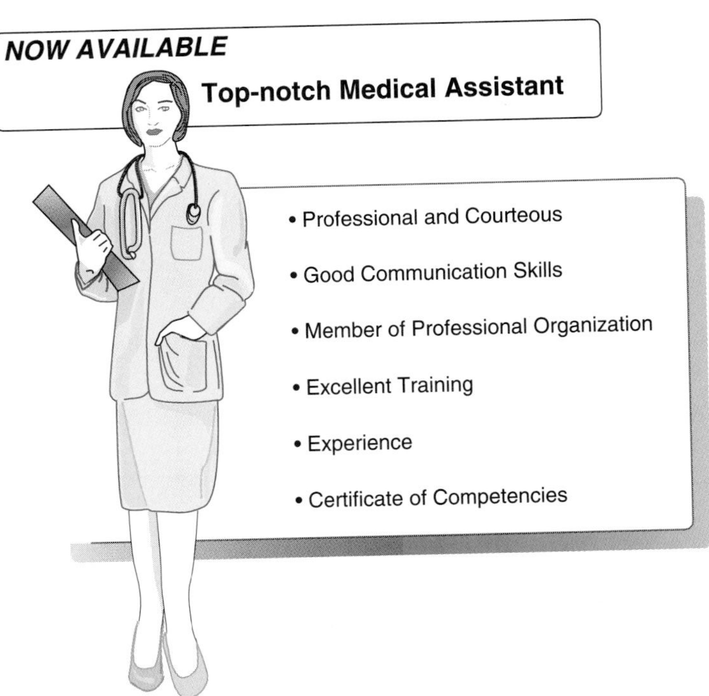
NOW AVAILABLE
Top-notch Medical Assistant
• Professional and Courteous
• Good Communication Skills
• Member of Professional Organization
• Excellent Training
• Experience
• Certificate of Competencies

FIGURE 2–3 Create a product that you can sell to employers with confidence.

To Do Now

Complete and continue to add to the exercises in which you describe your work style and preferences. As you go through your training, learn as much as possible about the various jobs for which you might qualify. There may be jobs you are unaware of that closely match your interests. It is not uncommon to rewrite objectives more than once before beginning the actual job search.

PRESCRIPTION FOR SUCCESS 2–5

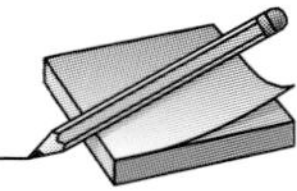

My Objective Is . . .

Write at least two sentences that describe your occupational objective as you see it now.

Education A list of all your education and training, with emphasis on health care training. (High school is usually omitted.) Grade point average and class standing (not all schools rank their students by grades) are included if they are above average. Knowing that you can put this information on your resume can serve as a motivator for doing your best academically.

To Do Now

Think about what you want this section to reflect about how you did as a student. Focus on learning as much as possible in your classes.

Professional Skills and Knowledge These include the skills and knowledge that contribute to successful job performance. The way you organize this section depends on your educational program and the number and variety of skills acquired. They can be listed individually ("Take vital signs") or as clusters of related skills ("Perform back office duties").

PRESCRIPTION FOR SUCCESS 2–6

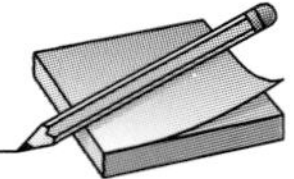

Tracking Your Progress: Developing a Skills Inventory

Use the following format to create an inventory form for each of your courses (Table 2–1). Fill these out as you progress through your program. (Skip this exercise if your school provides suitable lists.) Examples of skills to include:

Pronounce and spell medical terms correctly.

Accurately complete a medical insurance claim form.

Perform one-person adult CPR.

Set up dental trays for common procedures.

Transfer a patient from a bed to a stretcher.

TABLE 2–1 ***Course Inventory Record***

Course Title	**Skills Acquired**

Presenting lists of skills or clusters is particularly helpful if your previous work experience is limited and you want to emphasize the recent acquisition of health care skills as your primary qualification. It is also helpful if you have trained for one of the newer positions in health care that is not familiar to all employers. For example, "rehabilitation aides" are multiskilled workers who can work in several settings, including physical therapy, occupational therapy, and chiropractic. Highlighting your skills can help you present yourself and your potential contributions more clearly than simply a program or job title.

To Do Now

Find out if your school provides lists of program and course objectives and/or the competencies you will master. These are sometimes created in the form of check-off lists which instructors use to monitor the completion of assignments and demonstration of competencies. If these are not provided, prepare your own as you complete each course. Sources of information include handouts from your instructor, such as **syllabi** and course outlines; the objectives listed in your textbooks; and lab skill sheets. An extra benefit of tracking your progress in this way is the sense of accomplishment you gain as you see the results of your hard work. You will be amazed at how much you are learning!

Work Experience A list of your previous jobs that includes the name and location of the employer, your job title, and the dates of employment. You can maximize the value of this section even if you have no previous experience in health care. There are three ways to do this. The first is to think about all the duties and responsibilities you had in each job. Which ones can be applied to health care work? Consider the general skills listed in the SCANS report discussed in Chapter 1 that are applicable to a variety of work settings. Skills that are common to many jobs are called **transferrable skills.** Here are a few examples:

- Work well with people from a variety of backgrounds
- Create efficient schedules that reduce employee overtime
- Purchase supplies in appropriate quantities and at competitive prices
- Resolve customer complaints satisfactorily
- Perform advanced word processing
- Manage accounts receivable
- Provide customer service
- Provide appropriate care for infants and toddlers

Identifying transferrable skills is especially important when you are entering a new field in which you have little or no experience. There is a type of resume that emphasizes skills and abilities rather than specific job titles held. It is called a "functional resume," and the format is described in Chapter 9. At this point, start compiling a list of possible transferrable skills.

The second way to maximize the value of this section of your resume is to mention what you achieved in each job. In a phrase or two, describe how you contributed to the success of your employer. When possible, state these achievements in measurable terms. If you can't express them quantitatively, use active verbs that tell what you did. Here are some examples:

- Increased sales by 20%
- Designed a more efficient way to track supplies
- Worked on a committee that wrote an effective employee procedure manual that is still in use
- Trained five other employees to use office equipment correctly

A third way to add value to this section is to include your clinical experience. While you must clearly indicate that this was a part of your training and not paid employment, it serves as evidence of your ability to apply what you learned in school to practical situations. For many new graduates, this is their only real-world experience in health care. Students sometimes make the mistake of viewing their clinical experience as simply an add-on to their program, just one more thing to get through. They fail to realize the impact their performance can have on their career. Remember that clinical supervisors represent future employers. (In some cases, they *are* future employers.) Their opinion of you can help successfully launch your self-marketing efforts or cause them to fizzle. The inclusion of a positive clinical experience on your resume increases your chances of getting the job you want.

To Do Now

Start compiling a list of the skills acquired and results achieved in your previous jobs. Starting to do this now, rather than later when you are in a hurry to prepare your resume, gives you time to create a complete list. And *do your best* during your clinical experience in order to begin building a strong professional reputation.

PRESCRIPTION FOR SUCCESS 2–7

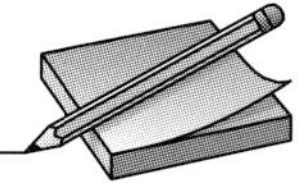

Transferrable Skills and Sources of Pride

Make a chart of the transferrable skills and accomplishments from previous jobs that can be applied to work in health care (Table 2–2).

TABLE 2–2 ***Record of Transferrable Skills and Accomplishments***

Job Title	Transferrable Skills	Accomplishments

Do *not* be concerned if your work experience is limited or you can't think of any achievements. Sometimes we don't recognize our own value. Review the SCANS list in Chapter 1 and be on the alert in your classes for skills to add. Just having a record of steady employment demonstrates a positive **work ethic.**

Licenses and Certifications Some professions require you to be licensed or have specific types of approval before you are allowed to work. Nursing is an example. Or there may be voluntary certifications and registrations, such as those earned by medical assistants. Approvals vary by state and profession. Most licenses and certifications require verification of training and passing a standardized exam. It is important that you clearly understand any professional requirements that are either necessary or highly recommended for your profession.

To Do Now

Learn as much as possible about your professional requirements. It is not advisable to wait until the end of your studies to start thinking about preparing for required exams. Ask your instructors about review classes, books, and computerized material. Become familiar with the kinds of topics on the exams and plan your studies accordingly. Knowing the format of the questions (multiple-choice, true-false, etc.)

is helpful. Increase your chances for success by preparing over time, which has proven to be more effective than last-minute cramming.

PRESCRIPTION FOR SUCCESS 2–8

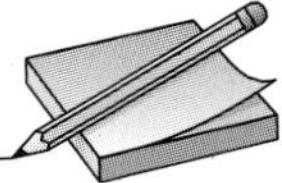

Don't Worry, Be Prepared

1. Are there licensing or certification requirements for your occupation?
2. Are there voluntary approvals for which you can test or apply?
3. Are written and/or practical exams required? What range of content is covered? How are the questions formatted?
4. Are content outlines, review books, software, and practice exams available?

Honors and Awards

This is an optional section. As mentioned in Chapter 1, your school may offer recognition for student achievements and special contributions. Your community and professional organizations may also give awards. Acknowledgments received for volunteer work can also be included in this category.

To Do Now

If you are motivated by the reward system, investigate what you might be eligible for and use these rewards as incentives for excellent performance. Keep this in perspective, however. Awards should serve as motivators, *not* indicators of your value. They are nice to have but certainly not essential for career success.

Special Skills

Special skills are those that don't fit into other sections but do add to your value as a health care professional. Examples include proficiency in desktop publishing and the ability to use American sign language.

To Do Now

Research the needs of employers in your geographic area. Do you already have special skills that meet these needs? Would it substantially increase your chances for employment if you acquired skills outside the scope of your program—for example,

PRESCRIPTION FOR SUCCESS 2–9

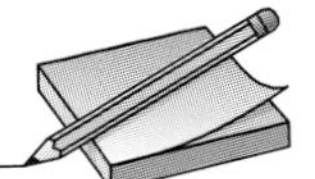

Special Skills Inventory

Create a form like Table 2–3 and fill in any skills you think are appropriate.

TABLE 2–3 ***Record of Special or Supplemental Skills***

Skill	How Acquired/Can be Acquired	How Applies to Health Care

to become more proficient on the computer? If (and *only* if!) time permits, you might decide to attend workshops in addition to your regular program courses, do extra reading, or take a course on the Internet.

Community Service and Volunteer Work

Include these activities if they relate to your targeted occupation or demonstrate qualities such as responsibility and concern for others.

To Do Now

If you are already involved in these types of activities, think about what you are learning or practicing that can help you on the job. If you aren't, consider becoming involved *if* you have a sincere interest and adequate time. Adult students face many responsibilities outside of class, and the additional activities mentioned in this chapter should be taken as *suggestions,* not must-dos. Mastering your program content takes priority.

Memberships in Professional and Civic Organizations

Professional organizations provide excellent opportunities to network, learn more about your field, and practice leadership skills. Participation in **civic organizations** promotes personal growth and demonstrates your willingness to get involved in your community.

To Do Now

Consider joining and participating actively in a professional or civic organization while you are in school. See if your school or community has a local chapter.

PRESCRIPTION FOR SUCCESS 2–10

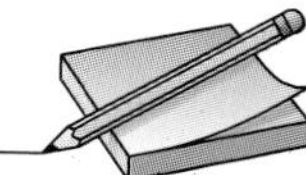

Opportunities for Growth

Create a chart like Table 2–4 to track activities that contribute to your personal and professional growth.

TABLE 2–4 ***Record of Special or Supplemental Activities***

Organization	Activities	Skills Acquired

Languages Spoken

In our multicultural society, the ability to communicate in a language other than English is commonly included on the resume. It is also customary to indicate how well you know any languages that you list (e.g., "Some conversational knowledge of Spanish").

To Do Now

Find out if there are many patients who speak a language other than English in the area where you plan to work. Consider acquiring at least some conversational ability. If your program offers these languages as elective courses, they would be good

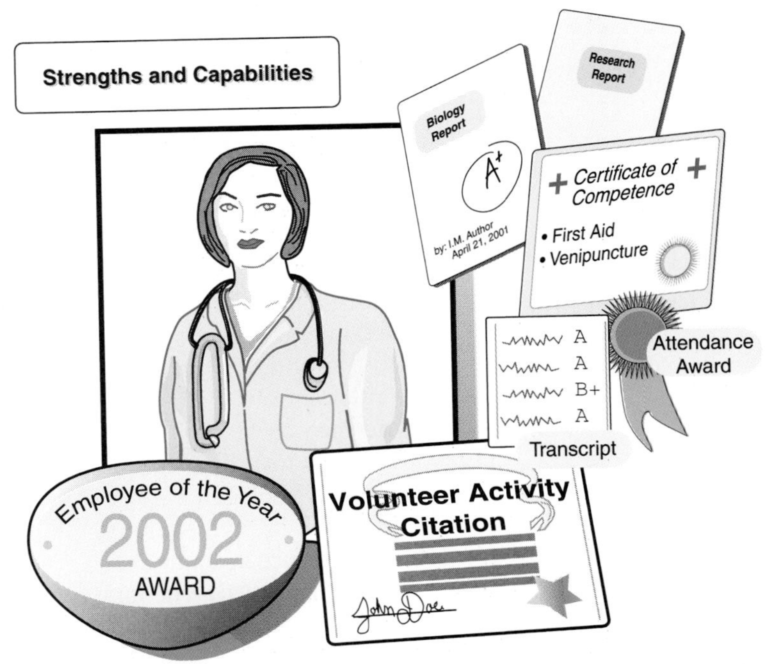

FIGURE 2–4 Resumes and portfolios provide organized and documented evidence of your strengths and capabilities.

choices. Patients benefit greatly, during the stress of illness or injury, when health care professionals know at least a few phrases of their native language. Speaking another language increases your worth to employers.

PORTFOLIOS

Resumes are the principal method of presenting the qualifications of job seekers. In recent years, **portfolios** have increasingly been used to supplement the resume. They consist of an organized collection of items that document capabilities and are presented to potential employers at interviews to support claims of competence (Fig. 2–4). Portfolios are recommended today as a means of gaining a competitive edge in the job search.

There are several reasons to start thinking about your portfolio now. It puts your class assignments in a new light because they have the potential of demonstrating your abilities to an employer. Strive to perform consistently at your highest level, producing work that can represent you well.

As you complete each course, save works that might be suitable for your portfolio. Store them in a folder or large envelope, where they will stay in good condition. In addition to written assignments, look for nontraditional ways to showcase your abilities. The items you collect need not be limited to evidence of your technical skills. It is appropriate to include confirmation of other traits, such as the SCANS competencies. If you start now, you are more likely to compile a good representation of skills and accomplishments, as well as avoiding the last-minute scramble.

There is no standard list of items that you should put in your portfolio, although only work that is done accurately and neatly should be included. Finalizing the contents and assembling your portfolio for presentation will be covered in Chapter 9. If the career services department at your school encourages the use of portfolios, ask if there is a list of items they want you to include. If not, the following list includes items that are appropriate for the health care graduate's portfolio:

1. Examples of Class Work
   Accurately filled out insurance form
   Accounting forms
   Perfectly typed/word processed letter

Lab reports
Medical history form filled out
Charting entries
Research report

2. Certificates of Completion or Achievement
   Verification of having completed courses, seminars, and workshops
   Proof of skill mastery, such as CPR, first aid, or the Burdick electrocardiographic (EKG) procedure, or documentation of the number of successful performances of an important procedure, such as venipunctures, injections, and x-rays
   Documentation of speed, such as for word processing or data entry
   Recognition of special achievements, such as honor or merit roll or perfect attendance
3. Grade Records or Transcripts
   Consider including these if your grades are above average. If they started out as average or even below-average and then improved as you advanced through your program, you might use them to demonstrate your persistence and progress.
4. Employer Review or Evaluation
   You can include these from your previous employment if they demonstrate attitudes or skills applicable to work in health care. A positive review from your clinical supervisor can be very valuable, because it is recent and relates directly to health care.
5. Recognition of Contributions
   Thank-you letters
   Verification of participation in activities such as walk-a-thons to raise money for worthy causes
6. Attendance Record
   Excellent addition if you have very good attendance
7. Honors and Awards
8. Licenses or Certifications (copies)
9. Photographs
   These materials document activities in which you had a major role, such as organizing a fund-raising activity or planning and coordinating a school picnic.

Promotion

Companies use promotional campaigns to give new products maximum exposure. They request personal testimonies, create advertising, and spread the word to as many consumers as possible about how the product will fill their needs. You will conduct a similar campaign when you conduct your job search. As with your resume and portfolio, you can begin to prepare now. We will discuss the promotional value of networking, references, and the job interview.

NETWORKING

Networking refers to meeting and establishing relationships with people who work in health care. It is an effective way to learn more about your chosen career. At the same time, it gets the word out about you and your employment goals. Opportunities for networking present themselves in settings such as professional meetings, career fairs, and health care facilities.

There are many ways to begin networking: at a professional meeting, introduce yourself to other members; after a seminar, write a thank-you note to an interesting

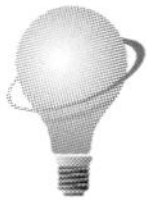

Take a Moment to Think

What opportunities are available to you now for professional networking?

speaker; at a career fair, ask a local employer for advice about what to emphasize in your studies. Be *sure* to follow up with a phone call or thank-you note to anyone who sends you information or makes a special effort to help you.

Another benefit you can gain from networking is to build your self-confidence as you introduce yourself to other professionals. You can improve your speaking ability and learn to express yourself effectively. These are valuable skills that you will apply later when you attend job interviews. Start now to create a web of connections to help you develop professionally and assist you in your future job search and career.

REFERENCES

References are people who will confirm your qualifications, skills, abilities, and personal qualities. In other words, they endorse you as a product. Professional references are not the same as personal or character references. To be effective, they must be credible (believable) and have personal knowledge of your value to a prospective employer. Your best references have knowledge of both you and the health care field. Examples include your instructors, clinical experience supervisors, and other professionals who know the quality of your work. Previous supervisors, even in jobs outside of health care, also make good references.

Recall the discussion in Chapter 1 about how you can become a health care professional by conducting yourself *as if you already were one.* Start now to project a professional image to everyone you meet. Become the person that others will be happy to recommend.

PRESCRIPTION FOR SUCCESS 2–11

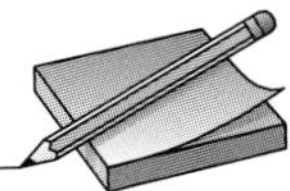

Planning Ahead

1. Who do you already know who would be a good professional reference?
2. What can you do now to help ensure that you have access to at least four positive recommendations when you begin your job search?

EMPLOYMENT INTERVIEW

Job interviews are your best opportunity to promote yourself to a prospective employer. Interviewers often ask for examples of how you solved a problem or handled a given situation. Start thinking now about your past experiences and begin to collect examples from your work as a student, especially from your clinical experience, that will demonstrate your capabilities. It is not too early to start preparing so that you can approach your future interviews as opportunities to shine, at ease and confident that you are presenting yourself positively. Job interviews will be discussed in detail in Chaper 10.

SUMMARY OF KEY IDEAS

1. Preparing for a new career is like creating and marketing a new product.

2. Plan ahead and avoid the rush.

3. Resumes serve as career preparation guides.

4. It's not too early to start your portfolio.

5. Networking is a valuable way to grow professionally and help ensure career success.

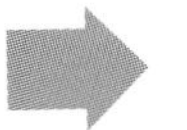

POSITIVE SELF-TALK FOR THIS CHAPTER

1. I have many qualities that will be valuable to my future employer.

2. I am acquiring new skills that will increase my employment value.

3. I set and achieve worthy goals for my life.

4. I am on my way to a great future.

BIBLIOGRAPHY

Binghang, Mindy and Sandy Stryker. *Career Choices.* Santa Barbara, CA: Able Publishing, 1990.

Covey, Stephen. *7 Habits of Highly Successful People.* New York: Simon and Schuster, 1989.

Covey, Stephen, Merrill A. Roger, and Rebecca R. Merrill. *First Things First.* New York: Simon and Schuster, 1995.

Levitt, Julie Griffen. *Your Career: How to Make It Happen,* 3rd ed. Cincinnati: South-Western Educational Publishing, 1996.

Yena, Donna. *Career Directions,* 3rd ed. Chicago: Irwin, 1997.

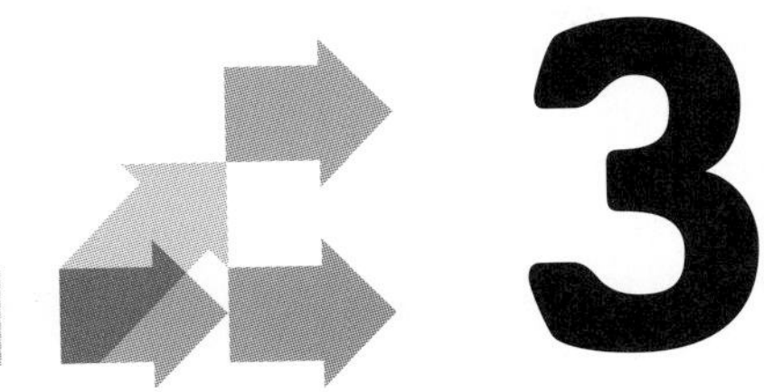

3

Developing Your Personal Skills

OBJECTIVES

THE INFORMATION AND ACTIVITIES IN THIS CHAPTER CAN HELP YOU TO:

- ➢ Identify your values and create a mission statement to support them.
- ➢ Set achievable goals to help guide your life.
- ➢ Recognize the importance of maintaining a positive attitude.
- ➢ Develop time management strategies to improve your personal efficiency.
- ➢ Create organizational techniques to make your life easier.
- ➢ Practice health habits that increase energy and reduce stress.
- ➢ Identify and use personalized learning strategies.
- ➢ Improve your ability to retain information.
- ➢ Understand the benefits of having a mentor.

KEY TERMS

Burnout: A physical and emotional state of exhaustion in which the person has difficulty handling work. It is often caused by overwork and feeling that one's efforts are not appreciated.

Insomnia: The inability to sleep well. It can be caused by worry and anxiety, as well as physical disorders.

Learning styles: Different ways of taking in and processing information. Recent studies show that not everyone learns in the same way.

Media: Distributors of news and advertising, especially television, radio, newspapers, and magazines.

Peers: People with whom you have something in common, such as other students and coworkers.

Relevant: Meaningful or important. For example, learning medical language is relevant for the health care professional.

Stamina: Energy that lasts for a period of time. Attending school, raising a family, and working require stamina.

Setting Up Your Mission Control

Embarking on a new career path is much like launching a space craft. Both students and astronauts are entering new worlds, and to be successful, their missions require careful planning and preparation. Final destinations must be clearly defined so that, once the journey is launched, its progress can be constantly monitored and adjusted as needed to stay on target.

Writing a mission statement is the first step in planning. Stephen Covey, author of personal success books, suggests writing a personal mission statement to determine what is really important to you. It requires you to identify the values that guide your actions. Many people, he points out, become sidetracked in life because they either lose sight of their basic values or fail to identify them clearly in the first place. A personal mission statement can help you choose an appropriate destination and then stay on track until you arrive.

Personal values consist of our beliefs about what is important in life combined with our understanding of right and wrong. They are the result of the teachings of family, school, religion, and friends and form the basis of our conscience. Values provide the foundation for making important life decisions: what we hope to contribute to the world, how we perform our work, and what we believe our obligations are to others.

A mission statement is not a list of goals or actions to take, but it serves as the basis for planning them. Thinking about your mission can help you clarify and state what is important to you: your basic beliefs about how you should live your life and what you want to accomplish.

Mission statements are usually written out, but there is no set format. You can write yours as a list, a series of paragraphs, or even a letter addressed to yourself. If you prefer, you can create a poster or collage, with each picture illustrating a value. The following example is the mission statement of a medical assisting student:

MY DECISIONS AND ACTIONS WILL BE BASED ON MY DEDICATION TO:

Maintaining my health and that of my family.
Balancing my work and family life so that neither is neglected.
Doing my best to master the professional skills of medical assisting.
Serving the needs of all patients I work with.
Continuing to learn about my profession.
Being loyal to my family, friends, and employer.
Keeping a positive attitude.
Seeking to understand rather than judge others.

Mission statements help you focus your attention on the deeper-level purposes in your life and serve as powerful motivators when you feel adrift or discouraged. For example, if you are committed to the well-being of your future patients, this value, rather than the need to pass a test, should guide your studying. Suppose you have an anatomy test tomorrow morning. It is 10:00 p.m. and you have just finished a day filled with classes, work, and family responsibilities. Studying the skeleton becomes more meaningful when placed in the context of your dedication to helping future patients. You are not simply memorizing a collection of bones. You are learning about the source of Mrs. Jones's painful arthritis, and the more you know and understand about the bones and joints, the more you will be able to help her. In another example, the better you understand how insurance claims are reviewed and processed, the better you can explain them to a confused client who is anxious about filling out the forms needed to cover his medical care.

Your actions as a student have an impact on future events that give what you do meaning beyond your immediate goal to complete assignments and earn grades (Fig. 3–1). Your future involves dealing with human beings who will be directly affected by what and how you are studying now. You should be guided by your highest values. Suppose that your mission statement includes "Provide high-quality care to all patients." You have an important exam for which you feel unprepared, and

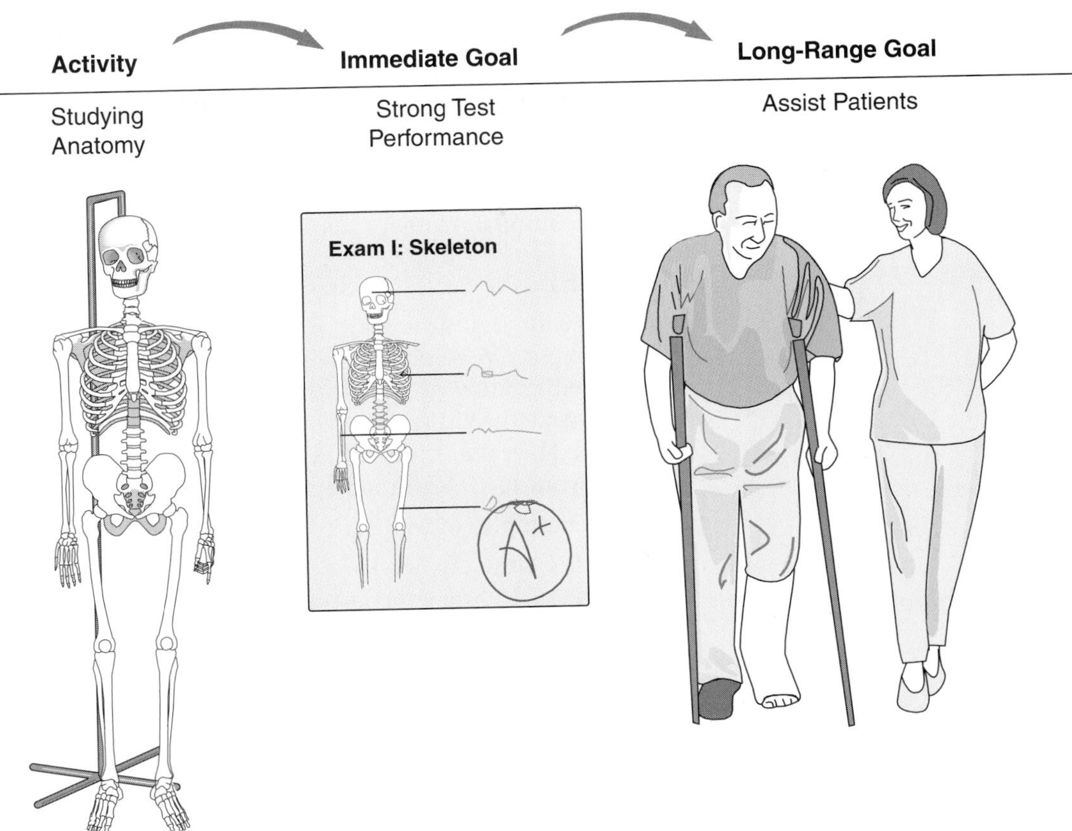

FIGURE 3–1 Keep your long-range goals in mind.

you are offered an opportunity to cheat. Cheating may take care of what you believe to be your most urgent need—getting a passing grade. But the consequence of this action—not learning the material—compromises your deeper-level purpose of competently serving the needs of future patients. A well-thought-out mission statement functions as the control center that keeps guiding you in the right direction toward achieving what is most important to you.

PRESCRIPTION FOR SUCCESS 3–1

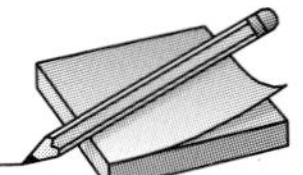

*Creating Your Professional Mission Statement**

Review your answers to Prescriptions for Success 1–1 in Chapter 1 and 2–1 in Chapter 2. Using your ideas and the following questions as a guide, write your mission statement for your life as a student and a future health care professional.

1. What do you most admire in other people?
2. How do you want to be remembered by people who matter to you?
3. Who do you most respect? Why?
4. If you could accomplish only three things in life, what would they be?
5. What makes you happiest? Why?
6. Which activities give you the most sense of purpose and satisfaction?

* Adapted from Covey, 1994.

Goals—Your Signposts to Success

The purpose of goals is to motivate, not to paralyze.—Maureen Pfeifer

Goals are based on your mission statement and provide guidance for your journey through life. Values provide the "why" for your actions, your mission statement the "what," and goals the "how." Goals serve as signposts, giving your life direction and measuring your progress on the road to success. Use them to motivate yourself and mark your accomplishments.

THE MARKS OF A GOOD GOAL

Good goals share the following characteristics:

- In line with your values: Do they agree with your basic beliefs?
- Reasonable: Do you have adequate time, energy, and knowledge?
- Measurable: How will you know if you have achieved them?
- Clearly stated: Will you understand your intention next month?
- Written: Have you thought them out and committed them to paper?
- Worth your time: Will they help you fulfill your mission?

Here are two examples of well-stated goals for a health care student:

1. Over the next ten weeks, I will learn the definition, pronunciation, and spelling of 150 new medical terms.
2. Within the next month, I will attend one professional meeting and talk with two people I have not met before.

MAKING GOALS WORK FOR YOU

1. Set them! The main reason people do not achieve their goals is that they fail to set them in the first place.
2. Develop an action plan outlining the steps needed to reach them.
3. Set reasonable deadlines for each step.
4. Identify and locate any resources needed to carry out your action steps (examples: people, materials, classes, equipment, money).
5. Don't forget to include your goals when you plan your daily activities. (Goals are often put aside in the scramble to meet everyday obligations.)
6. Periodically evaluate your goals and progress and make necessary adjustments.
7. Visualize yourself achieving them.
8. Use affirmations.
9. Work on them even when you don't feel like it. (Especially then!)
10. Don't give up!

Developing a Plan

Goals work only if you work steadily toward achieving them. Let's look at an example of a goal plan for mastering the 150 medical terms.

Goal:	Over the next ten weeks, I will learn the meaning, pronunciation, and correct spelling of 150 new medical terms.
Plan:	Learn 15 new terms each week. Study terminology four hours a week using flash cards, the workbook, tapes, and self-quizzes. Quiz myself at the end of each week.
Deadline:	15 terms each week. Achieve goal of 150 words at the end of ten weeks on ______ (date).
Resources:	Text and workbook; talk with instructors about suggestions for learning; check out tapes from the library; buy a medical dictionary.
Visualization:	See self in class receiving 100% on the medical terminology test. See self using medical terms correctly when talking with a coworker on the job.
Affirmation:	"I, ______, am mastering medical language easily and on schedule."

Ugh!! I don't really feel like studying these words. I'll just sit down and do a few at a time. Maybe this is the time for the anatomy coloring book?! The important thing is not to give up or procrastinate.

Goals vary in the time and effort required to achieve them. Write your long-term goals first; then prepare short-term supporting goals. Link them together in a progressive series so that each one supports the next. For example, Jaime's long-term career goal is to become successfully employed as an x-ray technician in a large city hospital. Here is his plan:

Long-Term Goal: Employment as an x-ray technician
Supporting Goals:
- Graduate from an approved x-ray training program.
  - Earn at least a B in all courses.
    - Take a study skills course.
    - Maintain perfect attendance for all classes.
    - Complete all homework assignments on time.
  - Receive a rating of at least "Above Average" on clinical experience.
- Pass the state licensing exam on the first try.

As we discussed in Chapter 2, you may have to set short-term stepping-stone employment goals as a means of achieving your long-term ideal job goal. For example, Jaime learns that the large urban hospital, Grand Memorial, where he wants to work, only hires technicians who have at least one year of experience. Furthermore, they prefer that technicians are able to perform specialized x-rays that are not included in most x-ray technology programs. Jaime adjusts his goals as follows:

Long-Term Goal: Employment in x-ray department at Grand Memorial
Stepping-Stone Goals:
- Receive a rating of "Excellent" on clinical experience.
- Improve communication skills.
- Work for at least one year in a facility that performs a variety of x-rays.
  - Complete three specialized x-ray courses.
  - Network with local professionals.
    - Become active in the x-ray professional organization's local chapter.

Jaime realizes that his clinical experience will provide a valuable opportunity to demonstrate his hands-on competence as a technician. It will serve him when he applies for his first job after graduation, as well as supplementing his work experience when he applies at Grand Memorial. His action steps to receive a top rating will include arranging reliable transportation (his old car is no longer dependable) and working on his oral communication skills, which he knows are a little weak. By planning ahead, setting goals, and identifying appropriate action steps, Jaime has greatly increased his chances of achieving what he really wants. He has avoided the frustration and disappointment of arriving at graduation without a Plan B to fulfill his employment hopes. Don't be discouraged if you find that a Plan C is also necessary!

In addition to promoting your own growth and progress, the ability to set appropriate goals and take action to achieve them increases your effectiveness as a health care professional. Patients often benefit from goal-setting: when they are recovering from an illness or injury, arranging to pay a large medical bill, or attempting to follow a weight-loss plan. By developing your own goal-setting skills, you can share this knowledge and help patients plan the steps necessary to achieve their goals.

PRESCRIPTION FOR SUCCESS 3–2

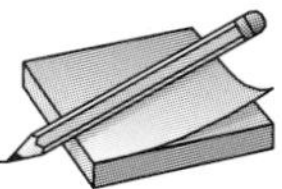

Name That Goal

1. Write one major career goal, three supporting goals, and two action steps for each supporting goal. Do they have the marks of a good goal?
   Major Career Goal ____________________
   - Supporting Goal 1 ____________________
     - Action Step 1 ____________________
     - Action Step 2 ____________________
   - Supporting Goal 2 ____________________
     - Action Step 1 ____________________
     - Action Step 2 ____________________
   - Supporting Goal 3 ____________________
     - Action Step 1 ____________________
     - Action Step 2 ____________________
2. Explain how your major goal relates to your mission statement and supports your values.
3. Plan deadlines for each goal and action step.
4. List the resources that will help you achieve Supporting Goal 1.
5. Create a visualization to help you achieve Supporting Goal 2.
6. Write two affirmations that will help you achieve Supporting Goal 3.

It's All in the Attitude

Man is not disturbed by the things that happened, but by the perception of things that happened.—Confucius

Your attitude can be your strongest ally or your worst enemy. It is more powerful than physical strength and more important than natural talents. It has helped people to overcome seemingly impossible difficulties. For example, survivors of concentration and prison camps attribute their survival to having a positive attitude. And the best thing about attitude is that it does not depend on other people or circumstances. Attitude is yours alone, one of the few things in life you have complete control over.

What exactly is this powerful possession? A good definition comes from Elkwood Chapman, author of best-selling books on attitude: "the way you mentally look at things." We hear about positive and negative attitudes to describe how people look at things. Is the weather partly clear or partly cloudy? Is a difficult class an opportunity to grow intellectually or a nightmare? Dr. Philip Hwang, a popular professor at the University of San Diego, tells his students that he prefers to interpret a popular offensive gesture as "half a peace sign." He *chooses* his reaction, and this is the key to the power of attitude: we have the opportunity to choose how we react to any situation.

"Well," you may say, "that doesn't make sense. If someone insults me or I'm having a bad day, it's natural to get angry or feel frustrated." It does seem natural, because we are in the habit of responding negatively to situations that are annoying or upsetting. But how does this benefit *you?* In most cases, nothing is gained except bad feelings. For example, if you develop a negative attitude about a class ("I'll *never* learn these 150 medical terms" or "She *really* can't expect us to perform twenty perfect venipunctures in two weeks!"), you are working against yourself. Your attitude, whether positive or negative, will not change the circumstances. Your negative attitude, however, will make it more difficult for you to concentrate on the task at hand, such as learning the vocabulary and mastering the procedure.

Let's look at another example. The guy who cuts you off on the freeway is at best inattentive and at worst a rude jerk. Why let a jerk ruin *your* day? In doing so, you give the jerks of the world far too much power. They may cut you off, but it doesn't make sense to give them the power to dictate how you feel. A negative attitude makes difficult situations even worse. Negativism is distracting, drains your energy, and interferes with your ability to concentrate. Choosing to approach life with a positive attitude releases you from the control of unpleasant people and circumstances and frees you to focus fully on your priorities and those actions that are in line with your mission and goals.

PRESCRIPTION FOR SUCCESS 3-3

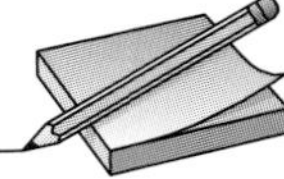

It's All How You Look at It

Scenario 1: Your medical terminology class is more difficult than you expected. You must memorize long lists of words and word parts and take quizzes twice a week. To make matters worse, the instructor is quite strict and does not seem very sympathetic. For each of the following options, indicate whether it reflects a positive or negative attitude. Then describe the probable outcome of each.

1. Be angry with the instructor and his "ridiculous" expectations.
2. Focus on how learning the terminology relates to your goal of becoming a health care professional.
3. Discuss the unfairness of the situation with your classmates.
4. Organize a study group with classmates.
5. Try using the memory techniques described later in this chapter.
6. Devote at least part of each day to worrying about this class.
7. Meet with the instructor privately and ask for suggestions about learning the vocabulary.
8. Look for ways to apply your learning style to master the vocabulary (discussed later in this chapter).
9. Skip class whenever possible; it's just too much to face every day, and besides, the instructor doesn't really help you learn.
10. Rethink your decision about becoming a health care professional.
11. Create and say affirmations about your ability to master the vocabulary.
12. Put off studying the words; it's a waste of time because you won't remember them anyway.
13. Think about the ways you will use medical terminology in your career.

continued

PRESCRIPTION FOR SUCCESS 3-3 *(continued)*

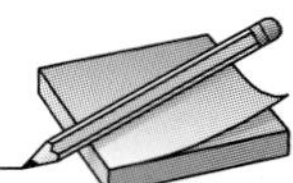

Scenario 2: You are working as a physical therapist assistant for a home health agency. Overall, you like your job and enjoy helping patients in their homes to regain mobility and strength following surgery and injuries. However, you have been assigned to work with a teenager who is recovering from a cycling accident. You find her very difficult to work with. She is rude and seems to resent your efforts to help her. List ten ways of handing this situation and label each as being either a positive (effective) or negative (ineffective) reaction.

1. __________
2. __________
3. __________
4. __________
5. __________
6. __________
7. __________
8. __________
9. __________
10. __________

DEVELOPING A POSITIVE APPROACH TO LIFE

1. *Do an inventory of the good things in your life.* What do I have to be thankful for? Good health? Friends? Family? Decent living conditions? Opportunity to attend school? Ability to succeed in school? My previous accomplishments and successes? Others?

2. *Keep things in perspective.* How important will this problem or situation be to me in one month? In one year? Does it threaten my survival?

3. *Fix your sights on your mission and goals.* Should I distract my focus and waste energy on negativity? How will a positive attitude help fulfill my mission?

4. *Distinguish between what you can and cannot change and concentrate your efforts on what you can change.* What action can I take? Which negative people and situations can I avoid? What changes can I make that will improve the situation?

5. *Ask yourself what will serve you best.* What attitudes and actions are most healthy for me? Are they in line with my mission? Will they further my goals and interests?

6. *Find sources of help and inspiration.* Who can give me support? Who can give me advice? Do I have deep-seated problems, such as depression or substance abuse, that require professional assistance?

7. *Visualize the satisfaction you will receive by overcoming a difficult situation.* How will this contribute to my personal growth? What can I learn from this?

8. *Challenge your negative beliefs.* Are they based on facts or on false perceptions?

TRIPPED UP BY YOUR THOUGHTS

The only thing we have to fear is fear itself.—Franklin Roosevelt

In Chapter 1 we discussed the self-fulfilling prophecy and its effect on teachers' perceptions of the ability levels of students. We saw that negative expectations can be just as powerful as positive ones, sometimes even more powerful. This is because our mental images, whether positive or negative, create our reality. It is important to understand that doubts and worries can actually *bring about* the outcome you fear. For example, Melinda believes that her supervisor dislikes her, so she avoids him and reacts defensively whenever he makes suggestions about her work. As a result of Melinda's behavior, chances are good that the supervisor *will* have a problem with her. Tripped up by her thoughts, she ends up creating what she expected and feared. Your attitude greatly influences your performance in school and your ability to secure and succeed in the job you want. Expect the best for yourself and you are likely to get it.

YOU MAKE A DIFFERENCE

Employers know that health care professionals with a positive attitude contribute to the success of their facility. This is a critical factor in promoting the well-being of patients and the spirit of teamwork among health care personnel. Patients seek health care in times of need, and they bring with them an assortment of fears and doubts. They want hope and encouragement, along with solutions to their health problems. Your cheerfulness, energy, and enthusiasm can make a difference in their progress and increase their satisfaction with the care they are receiving. Your good will is an important part of the example you set as a role model. Your positive attitude makes a difference in the lives of others.

A popular story illustrates the differences in attitudes in the workplace. Three stone workers were employed at a cathedral construction site hundreds of years ago. A visitor passing through asked one worker what he was doing. "I am mixing mortar. It's boring work," he answered. To the same question, a second worker replied, "I am building a wall. It's hard work." The third worker responded, "I am building a great cathedral to honor God. It's glorious work." Although all three were performing similar tasks, the third worker understood and appreciated the significance of his work. He had a positive attitude.

Make Time Work for You

Plan your work and work your plan.

Your success in life depends, to a great degree, on how you manage your time. Learning to use it to your advantage requires planning and self-discipline, but the payoffs are worth the effort. One fact of life is true for everyone: there will never be enough time for everything you want to do. Not accepting this fact can make you crazy and leave you wondering what happened and where all your time went.

The two keys to effective time management are prioritizing and practicing efficiency. *Prioritizing* means deciding what is most important and spending adequate time to ensure that it gets done. Your goals will determine your priorities. What do you most want to accomplish? Are you spending the majority of your time and energy on activities that will help achieve your goals? For example, if your goal is to graduate from a medical lab technician program with honors, are you spending the necessary time attending class, studying, and developing the work habits required of a lab technician? Or are phone conversations with friends and television viewing taking up a lot of your time?

Adult students have many responsibilities, and adding the role of student requires major adjustments. Determine which activities are critical to your success as a student and then focus on these. Some things may have to be postponed until you finish school and get your career underway. For example, washing the windows and waxing the car may have to wait. Attending classes and studying *must* take priority in your life.

Efficiency means planning and making the best use of time—getting the most done with the least effort. Examples of inefficiency include running to the grocery store to pick up a forgotten item, spending time looking for misplaced homework, and stopping for gas when you're already late for class rather than taking care of it the day before. It's easy to feel very busy and yet be inefficient. Pay attention to how you spend your time. A short break from studying to "rest your eyes" can stretch into an evening of lost hours in front of the television set.

PRESCRIPTION FOR SUCCESS 3-4

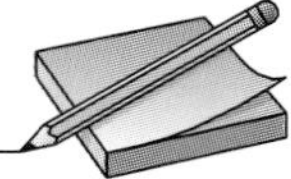

Where, Oh Where, Does the Time Go?

Keep a record of your activities for the next week. Create a chart that breaks each day into one-hour blocks. At the end of the week, answer the following questions:

1. How much time was devoted to school and learning activities?
2. How much time did you spend watching television?
3. On the telephone?
4. Doing other "escape" activities?
5. On "inefficiencies" (repeating, looking for, redoing, worrying, etc.)?

HELPFUL HINTS

There are many techniques for better organizing and using your time:

1. *List your priorities and goals.* Keep these clearly in mind as you plan your schedule and decide how to spend your time.

2. *Keep a calendar.* Many types of calendars are available, both paper and electronic. Select one that you can carry with you and that has room to list several items for each date. Next, collect all sources of important school and class dates: schedules, catalogs, and class syllabi. Write important items on your calendar, including days for quizzes and tests; due dates for assignments, projects, and library books; school holidays (for both you and your children); and deadlines for turning in required paperwork, such as financial aid and professional exam applications and for paying fees. Add important personal dates: birthdays of family members and friends, deadlines for bills and taxes, doctors' appointments, and back-to-school nights for your children. If you work, add any dates you need to remember: company potluck party, performance review, project deadlines. Create a calendar that works for you.

3. *Plan a weekly schedule.* Take a few minutes every week to plan ahead. This allows you to coordinate your activities with family members, plan ahead for important days (to avoid trying to find just the right birthday present on the way to the party), combine errands to save time, and plan your study time to avoid last-minute cramming. (More about that later.)

4. *Schedule study time every day.* This is your top priority! Give yourself a chance to succeed. Arrange not to be disturbed. Be sure that friends and family members know that when you are at your desk, the time is yours.

5. *Schedule around your peak times.* We all have individual body rhythms, specific times of the day when we feel most alert and energetic. Some people do their best work late at night. Others accomplish the most between 5:00 a.m. and 9:00 a.m. Class and work schedules cannot always accommodate your needs, but try to plan your most challenging tasks during your best hours.

6. *Do the hardest thing first.* When you have a number of things to do or subjects to study, try tackling the most difficult (or boring or tedious) one first. This way, you work on the one you like least when you are freshest. And completing unpleasant tasks gives you a surge of energy by removing a source of worry and distraction from your mind and rewarding you with a sense of accomplishment.

7. *Plan ahead.* Try to stay one—or even a half—step ahead. Use your calendar to anticipate and prepare for future events. Avoid wasting time. Call ahead to confirm appointments, get directions, or find out if the store carries what you need. If

your school requires you to wear a uniform and you often work late and have to rush, carry it in your car each day to avoid trips home and arriving late to class.

8. *Don't overorganize.* If you try to schedule every minute of each day, you are apt to become discouraged and give up planning altogether. Putting too much on your schedule will prevent you from concentrating on the most important tasks, and you will tend to ignore the whole schedule. And if you spend too much time scheduling, it will reduce the time needed to accomplish the very things that prompted you to try scheduling in the first place! Don't use planning as an excuse for not getting down to work. Aim for a happy balance.

9. *Be realistic.* We sometimes fail to schedule adequate time for what needs to be done. For example, thinking that you can complete a research paper in one weekend may be a serious mistake when you run into difficulties and the assignment is due on Monday. You will learn more about your work speed as you progress through your program. At the beginning, it is best to plan more time than you think you will need. On the other hand, spending so much time on one project or assignment that you neglect all others is not a wise use of time. Expecting absolute perfection is unrealistic and unnecessary.

10. *Plan for the unplanned.* Try not to schedule yourself so tightly that any emergency throws you into a panic. In the real world, children become ill and cars break down. Your schedule will sometimes include unplanned late night study sessions and early morning errands to cope with unexpected events and keep your priorities covered. Learning to be flexible is a valuable health care job skill.

11. *Avoid feeling overwhelmed.* Break work into small segments. (The thought of writing this book was overwhelming until the author broke it down into chapters, topics, and pages.) Plan deadlines and put them on your calendar. Ask for help and cooperation from family members and friends.

12. *Take occasional time-outs.* Sometimes doing less is actually doing more. Periodic rest breaks help you replenish your energy, maintain your perspective, and increase your efficiency. Work in at least a few minutes of daily private time and weekly time for something you enjoy.

13. *Learn to say "no."* Your schedule cannot always accommodate the requests of other people. It's difficult, but necessary, to turn down some of the demands on our time: social invitations, a request to help at the church rummage sale, or a three-day ski trip. Be sure to explain why you must refuse at this time and say that you will have more time after you graduate.

14. *Use down time to your advantage.* There are many pockets of time that usually go to waste: waiting for an appointment or to pick up the kids, using public transportation, or using an exercise bike. Use this time to study flash cards, write lists, review class notes, brainstorm topics for a research paper, review the steps involved in a lab procedure, or summarize the major points of a class lecture. (The author did about half of the work toward her last college degree while sitting in airports and on airplanes!)

PRESCRIPTION FOR SUCCESS 3–5

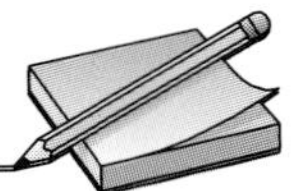

Beat the Clock

1. Based on your goals, which activities will receive the majority of your time and attention while you are in school? After you graduate?
2. Set up a personal calendar. Include all important dates for the next month.
3. Plan a schedule for the next week. Include items that must be completed each day.
4. Identify your peak times. How can you best use this time?

continued

PRESCRIPTION FOR SUCCESS 3-5 *(continued)*

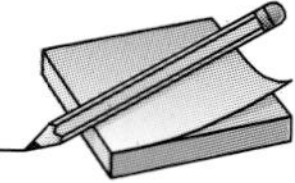

5. Plan one fun activity to do sometime this month.
6. Have there been requests that you declined (or should have declined) since you started school? How did you handle them? How can you handle them in the future?
7. Identify instances of down time in your life. How can you best utilize this time?

DEFEATING THE PROCRASTINATION DEMON

Procrastination is the cause of many missed opportunities. Putting off what needs to be done can result in late assignments, failed tests, and poor recommendations. Yet many of us fall victim to this self-defeating habit. It's natural to delay what we perceive to be difficult, tedious, or overwhelming. If procrastination is interfering with your efforts to succeed, you may find the following suggestions helpful:

1. Try to identify the reason for your procrastination. What is holding you back? Are you afraid of failing? Do you believe you lack the ability to do what needs to be done? Is the task so unpleasant that you cannot motivate yourself to start it? Is the project so large that you feel overwhelmed and the victim of "overload paralysis"? (If you find yourself continually procrastinating, you may want to ask your school counselor for help in finding the key to your behavior.)
2. Once the reason is identified, examine it carefully. Is it justified?
3. Identify sources of help: instructor, supervisor, friend. Do you need additional materials or more information to get started?
4. Break large projects into manageable pieces and plan deadlines for each. Develop a controlled sense of urgency (not panic) to encourage yourself to meet self-imposed deadlines.
5. Set a time to start, even if you simply work on planning what you are going to do. Accomplishing something, even a small amount, can inspire you to keep going.
6. Use affirmations such as, "I am capable of understanding how the endocrine system functions. My presentation to the class will be interesting and well organized."
7. Visualize yourself completing the work. Concentrate on the satisfaction you will feel.
8. Focus on your future. Think about how completing the work will help you achieve your goals.
9. Develop a positive attitude about your work. How are you approaching it? Concentrate your energy on the advantages of getting the work done rather than worrying about not doing it. Work up some enthusiasm for the project—how can you benefit from it?
10. When all else fails, just do something!

PRESCRIPTION FOR SUCCESS 3-6

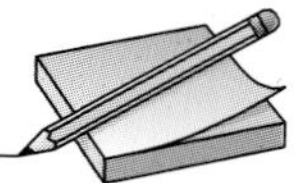

Defeating the Demon

Note: Students who never procrastinate may skip this exercise.

1. What are you now, or have recently, put off doing?
2. Why?
3. Which of the techniques listed do you think would help you most?
4. Develop a plan to get started, including the date you will begin.

Personal Organization: Getting It All Together

A vital key to success is learning to work smarter, not harder.

The purpose of personal organization, like time management, is to make life easier. Organizational techniques build consistency and predictability into your daily routines, saving you time and energy. Surprise-filled adventures are great for vacation trips, but efficiency is a better way to ensure academic and career success. Hunting for your keys every morning and arriving late for class is a waste of your time and a sign of inconsideration for your instructor and classmates. Lack of organization on the job can reduce patient satisfaction. No one wants to wait while the medical assistant scurries about to gather the equipment needed for an eye irrigation or injection.

Organization, however, should never become an end in itself. It doesn't mean keeping a perfectly tidy house, with clothes arranged according to color and season. It does mean surveying your needs and developing ways to avoid unnecessary rushing, repetition, and waste.

HELPFUL HINTS

1. *Write lists.* Most people today, especially students, have too many things on their minds to remember grocery lists, all the day's errands, who they promised to call, which lab supplies to take to class, and so on. Scraps of paper are easy to lose. Some students like to use commercial organizers. A small notebook also works and gives you a place to jot down phone numbers, addresses of stores, recommendations from friends, ideas you think of throughout the day, and so on.

2. *Carry a big bag.* A typical day may include classes, work, shopping, and returning a video. Start each day—either in the morning or the night before—by checking your calendar and to-do list to see what you need to take with you that day. If you go directly to class from work, pack your books, binder, uniform, and other necessary supplies. Take along your own fast food: fruit, granola bars, cheese and crackers. Always carry your calendar and lists.

3. *Stock up.* Running out of milk, shampoo, or diapers is a frustrating waste of time and energy. Even worse is discovering at 11:30 p.m., while finishing a major assignment that is due tomorrow, that your printer cartridge is empty and you don't have another. (The author knows that cartridges are well aware of deadlines and choose to dry up accordingly!) Keep important backup supplies on hand. A handy way to keep monitoring these is to keep a shopping list on the refrigerator and in your study area. Instruct everyone in the household to add to it as they notice supplies running low.

4. *Give things a home.* Keeping what you need where you can find it will save countless hours of search time. It will also prevent redoing lost assignments or paying late fees on misplaced bills. If your study area is a dual-use area such as the kitchen table, try keeping your books and supplies in one place on a shelf or in a large box where everything can stay together. This way you can set up an "instant desk" when it is time to study. Organize your class notes and handouts by subject in a binder. Color-coded files work well for keeping ongoing projects and notes from previous classes in order.

5. *Keep things in repair.* Life is easier if you can depend on the car and other necessities. If money is tight, focus on keeping the essentials in working order and look for ways to economize elsewhere.

6. *Think ahead.* Work on preventing "urgencies" by using your personal calendar to keep on top of due dates, birthdays, and other time-sensitive events. Plan what you can do today to smooth the way for tomorrow.

7. *Cluster errands.* Modern life requires trips to the grocery store, the mall, the children's school, the post office—you name it, we go there! Save time and transportation money by doing as much as possible on each trip. Look for shopping centers that have many services to avoid running all over town.

8. *Handle it once.* This is a popular technique recommended for businesses. If you find that mail, bills, announcements, and other paperwork accumulate in ever-growing piles, try processing each item as it comes in. Sort the mail quickly each day and do something with each piece: discard the junk, pay the bills (or file them together for payment once a month), answer letters with a short note, read messages and announcements, and place magazines in a basket to be looked over during your next time-out. Handle other papers that come into the house—permission slips for the kids, announcements from work—the same way.

9. *Get it over with.* Certain unpleasantries come into everyone's life: parking tickets, dental work, court appearances. It's easy to get caught up in worrying about them. A good strategy is to get them over with as quickly as possible: pay the ticket, make an appointment with the dentist, and prearrange an absence from class to make the court date. Seek help if you need it, and do your best to take care of what needs to be done. Putting these things off can drain your energy and interfere with your concentration.

10. *Plan backups.* Prearrange ways to handle emergencies: a ride to school if the car breaks down, child care to cover for a sick babysitter, a study buddy who will lend you notes when you cannot attend class. Backups are like insurance policies—you hope you won't need them, but if you do, they're good to have. Whenever possible, plan backups for your backups.

If getting organized seems like a waste or time, too much work, or just "not your style," consider the alternative: using even *more* time and energy in unproductive ways that end up in frustration and inconvenience. You can start now to help yourself get it together using skills that will be valuable in any future health care position.

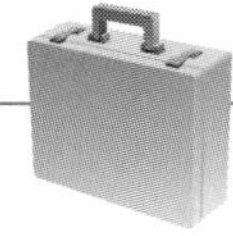

ORGANIZATION ON THE JOB

A typical job description for a medical assistant includes many organizational duties that correspond closely with the techniques suggested in this section:

1. Sort and handle the daily mail. **(Handle it once.)**
2. Monitor warranties on equipment, and call for maintenance and repair. **(Keep things in repair.)**
3. Inventory and order administrative, laboratory, and clinical supplies. **(Stock up.)**
4. Organize and store supplies and equipment. **(Give things a home.)**
5. Schedule and monitor patient appointments. **(Think ahead.)**
6. Complete all tasks as directed by the physician. **(Write lists.)**

CHILDREN IN THE HOUSE

Here are tips* for students who have young children:

1. If your children are old enough, work on homework together.
2. Have young children "help" you by drawing, coloring pictures, filling in sticker books, or performing other "desk work."
3. Exchange babysitting services with friends and family members, arranging to take the responsibility when your study load is lightest.

* Adapted from Ellis, 1994.

4. Organize a study group of classmates who have children. Contribute to a babysitting fund, and hire someone to watch all the children while you study together.
5. Explain to your children why you are in school. Show them a picture of a health professional, and tell them about your future job and how you will be helping people.
6. Ask your school if they have family days or picnics when children can see where their parents are spending so much time now.
7. Try to turn your study time into a positive experience for the kids by saving their favorite videos, toys, and other activities for the times when you are busy.
8. Investigate community and religious activities such as day camps, sports teams, and craft classes. Some organizations offer reasonably priced activities.
9. Plan to spend some time with your children each day just doing something fun, even if only for a few minutes. Let them choose the activity.
10. Tell them how much you appreciate their cooperation.

Your Health: Who's in Charge?

Good health and at least a moderate level of fitness will increase your energy and productivity and improve your outlook on life. Most people know about the importance of good nutrition, the dangers of smoking, and the need for regular exercise and sufficient sleep. But knowing is not the same as doing. Many of us continue to practice poor eating habits, avoid exercise, smoke, get too little sleep, and ignore common sense. Why do we avoid doing what is "good for us"? Let's begin to explore this by looking at four examples: exercise, fast food, smoking, and drinking.

If you're too tired to exercise, your fatigue is due partly to the fact that you don't exercise! People who exercise regularly tend to have more energy and **stamina** than those who do not. It can be argued that they actually make up the time spent on physical activity because they are able to concentrate better and work more efficiently. (Remember: "work smarter, not harder.") A brisk walk after a frantic day is an exceptional bargain: it costs nothing, renews your energy, settles your nerves, and gives you a sense of well-being.

The term "fast food" is a contradiction because while the food may be served and eaten quickly, it can actually slow you down and decrease your efficiency. This is because fats, a major component of fast foods, are digested slowly and tie up body energy in this process. Further, much of the fat we eat is stored by the body for future needs, and because many of us take in more potential energy (calories) than we need, we accumulate more stored energy than we use (fat). The energy that you could devote to studying, working, and moving through your day is being used to digest, store, and pack fat. In an effort to save time, we actually lose it. (Appearance is *not* a consideration here. The author believes that the current emphasis on extreme thinness for women is sexist and unhealthy.)

Smoking is a tricky habit because many smokers believe that cigarettes are "calming" and "settle the nerves." The fact is, cigarettes themselves are what *create* the need for calming. They are the *cause* of unsettled nerves. We commonly hear smokers speak of their "need" for a cigarette. They are right—they do need it to alleviate the physical craving (withdrawal symptoms) experienced when the nicotine in the body dips below the level to which the smoker is accustomed. The symptoms include anxiety, irritability, and the inability to concentrate. Smoking detracts from the smoker's quality of life by creating a continuous need that demands time, attention, and money. This is in addition to the health risks that everyone knows about. Keep in mind that smoking is prohibited in all health care facilities. Even having the odor of tobacco on your body or clothing is unacceptable because many patients find it offensive.

Drinking alcohol is an accepted custom in many cultures. Current research even indicates that drinking moderate amounts of alcohol may help prevent certain types of heart disease. For many persons, it is an important part of relaxing and enjoying social activities. Alcohol becomes a problem, however, when it is used excessively or to seek relief from life's problems. Rather than providing solutions, it adds a new problem. Like other escape activities, such as overeating and illegal drug use, alcohol simply diverts attention from addressing the real problems, such as stress, loneliness, boredom, and depression.

Many of our eating, drinking, and smoking habits are the result of the marketing campaigns of industries that earn billions of dollars annually by promoting the use of their products. Advertising focuses on convincing us that certain products will enhance our lives: we will have more fun, enjoy the rich taste, and receive other positive benefits. The major benefits, in fact, are the dollars that go into the pockets of the producers of these products. We become dependent on habits that do not benefit us but that are difficult to discontinue.

Doing the right things for your health may seem restrictive, boring, and a way to take all the fun out of life. Just the reverse may be true. Feeling well, energetic, and enthusiastic is not boring. On the contrary, life is easier and more fun when you have the physical and mental reserves to do everything that is important to you.

Consider the effect of your lifestyle choices on your mission and goals.

- Are you working for or against yourself?
- Do your health habits increase your mental alertness and ability to succeed in school?
- Are they distracting you from doing your best?
- Are you neglecting your health at the very time when you should be doing your best to take care of yourself?

As pointed out in Chapter 1, an important expectation of health care professionals is that they serve as positive examples in promoting sound health habits among both patients and the public. How do you rate as a role model?

HELPFUL HINTS

If you want to make changes in your health habits but feel overwhelmed by the idea, review the following suggestions; see also Boxes 3–1 and 3–2.

1. *Start small.* Choose one area you want to improve and begin slowly. Take a short walk every other day. Pack a lunch instead of eating chips or a candy bar. Eat breakfast, even a small one. Choose one activity, such as talking on the phone or driving, during which you won't smoke.

2. *Be patient.* Television programs in which problems are solved in thirty minutes and advertising that promises quick weight loss and tight "abs" in just eight minutes a day have conditioned us to expect instant solutions. Real life is not that way, and it may take time for you to see results from your efforts.

3. *Recognize your own power.* You are in control of your choices. Select products and activities because they are what *you* want, not because of the influence of friends or the **media.**

BOX 3–1. EASY WAYS TO EAT HEALTHY

1. Eat fruits. They taste great and come in their own wrappers!
2. Take appropriate vitamins.
3. Plan food to go. Pack healthy lunches and snacks.
4. Avoid fad diets. In the long run, almost no one keeps weight off. In the short run, you are shortchanging your body of what it needs.
5. Eat a balanced diet. Make selections from all the food groups, as recommended, by the U.S. Department, of Agriculture (Fig. 3–2).
6. Shop at farmers' markets and outlets that offer fresh fruits and vegetables at lower prices than most supermarket chains.

BOX 3–2. EXERCISE FOR FUN AND RESULTS

If a walk seems boring, go with a friend, family member, or pet. See if your area has a book describing interesting walks, or choose another form of exercise that you enjoy and that fits your budget. Many communities sponsor organized sports and offer inexpensive access to swimming pools, basketball courts, and ice skating rinks. When you're already busy, it's best to stay with something simple (Fig. 3–3).

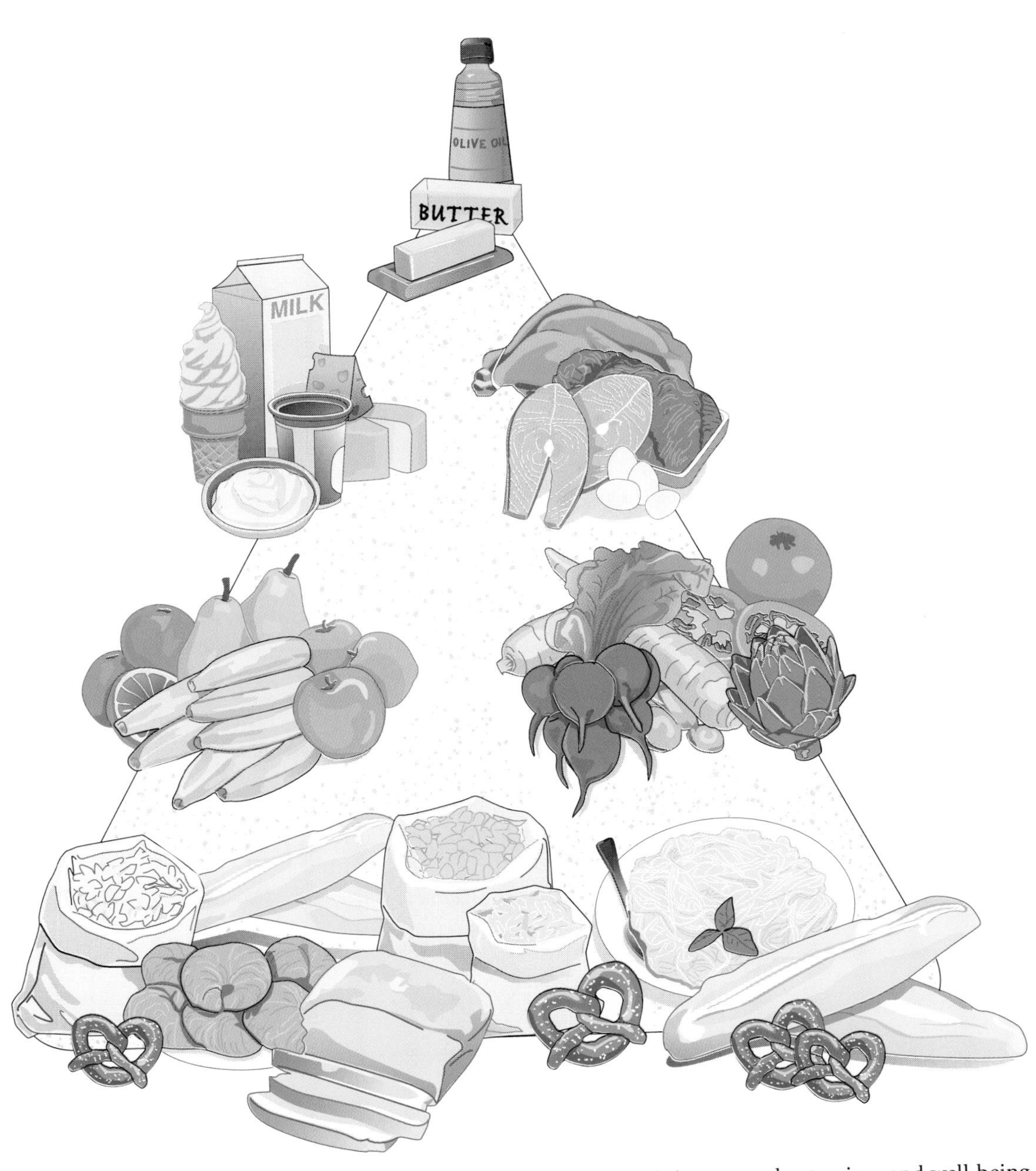

FIGURE 3–2 A healthy diet is essential for maintaining strength, stamina, and well-being.

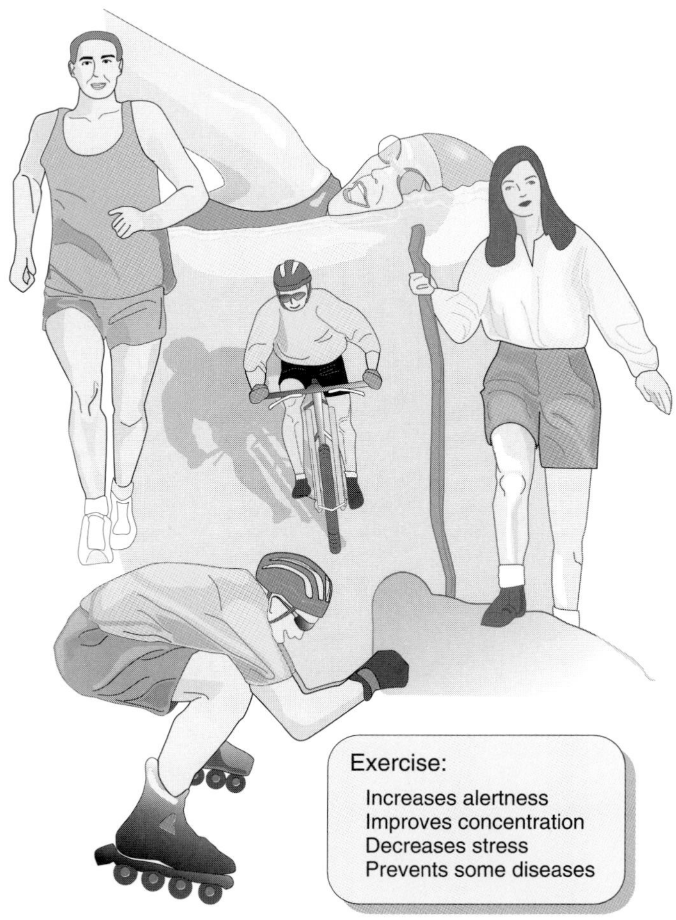
Exercise:
Increases alertness
Improves concentration
Decreases stress
Prevents some diseases

FIGURE 3–3 Exercise benefits the mind and the body.

4. *Use the tools.* Employ goal-setting, visualization, and affirmation techniques.

5. *Seek support.* There are organizations for every type of problem, and many charge nothing or only a small fee. Check with your school's student services to learn what is available in your area.

6. *Read about it.* Bookstores and libraries are filled with books and magazines about health issues. The Internet is another good source of current information.

7. *Focus on the benefits.* Identify what these will be for you.

8. *Think long-term.* Consider how action taken now will contribute to your future success. Keep the payoffs in mind.

PRESCRIPTION FOR SUCCESS 3–7

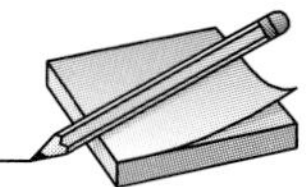

What's Your Excuse?

Write a positive argument against each of the following excuses.
Examples:

If I quit smoking, I'll look like a blimp.

If you don't smoke, you will probably feel more like exercising, and this will help control your weight. Also, food may taste better and you will

PRESCRIPTION FOR SUCCESS 3–7 *(continued)*

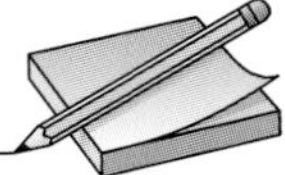

find that because you enjoy it more, you actually need to eat less to be satisfied. Finally, you don't have to eat. You have a choice, remember?

Fast food is the only thing my kids will eat.

It may indeed be more difficult if you have other people's habits to change in addition to your own. Children's habits can be changed if you introduce gradual changes into their diet. If possible, include them in cooking and meal planning so that the entire experience becomes a family project.

Pack a lunch? Are you kidding? With all that I have to do? I'm just too busy.

I've tried eating right before and I didn't really see any benefits.

Life is short—why should I deprive myself?

It's too expensive to buy fresh foods and go to a gym.

Smoking is one of my only pleasures.

By the time I get everything else done, I'm just too tired to exercise and cook balanced meals. Give me a break!

Exercise is totally boring.

I'm stressed out enough with school and work; there's no way I can worry about this stuff now!

Can you think of any other excuses that apply to you? What is your response?

What Is This Thing Called Stress?

We hear a lot about stress these days. One friend says, "I'm so stressed over this exam." Another exclaims, "I just can't take any more of this stress." "Stress" refers to our physical and emotional reactions to life's events. These reactions can either help or hurt us, depending on the circumstances. "Good stress" motivates us when we are called upon to perform beyond our usual comfort zone. For example, if you witness a car accident and stop to help the victims, your body experiences certain reactions: your heart rate speeds up, your blood pressure rises, and the blood vessels in your muscles and the pupils of your eyes dilate. These changes increase your energy, strength, and mental alertness. You are better able to deal with the situation. You can draw upon these natural reactions to help you in important, although less dramatic, situations such as taking a professional licensing exam, giving a speech in class, or planning a wedding. This is making use of good stress to maximize your performance. The excitement experienced when you pass the exam and start a new career or get married and begin a new life with the person you love is also a form of good stress. Stress can serve a useful purpose in our lives.

Pressure and worries experienced over long periods of time can create "bad stress." This causes responses that actually *decrease* your ability to cope with life's ups and downs. In a sense, your body wears itself out as it repeatedly prepares you to handle situations which are never resolved. Signs of long-term stress include **insomnia,** headaches, digestive problems, muscle tension, fatigue, frequent illness, irritability, depression, poor concentration, excessive eating and drinking, and use of illegal substances. It's easy to see that these don't work in your favor and are likely to *increase* your stress level. You can become caught in a vicious cycle of ever-increasing stress that results in the hopeless feeling that there is no way out. Your mental images are dictated by worry and fear and may bring about, as we have discussed, the very thing that you fear.

DEALING WITH LONG-TERM STRESS

The first step in dealing with long-term stress is to identify its source. The following list contains some of the common reasons for stress experienced by adult students:

1. Financial difficulties.
2. Family problems: nonsupportive partner, abuse, children's behavior.
3. Poor organizational skills.
4. Inability to manage time; having too much to do.
5. Lack of self-confidence and poor self-esteem.
6. Feeling unsure about study skills and ability to learn.
7. Loneliness.
8. Health problems, pregnancy.
9. Believing that instructors are unfair or don't like them.
10. Poor relationships with **peers.**
11. Believing that assignments and tests are too difficult or not **relevant.**
12. Difficulty following school rules and requirements.

The second step in handling stress is to examine the source to see if it's based on fact or fiction. For example, if you worry about failing your courses because you are not "smart enough," this may be based on a false belief about yourself. It is very likely that you are intellectually competent. But believing that you aren't can create stress that discourages you from even trying. After all, what's the point of making a lot of effort if you're going to fail anyway? (The self-fulfilling prophecy at work!) Seek guidance from your instructor or student services.

Finally, look for a practical solution. What are your options? Can you distance yourself from the stressor (for example, a negative friend who constantly asks why you are returning to school at *your age*)? Get help to resolve the problem (free financial counseling for budget and credit problems, tutoring in a difficult subject)? Empower yourself (math refresher course, speed reading tapes)? The important thing is to face the stressor and take control. Convert bad stress into good stress by using it as a signal that you have issues that may prevent you from achieving your goals and attaining the success you want and deserve. Then take action to deal with the issues.

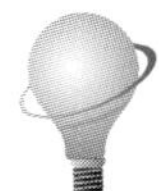

Take a Moment to Think

1. Do you believe you may be experiencing long-term stress?
2. If yes, what are the signs?
3. If yes, can you identify the cause or causes?

REDUCING STRESS

The very nature of being a student and working in health care brings a certain amount of ongoing stress that cannot be avoided entirely. Many of the practices that promote good health are excellent for relieving stress: exercise, adequate sleep, eating complex carbohydrates, and avoiding excessive caffeine. Here are some other things you can try:

1. *Practice mentally.* If the stress is caused by an upcoming event such as a job interview, you can anticipate and mentally practice the event. Athletes use this technique to prepare for the big game. They "see" themselves performing the perfect tennis serve or drive down the fairway. Employ your stress to motivate you to prepare in advance.

2. *Use time management and personal organization strategies.* Try the techniques suggested in this chapter to help you take control of your life. Prevent the disorder that has you feeling as if you're racing downhill with no brakes.

3. *Seek the support of others.* People do better when they have the support of others. Studies have shown that students who have just *one* other person who really cares if they graduate are more likely to finish school than those who have no one. Seek the help of trusted friends, family members, classmates, or school personnel for listening and sharing.

4. *Perform relaxation exercises.* Meditation, yoga, deep breathing, and muscle relaxation can relieve physical discomfort and promote emotional well-being (Box 3–3).

5. *Take some time for hobbies and fun.* Even short breaks can increase your ability to deal with stress.

6. *Adjust your attitude.* Focus on your goals, acknowledge all progress, and concentrate on the benefits you will receive.

7. *Use school and community resources.* Refer to the chart you prepared in Prescription for Success 1–11. Community service information may be available from student services, your religious organization, or the local community center.

8. *Make use of this book.* Chapters 4 through 7 contain many suggestions for developing effective study skills. Try them out and use the ones that work best for you.

BOX 3–3. RELAXATION EXERCISE

Eliminating muscle tension prevents anxiety and fatigue. Try this simple exercise to help you relax. Using these techniques can prevent muscle tension from reaching the point of causing headaches and other pain.

1. Sit comfortably in a place where you won't be disturbed. Choose a chair that supports your back and allows you to place your feet flat on the floor.
2. Close your eyes.
3. Begin at your toes and tense each group of muscles. Hold for a few seconds and then release. Work from the bottom of the body to the top, tensing and relaxing each area. Pay special attention to the shoulders and jaw muscles, common areas of tension.
4. As you proceed, focus on the feelings of tension and then letting go.
5. When you finish, sit quietly and say to yourself "I am relaxed."

PRESCRIPTION FOR SUCCESS 3–8

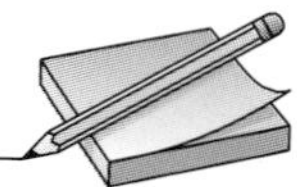

Personal Stress Relievers

If you identified sources of stress in the preceding "Take a Moment to Think" section, list at least three strategies for dealing with them.

1. ______________________________
2. ______________________________
3. ______________________________

Good stress can serve the health care professional by providing extra energy and increased mental alertness to handle emergency situations properly, provide competent patient care, and maintain a busy schedule. Assisting a fallen patient, performing first aid, and getting through a hectic day of unplanned interruptions can drain your personal resources. It is important that you incorporate stress-reduction techniques into your daily life. Tragic results of excessive buildup of stress among health care workers include **burnout,** addiction to pain killers, and alcoholism. Start now to learn effective stress management, converting stress from an enemy to an ally.

Learning to handle stress will benefit not only you, but your future patients as well. Illness and injury are major stressors, and an important part of patient education is helping patients deal with both physical and emotional stress.

Learning for Life

Learning means much more than getting by in school and remembering information long enough to pass tests. It means acquiring information and mastering skills that you store mentally and are able to retrieve and use when you need them on the job. Further, it means being able to *apply* what you have learned to solve problems

TABLE 3–1 Three Major Learning Styles

Learning Style	How Student Learns Best	Most Effective Learning Activities
Auditory	Through *hearing.* Remembers information from lectures and discussions better than material read in textbook. Prefers music over art, listening over reading. Understands written material better when one reads aloud. May spell better out loud than when writing. Misses visual cues. Prefers doing oral rather than written reports.	Lectures, tapes, music, rhymes, speaking
Visual	Through *seeing.* Remembers information presented in written form better than in lectures and discussions. Often needs people to repeat what they have said. Takes notes when oral instructions are given. Prefers art to music, reading to listening. Understands better when the speaker's face is seen. Prefers doing written rather than oral reports.	Reading, pictures, diagrams, charts, graphs, maps, videos, films, chalkboard, overhead projections
Kinesthetic (hands-on)	Through *doing.* Remembers information acquired through activities. Reads better when moving lips and saying words silently or moving finger along the page. Enjoys moving around while studying. Likes to touch things, point, use fingers when counting or calculating. Prefers doing a demonstration rather than an oral or written report.	Lab activities, skills practice, experiments, games, movement, building models

and make informed decisions. Let's look at an example. If you are learning about the skeleton, you are not simply memorizing the names of the bones and joints. You are acquiring information to help real patients with real problems. Your purpose for learning is far more important than simply studying to earn a grade. Your future patients will depend on your knowledge, and they deserve your best efforts to learn now.

HOW DO YOU LEARN BEST?

If you ever feel that you just can't follow your instructor's lectures or find that your class notes are a confusing jumble, you are not alone. It is possible that you learn better when instruction is presented visually or through hands-on experience. Recent research has demonstrated that people learn in different ways, called **learning styles,** and that by identifying your own preferred learning styles you can be more successful in your studies. The three learning styles most commonly discussed are grouped by the three senses used when acquiring and processing new information: auditory, visual, and kinesthetic (hands-on). See Table 3–1.

In addition to the senses, other factors influence how you learn. The following sets of approaches, combined with your sensory preferences, make up your set of learning styles:

1. *Deductive:* Learning the facts helps the deductive learner understand generalizations (the big picture). Prefers to first memorize dates, study individual events, and know the details. For example, would rather study the parts of the circulatory system before learning how they work together to circulate the blood.

OR

2. *Inductive:* Understanding the big picture provides a framework for learning the details. Wants to know the purpose and function of the human cell before learning the individual components.

---

1. *Linear:* Learns best when material is organized in a logical sequence. Likes to do things in order, building on material previously learned.

OR

2. *Global:* Likes to work with all the facts, regardless of the order. Interested in forming relationships within the material.

---

1. *Individual:* Prefers to work alone. Likes to figure out problems and do all the work on assignments and projects.

OR

2. *Interactive:* Likes to work with another student or in groups. Wants to share own ideas and hear those of others.

It is important to realize that one way to learn is not better than the others. The purpose of discovering your learning styles is to help you study more effectively. Each of us has a unique set and employs a combination of methods to learn, as in the following example of a student who is studying psychology:

1. Prefers to receive new information from a class lecture (auditory);
2. Reviews by studying notes alone (individual); and
3. Concentrates first on memorizing the important facts (deductive).

PRESCRIPTION FOR SUCCESS 3–9

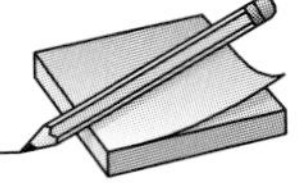

What Are Your Styles?

Describe all the learning styles you believe apply to you.

DEVELOPING LEARNING STRATEGIES

Identifying your preferred ways of learning does not mean that you will avoid the others. This would be impossible in a health care program that includes both theoretical and practical knowledge and skills. And instructors use a variety of approaches to teaching. Some will match your learning styles; others won't. For example, when teaching students how to take a blood pressure, the instructor might introduce the topic with a lecture (auditory); give a reading assignment (visual); demonstrate and describe the procedure (auditory and visual); assign a worksheet (individual); and have partners practice on each other (kinesthetic and interactive). In her lecture, she might list the individual steps first (deductive) or explain the purpose and significance of blood pressure before explaining how to take it (inductive). The good news is that you can learn in a variety of ways and benefit from your strongest methods while developing your weakest. Table 3–2 gives examples of study techniques applied to a specific assignment: learning the names and locations of the major bones. See also Figure 3–4.

TABLE 3–2 Developing Learning Strategies

Learning Style	Learning Strategies
Auditory	1. Say the names of the bones out loud. 2. Listen to a tape of the names and locations of each. 3. Make your own tape of the names and locations. 4. Create a song, rhyme, rap, or jingle. Silly is good ("There are fourteen phalanges in my little handies") 5. Clap or tap out a rhythm as you repeat the words. 6. Make flash cards and say the words and/or definitions out loud. 7. Create sound-alike association. Remember, silly is okay ("The cranium holds the brain-ium").
Visual	1. Look at photos or drawings of the bones as you study their names. 2. Label a drawing of the skeleton. 3. Color the bones on a drawing. 4. Create mental pictures of associations (a crane lifting a huge cranium). 5. Put up a labeled drawing of the skeleton where you will see it often—the bathroom mirror, your bedroom wall, near your study desk. 6. Make flash cards that have a picture of the bone on one side and the name on the reverse.
Kinesthetic	1. Point to or touch each bone as you learn its name. Use drawings, a model (inexpensive anatomical models are sold in toy stores), or your own body. 2. Make two flash cards for each bone: one with the name, the other with the location. Mix the cards, then study by sorting and matching each set. 3. Stand, move, or walk around as you study. 4. Associate movements as you learn. For example, lift and bend your arm when studying the humerus, ulna, and radius. 5. Write the name of each bone several times.
Deductive	Start by learning the name and location of one bone at a time.
Inductive	Start by looking at the relationships and connections between the bones. Think about how each contributes to body function.
Linear	Study the bones in a logical order that makes sense to you: by area (extremities—arms and legs), from top to bottom (shoulder to hand), etc.
Global	Study from a labeled diagram that includes the entire skeleton or all the bones of a given area.
Individual	Use the suggested learning techniques by yourself. Set goals for how many bones you'll learn each day. Create a reward system for yourself.
Interactive	Form a study group with classmates. Ask a friend or family member to quiz you. Organize a group or class competition.

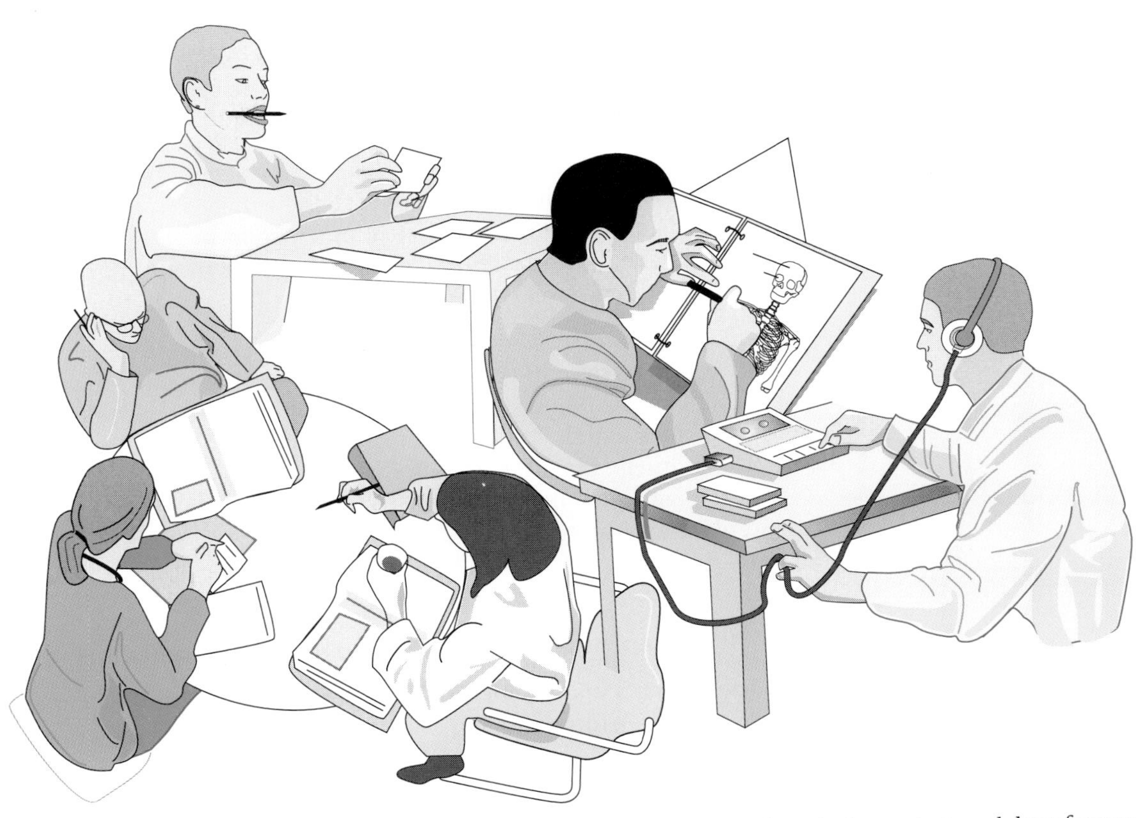

FIGURE 3–4 Identify and use the study techniques that work best for you.

PRESCRIPTION FOR SUCCESS 3–10

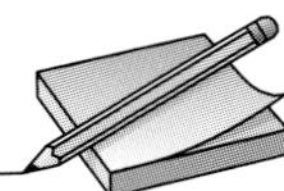

Make Your Learning Styles Work for You

Using what you have learned so far about your preferred styles of learning, list five strategies that you believe would help you to learn the name and purpose of a list of twenty-five vitamins.

1. ______
2. ______
3. ______
4. ______
5. ______

DOWN MEMORY LANE

Memorizing is not the same as learning, but it is an important component of the learning process. While you may be able to rely on your short-term memory to complete assignments and pass tests, it is the material that is stored in long-term memory that will serve you throughout your studies and afterward on the job. There are many ways to improve your memory:

1. *Understand first.* Experiments have shown that it is much more difficult to remember nonsense syllables or lists of unrelated numbers than material that has meaning. In other words, it is very difficult to remember what you don't understand in the first place. Ask questions in class, look up words you don't know when read-

ing, and use what you discovered about your learning styles to increase your understanding of the material presented in your courses.

2. *Repeat, repeat, repeat.* The *very best* way that has been proven to help people remember new material is repetition over an extended period of time. In fact, the length of time information is remembered is often in direct proportion to the length of time over which it is learned. Review new material as soon as possible after it is presented and continue to review it on a regular basis, at least weekly. (If your program is divided into classes that are less than one month long, you should review at least three times a week.)

3. *Use strategies based on your learning styles.* For example, listen to or say new math formulas over and over (auditory); review them daily in written form (try posting them on the bathroom mirror) (visual); and write each new formula at least ten times (kinesthetic). Use your imagination. Studying does not necessarily mean working quietly at a desk. Create rhymes or funny images. Make up movements associated with each item you have to remember. One method, called "pegging," has you place imaginary pegs around the house. On each one, "hang" a fact or idea you must remember. As you walk through the house each day, review the material on each peg.

4. *Organize information.* Put new material in an order that makes sense to *you.*

5. *Relate to your experience.* Connect new information to something that you already know. Before studying something new, quickly jot down what you know about a topic and look for ways to make connections.

6. *Relax.* The memory does not work well when your body is tense and your mind is distracted with worry and other sources of interference. Try doing a relaxation exercise before starting a study session.

7. *Remove distractions.* Studying for mastery requires concentration. Find a place where interruptions are limited and where you can use your chosen techniques. (Auditory learners who plan to use singing and tapping should probably not study in the school library!)

8. *Break up your study sessions.* Most people can't concentrate fully for long periods of time. The great thing about reviewing over time, rather than at the last minute, is that you can take time for short breaks.

9. *Overlearn.* Continue to review and repeat material you already know. This firmly locks it into long-term memory.

10. *Quiz yourself.* Make up your own quizzes and tests. Review one day and take the quiz several days later to evaluate your retention.

11. *Keep your goals in mind.* Remind yourself why you are learning the material and how it will benefit both you and others.

PRESCRIPTION FOR SUCCESS 3-11

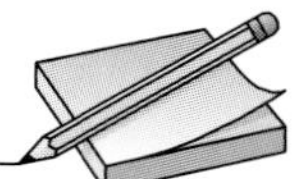

Select among the eleven suggestions for improving your memory and use them to memorize all eleven. Test yourself one week from today. How many did you remember?

THE PERILS OF CRAMMING

Cramming is a well-known student activity consisting of frantic last-minute efforts, sometimes fortified with coffee and cigarettes, to complete assignments or prepare for tests. The major problem with cramming is that it serves only the immediate goal of meeting a school deadline. True learning rarely occurs. The conditions required for learning, such as the opportunity for repetition over time, are absent. Most of what is crammed is forgotten within a few days—or hours! Work in health care demands a higher level of competence than you are likely to achieve as a result of cramming. Do your future patients deserve your best efforts to learn or are the bits you may remember after a night of cramming good enough? This is an important consideration for students who claim that cramming works well for them because they can study *only* at the last minute when the deadline is close. This is true *only* if simply passing the test is the *only* goal.

Another problem with cramming is that it leaves you with few options. If you are writing a paper the night before it is due and you discover that the information you have is inadequate (and the Internet is not available), you have no time to consult other sources. If you are studying for a test and realize that there are several points you don't understand, it's too late to ask the instructor to explain them.

Finally, cramming adds more stress to an already busy life that requires you to balance your responsibilities as an adult with your role as a student. If it costs you a night's sleep, it depletes your energy supply and can interfere with your ability to concentrate. You set up a nonproductive cycle that results in a continual game of catch-up and the danger of creating ongoing stress.

The reality is that things happen, you get behind, and you run out of time. Almost every student finds it necessary to cram at least once. Here are some tips* to make the best of a bad situation:

1. Don't beat yourself up and waste energy feeling guilty. You'll only distract your attention from what you have to do. Just make a mental note to avoid the need for future cramming.
2. Do a very quick visualization in which you see yourself accomplishing what you need to do in the time you have available.
3. Minimize all distractions. Can someone help you by watching the children?
4. Focus on the most important material. Which material is most likely to be emphasized? What are the principal requirements of the assignment?
5. Use the learning and memory techniques described in this section. Draw on your learning style to help you organize the major points so that they make sense to you; read material aloud; and walk around the room as you concentrate on definitions.
6. Try to stay calm. Physical tension distracts from mental effort. Breathe deeply, stretch, and do a quick relaxation exercise.

Mentors Make a Difference

People seldom improve when they have no other model but themselves to copy.—Oliver Goldsmith

A mentor is like an advisor that you choose for yourself. It is someone you admire and who has the experience and background to give you sound advice about your studies and career. This is a person you respect and see as a positive role model. You must be able to count on your mentor to meet with you periodically to answer your questions and share your feelings and concerns. There are many other ways a mentor can help you:

1. Inform you about the current state of your targeted occupation.
2. Advise you about what you should emphasize in your studies.
3. Give you encouragement.
4. Introduce you to other professionals.
5. Help you learn professional behaviors.

Your chances of succeeding are greatly increased when someone you respect cares about your progress. This has been proven in both school and business set-

* Adapted from Ellis, 1994.

tings. Where can you find such a person? It can be an instructor, school staff member, or administrator, or it can be someone who works in health care who you already know or meet through your networking efforts. You might find a graduate of your school who is working successfully. The important thing is that this is someone with whom you feel comfortable.

Once you have identified a person you would like to have as your mentor, ask for an appointment. Let him or her know you want to talk about mentoring. At the meeting, explain that you are changing careers, have set professional goals, and would like this person to serve as your mentor and give you guidance. Ask how much time he or she has to meet with you. (Once a month or every other month should be adequate.) If the first person you approach does not have the time or is not comfortable serving as a mentor, don't get discouraged. Continue your search—it will be worth the effort.

SUMMARY OF KEY IDEAS

1. Mission statements express your values and purpose in life.
2. Let your goals be your guides.
3. Never underestimate the power of attitude.
4. If managed well, time can work for you.
5. Work smarter, not harder.
6. Good health can improve the quality of your life.
7. You can use stress to work for instead of against you.
8. Learning how to learn is as important as what you learn.
9. A mentor can help you succeed.

POSITIVE SELF-TALK FOR THIS CHAPTER

1. I have worthy goals and am on track to achieve them.
2. I manage my time efficiently.
3. I am well organized and in control of my life.
4. I live a healthy life and enjoy a high level of energy.
5. I use effective study strategies based on my learning styles.

BIBLIOGRAPHY

Chapman, Elkwood. *Life Is an Attitude!* Menlo Park, CA: Crisp Publications, 1992.

Covey, Stephen, Merrill, A. Roger, and Rebecca R. Merrill. *First Things First.* New York: Simon and Schuster, 1995.

Ellis, Dave. *Becoming a Master Student.* Boston: Houghton Mifflin Company, 1994.

Hwang, Philip. *Other-Esteem.* San Diego, CA: Black Forrest Press, 1995.

O'Toole, Maria, ed. *Miller-Keane Encyclopedia & Dictionary of Medicine, Nursing, & Allied Health,* 6th ed. Philadelphia: W.B. Saunders Company, 1997.

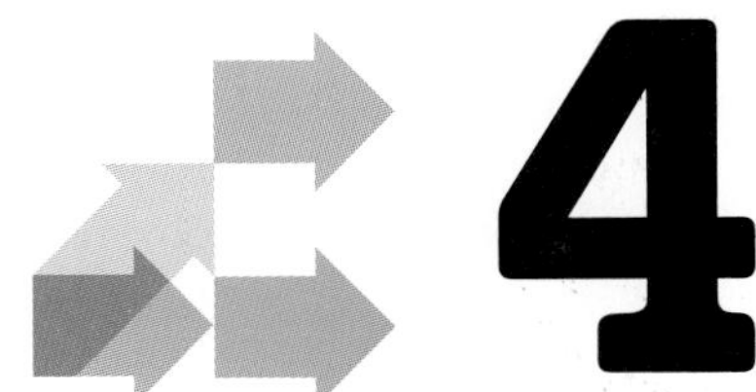

4

Developing Your Paper Skills I: Intake of Information

OBJECTIVES

THE INFORMATION AND ACTIVITIES IN THIS CHAPTER CAN HELP YOU TO:

- ➢ Understand the importance of developing good note-taking skills.
- ➢ Use effective listening techniques to take advantage of learning opportunities.
- ➢ Develop a note-taking format and techniques that work for you in class and on the job.
- ➢ Convert your class notes into powerful learning tools.
- ➢ Use previewing and reviewing to learn as much as possible from your reading.
- ➢ Locate reliable sources of information for use in school and on the job.

KEY TERMS

Active listener: One who listens purposefully and attentively; focuses on what the speaker is saying; asks questions and clarifies, when necessary.

Appendices: Sections at the end of a book that contain supplementary information. (Singular form is "appendix.")

Concept: A general idea or reference to a unit of knowledge. For example, lab safety is an important health care concept.

Cornell system: A method for taking notes that recommends leaving space for follow-up notes and summaries.

Database: Computerized records that organize and store large amounts of related information. Key words are entered to locate specific topics and information.

Edit: To correct, organize, and add to written materials.

Glossary: An alphabetical list of words with their definitions. Usually located at the end of a book, it serves as a mini-dictionary.

Internet: A system that connects millions of computers so that they can share information. It provides access to all types of resources and services.

Key terms: In note taking, words that identify the most important concepts and ideas in a lecture.

Logical: In an order that makes sense, that is, that follows some sort of pattern and shows relationships. For example, a logical way to learn human anatomy is to group the various body parts that work together or that perform similar functions.

Objective: Statement of what students should know or be able to do as the result of a given learning activity.

Preface: An introduction placed at the beginning of a book before the first chapter.

Preview: To look over a written selection before reading it carefully.

Rationale: An explanation or reason for something. Rationales often accompany medical procedures in textbooks so that students will understand why an action is important.

Research: To gather information. Research uses many sources. It is not limited to books and journals.

Tactfully: Making an effort not to offend another person. For example, if you need to inform a patient that his ideas about nutrition are incorrect, you should do it tactfully.

Web sites: The specific "places" that you see on the computer screen when you are connected to the Internet. They represent the offerings that have been placed on the Internet and may contain advertising, information, opportunities to make purchases, schedules, etc.

Prospering in the Information Age

We are in the midst of the Information Age. All types of businesses and services depend on the production and efficient communication of huge amounts of information. In health care this involves keeping track of medical advances, fulfilling patient record-keeping requirements, and exchanging data between health care providers. Information will also play a significant role in your education. The majority of the time you spend in school will be devoted to the intake of information through listening, note taking, and reading. It makes sense, then, to learn to take notes and read in ways that maximize your learning. Good intaking skills are also needed by successful health care professionals.

The ideas in this chapter draw on many of the concepts presented in Chapter 3 in the section called "Learning for Life." Keep in mind that the techniques you learn here will help you succeed in the future. You are doing much more than simply learning how to get through your classes.

Note Taking: Now and on the Job

Taking good notes combines the art of listening and the act of selective writing. Be optimistic about your ability to learn to take good notes. You actually have a big advantage because you can listen at a rate several times faster than the rate at which the average person speaks!

Note taking is a skill that health care professionals use on many occasions (Fig. 4–1). When patients explain their health background, symptoms, and reasons for seeking care, the information must be recorded correctly. Patient records serve as the basis for giving appropriate and consistent care, so it is critical that they be both accurate and legible. In addition, they serve as legal documents and are used in court cases to defend the actions of health care providers.

The most common teaching methods for health care courses are lecture, instructor demonstrations, and hands-on activities in the lab or at the clinical site. The first two require students to take notes that they use as study aids. You will have many opportunities to practice this important skill, which will serve you now and later on the job.

WHY TAKE NOTES?

Some students find taking notes difficult or tedious and wonder why they should even bother. Why not just look in the textbook later and find the information? There are several important reasons for taking notes in class, in addition to learning to take good notes because it is an important health care skill.

1. Taking notes forces you to attend class, pay attention, process the material mentally, and selectively write down what you hear. It converts you from a passive to an **active listener.** Increasing the number of ways you interact with new material greatly increases your chances of understanding and remembering it.

PATIENT HISTORY

Soc Sec Number 203-46-7809

Patient Name Sean D. Austin DOB 03/03/83
Address 1234 Crown Ave. City Dayton State Ohio ZIP 24354
Home Phone (937) 123-4567 Work Phone Emergency Phone (937) 545-4415
Status M (S) W D Spouse's name — Referring Physician
Occupation student Employer Phone
Primary Insurance Anthem BC/BS Policy Holder John Austin Policy No. AN232435545

Chief Complaint (L) shoulder pain p̄ playing basketball this AM.
Present Illness soreness and immobility (L) shoulder x 8 hours; strained upon collision w/ another player

HT	62"	Sc Fever	—
Weight	112#	Rheum Fev	—
Past yr + –	8#	Measles	+
Temp	98.4°F	Mumps	—
Pulse	72	Rubella	—
Resp	12	Chicken Pox	+
BP	108/64	Asthma	—
LMP	NA		

FAMILY HISTORY

Heart	Father	Mother	Brother	Brother	Sister	Sister	MGM	MG
Heart	—	+	—	—			+	—
Bld Pressure	—	—	—	—			—	—
Diabetes	—	—	—	—			—	—
Bld Diabetes	—	—	—	—			—	—
Asthma	—	+	—	—			—	—
Epilepsy	—	—	—	—			—	—
Stroke	—	—	—	—			—	—

SURGICAL HISTORY

Surgery	Year	Physician	Surgery	Year	Physician	Surgery
Adenoidectomy	1986	Smith				
BTTI	1986	Smith				

REVIEW OF SYSTEMS

HEENT

Head	Acne	—						
Eyes	Vision	—	Glasses	—	Pain	—		
Ears	Hearing	—	Pain	—	Discharge	—	Tinn	
Nose	Obstruction	—	Discharge	—	Epistaxis	—	Sinu	
Throat	Teeth	—	Tongue	—	Gums	—	Thro	
NECK	Swelling	—	Stiffness	—	Hoarseness	—		
BACK	Pain	—						
LUNGS	Cough	—	Hemoptysis	—	Sputum	—	Pair	
HEART	Chills	—	Fever	—	Nightsweats	—	Whe	
GI	Pain	—	Dyspnea	—	Edema	—	Palp	
	Appetite	good	Diet	"normal"	Nausea	—	Vomit	—
	Diarrhea	—	Constipation	—	Jaundice	—	flatulence	—
GU	Belching	—						
	Frequency	—	Dysuria	—	Burning	—	Nocturia	—
MENSES	Incontinence	—	Hematuria	—	Discharge	—	Vaginal irritation	—
PREG HX	Menarche	—	Regularity	NA	Duration	NA	LMP	NA
LIBIDO	Cramping	—	Menorrhagia	NA	Metrorrhagia	NA		
EXTREM	#Pregnancies		Miscarriages	NA	Abortions	NA	Live births	NA
ENDO	Frequency	—	Satisfaction	NA				
SKIN	~~Joint pain~~	—	Weakness	—	Varicose veins	—	(Swellling)	
NEURO	Hair		Nails	—	Sensitivity to temp	—		
HABITS	Dryness	—	Perspiration	—	Itching	—	Eruption	—
STRESS	Paralysis	—	Tingling	—	Numbness	—	Tremor	—
	Faint	—	Dizziness	—	Memory loss	—	Convulsion	—
	Sleep	8hr/night	Caffiene	16oz/day(pop)	Smoking	—	Alcohol	—
	Home	some	Work	—	Finances	—	General disposition	"easy going"

WHILE YOU WERE OUT

FOR: Pt Billing DATE: 05/04/00 TIME: 10:20 am
FROM: Bonita Henderson
OF: (Dr. Arewells Pt)
PHONE NUMBER: (771)- 423-6740
FAX: ( )-
RX REFILL: PHARMACY: RX#:
REMARKS: ☒ telephoned ☐ needs to talk to you ☐ will call back ☐ will call again ☐ stopped by ☐ needs to see you ☒ please return call ☐ urgent
MESSAGE: Questions about her April bill and insurance
taken by: G. Chester, CMA

CHARTING NOTES

02/10/97	9am c/o sore throat. T—99⁴F, P—72, R—18, BP—120/68,
	Throat culture obtained. Amoxicillin 500 mg P.O. given to pt.
	P. Dunham, CMA

FIGURE 4–1 Record keeping and note taking are important health care skills. (From Chester, Gail. *Modern Medical Assisting.* Philadelphia: W.B. Saunders Company, 1998. pp. 79, 458, 586, used with permission.)

2. Your instructors are likely to present information that is not in the textbook. They may have examples and additional techniques from their work experience or new information from a seminar they have just attended.
3. Some of the information in the textbook may be outdated. While publishers do their best to ensure that textbooks contain the very latest information, it

usually takes over a year from the time a book is written until it is ready for distribution to students. In a fast-changing field like health care, there is a continuous flow of new developments, and your instructors can provide you with the latest updates.

4. There may be information that does not apply to your geographic area. The scope of practice of professionals varies across the country. For example, some states allow medical assistants to take an active role in taking x-rays. Therefore, many textbooks include information about positioning patients for x-rays. In the state of California, only graduates of approved x-ray programs who have also passed a state exam are allowed to perform these procedures. Classroom instructors give you the rules and regulations of the area in which your school is located.
5. Your instructors can assist you with difficult sections of the textbook, presenting the material in such a way that you understand it. They may break it down into manageable chunks, provide examples, or explain it in different words. You can ask instructors questions, a definite advantage over the textbook.
6. Health care programs cover a vast amount of information. Your instructors' lectures can help you identify the most important points and give you clues about what will be included on tests.
7. You boost your personal efficiency. Taking notes saves you the time of looking up the information discussed in class that does not appear in your regular textbook.
8. Notes serve as powerful tools for studying and mastering important information needed for tests and job success. Later in this chapter, you will learn techniques for converting your notes into study aids.

ACTIVE LISTENING: PREREQUISITE FOR GOOD NOTE TAKING

Good note taking requires good listening habits. You cannot record what you do not hear. It is sometimes difficult to pay attention in class when you're tired, there are distractions, the instructor speaks too quickly or not clearly, or you find the subject matter boring. However, listening is one of *the* most essential skills for the successful health care professional. In fact, poor listening skills can doom your professional life to failure. The classroom provides the perfect opportunity to learn information and a critical life skill at the same time. The following suggestions can help you improve your ability to listen:

1. Develop a positive attitude toward listening. Doing it well increases your chances for success in life. Review your goals and focus on how being a good listener will help you achieve them.
2. Leave your mental baggage at the classroom or health care facility door. Try to enter the class and your job with a clean slate for listening and learning. If you are having a bad day and your mind is distracted, look at class as an opportunity to learn and have a productive experience.
3. Choose where you sit carefully. Find a place where you can both see and hear the instructor. Avoid sitting near people who talk or continually ask you questions during class. The distraction will disrupt your attention and can make you tense. (And don't *you* be the talker!)
4. Concentrate on the content of the lecture, not the way it is delivered. It is easy to let the appearance, mannerisms, and voice of instructors distract you from what they are saying. This breaks your concentration and interrupts your intake of the information. If the problem is interfering with your learning (e.g., the instructor speaks too fast or mumbles, so that you cannot understand what he or she is saying), meet with the instructor privately and **tactfully** explain the situation. Learning to focus on content is an important health care skill because patients will come to you with all kinds of physical and emotional conditions, and each merits your full attention.

5. Reel in your wandering mind. Do your best to stay with the instructor mentally. If your mind does wander, remind yourself where you are, your purpose for being there, and come back to class. If you think of something important, jot a quick note to yourself so that you can take care of it later. This frees your mind to focus on the class.
6. Keep your mind open and suspend judgment. There are times when we stop listening because our thoughts get in the way. This can happen when we disagree with something we hear. Perhaps the instructor says something that conflicts with what you've read in the textbook, your personal experience, or what you learned from another instructor. Write down the point of disagreement. After listening to the remainder of the presentation, ask the instructor to clarify the point (either in class or in private). Very often there are several "right answers" or ways to perform a technique. It may be that you heard or interpreted the information incorrectly. If the instructor did make a mistake, show respect. Enjoying "being right" in front of the class is unacceptable classroom conduct. On the job, it could result in insubordination and is generally not tolerated.

Learning Styles and Listening

Obviously, auditory learners have the edge when it comes to lectures. However, they can get caught up in the listening and find it difficult to take adequate notes. This can be a problem because even good listeners won't remember every important point presented.

Visual learners may have more difficulty paying sustained attention and comprehending long lectures. Here are some techniques that can help them benefit from lectures:

1. Complete any reading and homework assignments related to the lecture. Knowing something about the topic, rather than starting out cold, gives a framework to guide your listening.
2. Avoid sitting near visual distractions that attract your attention, such as a window with an interesting view or pictures and displays that are not related to the topic being discussed.
3. Watch the instructor. Note movements, gestures, and facial expressions and see how they reinforce the material being presented.
4. Pay attention to anything shown on the board, on the overhead, or through other visual aids. This will help you better comprehend the lecture.
5. Ask the instructor to write down words or phrases that you cannot understand orally.
6. If an instructor never uses the board or overheads, talk with him or her outside of class about adding them to the presentations. Explain that you want to learn as much as possible in class and that this would help you better understand the lectures.
7. During lectures, refer to your textbook or handouts if they relate to the material.

Kinesthetic (hands-on) learners can benefit from the physical activity involved in taking notes. Further suggestions to improve listening include the following:

1. Think of applications for ideas you hear during lectures. (But be careful not to get too carried away and miss the next thing the instructor says!)
2. Imagine yourself interacting physically with the topic: performing procedures, feeling materials, or operating a machine.
3. Make slight movements that do not disrupt others: count off steps on your fingers, stretch your legs slightly, take occasional deep breaths, or move your hand down the page of your text or handout as the material is being explained.
4. Take enough notes to keep yourself busy, but not so many as to miss the important points as the instructor moves on.

PRESCRIPTION FOR SUCCESS 4-1

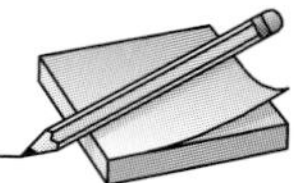

My Listening Habits

1. Do you sometimes find it hard to concentrate during lectures?
2. If you answered yes, is there a pattern to the breaks in your concentration? (For example, you are distracted by something visual or your private thoughts; you don't understand everything your instructors say; it is difficult to follow long periods of speech; etc.)
3. Which of the suggestions given in this section do you think might help you?
4. You can develop your listening skills by practicing awareness. One way is to listen to the news on the radio for several minutes at a time. Pay attention to when your mind wanders or you lose track of what is being said and record it with a check mark. Track your progress over the next few weeks on the following chart. (You can try the same technique in your classes if you don't have time to listen to the radio and *only* if it does not distract your attention further from the lecture.)

Listening Track Record

Event	Date	Lost Attention

ADVANCE PREPARATION FOR TAKING GOOD NOTES

Preparing for classes is an important part of listening and taking good notes. Advance preparation, according to many instructors, is the *key* to benefiting from class sessions. If you forget about class between meetings and just show up each time as the instructor begins to speak, you will lose out on a good part of your educational investment. To obtain maximum benefit from your in-class experiences, try the following suggestions:

1. Complete any assigned reading and other homework. There is nothing more frustrating than trying to follow a lecture that assumes you know something about the subject—and you know nothing! Give yourself every advantage by anticipating what the lecture might cover and preparing questions from your reading. Increase your alertness by listening for the answers to your questions. Ask the instructor any unanswered questions at the end of class.
2. Review your notes from the previous lecture. This gives you an opportunity to set the stage for a continuation of the subject and to highlight questions or points that you need to have clarified.
3. Arrive at class a few minutes early. This gives you a chance to choose an appropriate seat, quickly look over your notes from the last class, and prepare yourself to take notes.
4. Attune your attitude to learning. Decide that you will benefit as much as possible from every class. Expect to acquire information that will help you now and in your future work.
5. Take all necessary supplies to class: a binder with extra paper, pencil, or pen, textbook, and handouts. (Make sure they're in the "big bag" discussed in Chapter 3.)

NOTE-TAKING MATERIALS

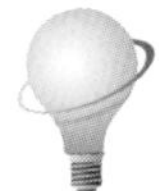

Take a Moment to Think

1. How do you keep and organize your notes?
2. Can you quickly find what you need to study?
3. Does your system need improvement?
4. Are you willing to try something new?

There are a variety of ways to take and organize notes. Base your choice on your learning styles and personal preferences, your instructors' lecture styles, and the number and type of handouts distributed in your classes.

Taking notes in class is the first step in creating a personalized learning tool. Your notes are not completed when the instructor finishes the lecture. You will **edit** them to increase their value as a learning tool and then review them regularly.

Notes are useless, however, if you cannot find or identify them, so good organization is critical. Looseleaf binders receive the highest marks from instructors because they are the most flexible and easiest to organize and keep in order. You can add new information in any order you wish, which cannot be done in spiral notebooks. This includes class notes, revisions of your notes, handouts, assignments, reference sheets, and check-offs of skills. Binders offer the best protection against weather and keep papers flat and neat. Portfolios and other types of folders with pockets tend to get messy and torn.

You can purchase several binders with thin vinyl covers and use one for each class. Alternatively, you can divide a large binder with indexed dividers. Each class can also be subdivided for class notes, handouts, reading notes, and assignments. Periodically review and tidy up your binder as needed.

Regardless of how you organize your binder, the important thing is to keep your notes for each class together and in order. Label the outside cover with the name of the class or classes. If you are using more than one binder, color-code or mark them in such a way that you never arrive at anatomy class only to discover that you have your pharmacology notes! Label the individual pages with the name of the class and the date.

PRESCRIPTION FOR SUCCESS 4-2

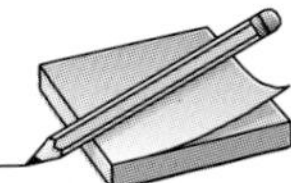

Get Organized to Take Great Notes

1. If your current note-taking system needs improvement, what steps can you take to improve it?
2. What materials do you need?
3. Set a date by which you will have your system in place.

THE CORNELL SYSTEM

The **Cornell system** is a method for laying out and editing your notes to get the most benefit from them (Fig. 4-2). It was devised by Professor Walter Pauk, who wanted to help his students improve their study habits (Pauk, 1997). A key feature of the system is leaving enough blank space on the page to add specific kinds of information when you review and edit your notes. To do this, set up each page on which you will take notes by drawing a line about two and one half inches in from the left side. Then draw a line about two inches from the bottom.

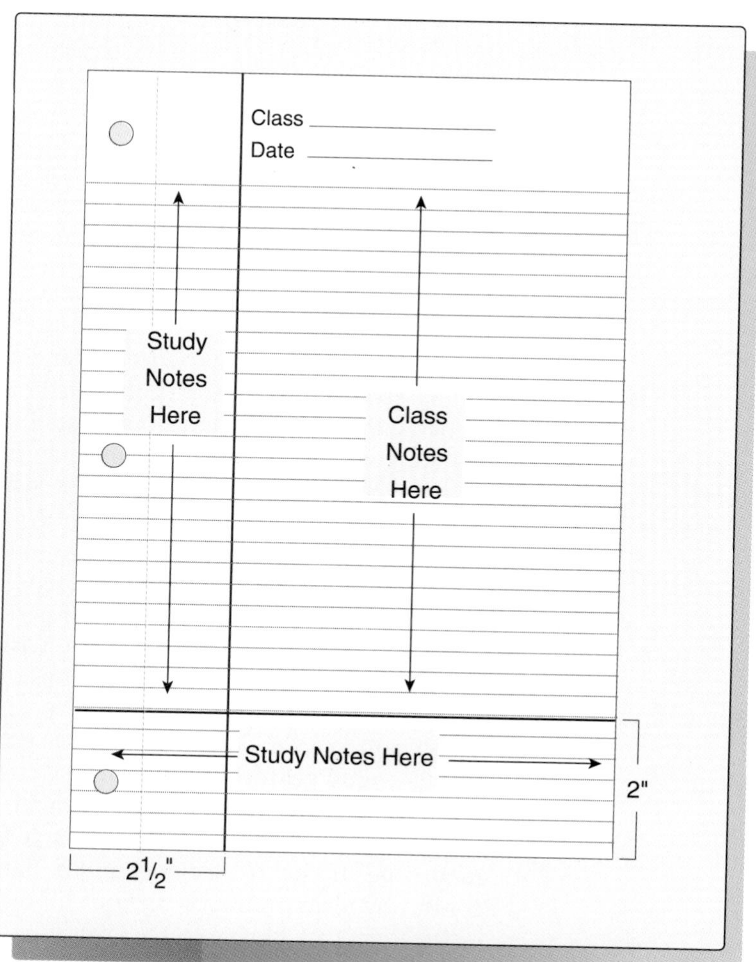

FIGURE 4–2 Page design for the Cornell system of note taking.

The large space in the center is for recording notes during class. The left side is used after class to write key words, headings, questions, and other notes. The bottom space is reserved for writing short summaries of the contents of the page. We will discuss how to use these spaces later in this chapter.

DECIDING WHAT TO RECORD

Instructors can say a lot during a lecture, and sometimes it can be difficult to decide what to write down. If you feel this way, you're not alone. Students report that this is the hardest part of note taking. And it is especially true when a subject is new and you lack the background to help sift the must-know from the interesting-to-know. You need to write down enough so that you understand your notes later. But if you try to record every word, you will miss half of what the instructor says. The following guidelines can help you get the most important content from class lectures:

I. We have said it before, and it is worth repeating: do the reading and assignments before going to class—even if it is not required. This will give you a preview of the topic. Your textbook has headings and other ways of emphasizing the major points of a subject. Use these to develop a mental framework. If you find the subject especially difficult and have the time, consider outlining your chapters before the lecture. Check the course syllabus or outline to find out the topics for each day's lecture. If they are not given there, ask the instructor.

II. Listen for the main ideas. Your prereading is an excellent way to help you identify these. Listen carefully to the instructor. She may list important points; introduce them and then provide details and examples; or tell you what is most important. Try not to get discouraged if you find this difficult. As you become familiar with the material and health care topics in general and take quizzes and tests, you will find it easier to identify the major points.

III. Listen for organizational patterns. There are some common ways that health care topics are presented, and recognizing these can help you follow your instructor more easily and improve your note taking.
   A. Clusters of information: topics are divided into chunks of related material. A lecture covers one chunk before moving on to the next. Examples: the human body parts and functions are usually grouped by systems: skeletal, digestive, and reproductive. Appointment scheduling for the medical office is usually organized by the different methods used to set them.
   B. Procedures: these are often explained in a step-by-step sequence. Examples include how to measure an infant and how to perform one-person, adult CPR.
   C. **Concepts** or procedures with **rationale:** material is introduced, and then important reasons are given to explain and support it. Examples: legal reasons for maintaining patient confidentiality; why standard precautions must be followed.
   D. Definitions: in addition to medical terminology, each area of health care has its own vocabulary. Lectures may be organized around explanations of new terms. Example: discussion of terms related to medical insurance billing.
   E. How things work: descriptions and explanations. Examples: parts and operation of the microscope; safe use of the autoclave.
   F. Lists: descriptions or explanations of a number of items of equal importance. Examples: purpose and interpretation of a series of lab tests; different medications and their use.
   G. Patterns created by the instructor: material presented in a specific order. Example: anatomy and physiology course in which body systems are always presented in the same order—names of parts; purpose and function of each part; common disorders; causes; diagnostic tests; treatments; prevention.
   H. Verbal signals: certain words tell you where the lecture is going. Examples: "Let's go on to . . ." signals the transition to a new topic. "Therefore" and "In conclusion" let you know that a summary statement is coming." "First," "second," and so on advise you that there will be a list of items of equal importance.

IV. Listen and watch for clues from the instructor. Instructors plan their lectures to help students learn the subjects they are teaching. They want you to succeed. As a result, they often give clues, both consciously and unconsciously, about what is important in their classes; this is important for your career success as well as for passing the class. Here are some common instructor behaviors that say "Write this down!"
   A. Saying, "This is important" or "You must know or be able to do this when you are working in the field" or "Write this down" or "This will be on the test." (They really do say these things. That is why missing classes or daydreaming when there can endanger your chances for success.)
   B. Emphasizing certain words or concepts by saying them loudly, writing them on the board or overhead, or repeating them. (It is a good idea to copy everything the instructor writes down.)
   C. Expressing extra interest or enthusiasm. This may indicate an area the instructor believes to be especially important.
   D. Asking questions of students during the lecture. These are usually points that the instructor considers to be important.

V. Mentally ask yourself questions, based on the topic, and then listen for the answers.
   A. Why is this important?
   B. How does it work?
   C. What are the main parts?
   D. Why is it done this way?
   E. How is it done? How will I do this? When will I do this?
   F. How will I apply this in my work?
   G. How will this knowledge help me be a better health care professional? How will it help me to help patients?

Learning to listen for clues and patterns when others are speaking is a useful job skill. For example, it is important to understand instructions given by busy supervisors who may not have time to repeat or clarify what they say. (Nonauditory learners may find that thinking of questions is too distracting; they have enough to do just following the lecture. As with all the suggestions given in this book, select only the ones that work for *you.*)

If you continually miss the major points of lectures, see the instructor outside of class. Ask for suggestions to improve your listening, follow the style of lecturing, and take better notes. If English is your second language and you have difficulty understanding spoken and/or written English, seek help from your instructor or the administration at your school.

PRESCRIPTION FOR SUCCESS 4–3

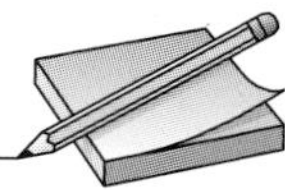

Applying What You've Learned

1. Review the notes you have taken for this or any other class:
   A. Do you believe that you heard, understood, and recorded most of the main ideas?
   B. If you have taken any tests, did your notes reflect the content of the test? If not, why do you think content was missing?
2. Practice listening for organizational clues in your classes during the next week. Choose two lectures and take a couple of minutes afterward to note how they were organized.

Class/Subject 1 *How lecture was organized*

___ Clusters
___ Procedures
___ Concepts with rationale
___ Definitions
___ How things work
___ Presentation patterns
___ Other (explain)

Class/Subject 2 *How lecture was organized*

___ Clusters
___ Procedures
___ Concepts with rationale
___ Definitions
___ How things work
___ Presentation patterns
___ Other (explain)

PRESCRIPTION FOR SUCCESS 4-3 (*continued*)

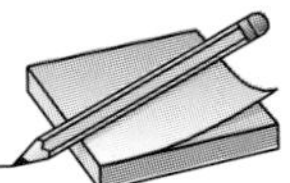

3. Do your instructors give clues about what they consider to be most important in their lectures? Choose two lectures (from different instructors, if possible), listen and observe carefully, and check any behaviors you notice.

Class/Subject 1	*Class/Subject 2*	*Behaviors/Clues*
____	____	Tell you directly that something is important
____	____	Emphasize words
____	____	Say words louder
____	____	Write on board or overhead
____	____	Show enthusiasm
____	____	Ask questions
____	____	Other (explain)

DECIDING HOW TO RECORD

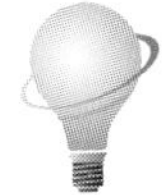

Take a Moment to Think

1. What note-taking format do you currently use?
2. Does it seem to work for you? Why or why not?

There are several formats you can use to organize lecture content as you record it. Consider your learning style, the instructor's manner of lecturing, and the subject matter when you choose a format. You may prefer one method and decide to use it in all of your classes. The important thing is to become proficient so that when you are in class, you can focus more on content than on how you are recording it. Write the notes you take in class in the large center space on your Cornell system pages. Five of the most common methods for taking notes are shown here, each illustrating its own format.

Informal Outlines

How to use
  Create indentations to organize ideas
  Write phrases
  Don't use numbers or letters
When to use
  Student is linear thinker
  Lecture is easy to follow
Advantages
  Helps you organize thoughts
  Keeps materials in logical order
Disadvantages
  Difficult if lecture is disorganized, rambling
  May distract from lecture content
    Trying to make neat outline
  Holistic thinkers need time to formulate outline

Paragraphs Writing in paragraphs helps when lecture hard to follow. Use phrases. Create paragraph for each main idea. Mark important points during lecture. Organize later by creating outline.

Difficult for some. Must write quickly and neatly. Must decide what to write. Advantage for kinesthetic learners—involves activity. Lots of writing.

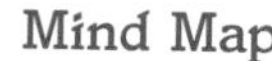

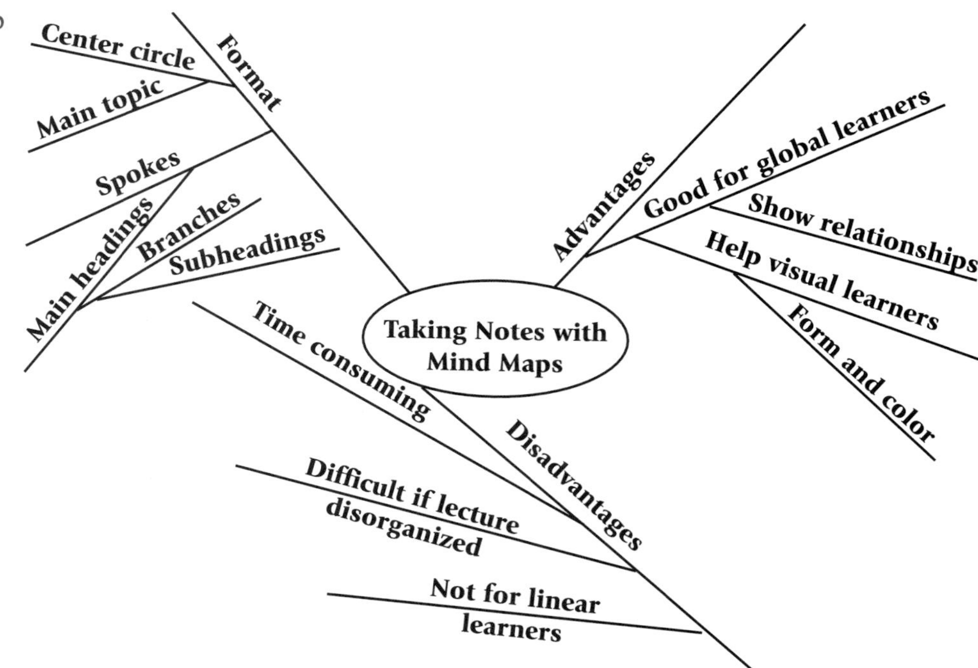

Key Words

Main ideas
Relationships
Supporting facts
Auditory learners
Reminders
Fill in later
Difficult material—may miss facts
Easy to forget!

Write It All A few students are successful with writing everything down. They are more comfortable knowing they haven't missed anything the instructor says. Must use shortened sentences, phrases, and abbreviations, but they try to record all that instructor says. Might work well for kinesthetic learner, who needs activity, or for students who have trouble concentrating and find that this method helps them concentrate. Method not recommended for everyone because if you don't write fast you can get behind and get very frustrated. Usually unnecessary to write everything down. Lose important ideas in details.

Following are examples of notes taken in the various styles, based on the following lecture segment from *Modern Medical Assisting* by Chester (1998, pp. 52–53).

Lecture Segment on Fear and Anxiety

To understand the effects that fear and anxiety have on your patients, it is important to know that they are two very different emotions: fear is reacting emotionally to a *known* threat. Anxiety is reacting emotionally to an *unknown* threat.

Fear can be a strong motivational factor for many patients. Fears can be positive emotions if they cause a person to take constructive measures, such as seeking medical consultations for symptoms he or she is experiencing. However, if the fear causes a person to avoid seeking medically necessary help, these emotions can be destructive. Fear of pain or death are two very strong emotions for most people. The fears that an individual possesses may be a result of a direct or an indirect experience. A direct experience would be the result if the patient has experienced a situation such as touching a hot stove. An indirect experience would be when a person hears "horror" stories of experiences from well-meaning friends or relatives. Most of the time stories become exaggerated as they are told for the second, third, and fourth time. Perhaps the procedure that Aunt Bessie's best friend's brother had done is not even the same procedure as is scheduled for your patient.

Another way in which patients can experience indirectly is through watching television and reading books or magazines. Try to understand what the basis of a patient's fear is so you can help alleviate the fear. In this way you can make the experience a much more positive one. This results in better patient rapport, which will help the patient face future fear and anxiety in a more positive manner. These two emotions will be responsible for many of the patient reactions that you will observe in your medical office.

Each person's fears are very real to him or her, and these fears need to be treated with kindness and reassurance. Once a patient sees that your service can be of benefit and aid him or her toward better health, appearance, or perhaps success, the patient's fears are likely to disappear.

INFORMAL OUTLINE

- Patient emotions
  - Fear = reaction to known threat
  - Anxiety = reaction to unknown threat
- Fear
  - Strong emotion
    - Pain and death
  - Both positive and negative types of fear
    - Positive
      - Motivates person to seek medical care
    - Negative
      - Avoid care
      - Destructive
- Fear is result of experience
  - Direct when happens to person
    - Touch stove
  - Indirect when happens to others
    - Hear or read about
      - Stories from family, friends—exaggerated
      - TV
      - Books and magazines
- How medical assistant can help
  - Try to understand basis for fears
    - Recognize importance to patient
    - Treat kindly
    - Give reassurance
- Results of medical assistant's actions
  - Better rapport with patients
  - Help patient face future fears

PARAGRAPHS

Fear & anxiety diff emotions. Fear is react to known threat. Anxiety is react to unknown.

Fear strong motiv factor. Can be pos. & encourage to seek med care. Can also cause avoidance and therefore be destruct. Fear/pain & death strong emot for most people. Fear result of direct or indir exper. Dir is when person has exper himself. Ex = touch hot stove. Indir when hears about from others. Ex = stories from friends & relatives, TV, mag. Exaggerated.

Try to underst pt fear. Help alleviate. Make exper pos. Results = better pt rapport, help pt face future fear better.

MIND MAP

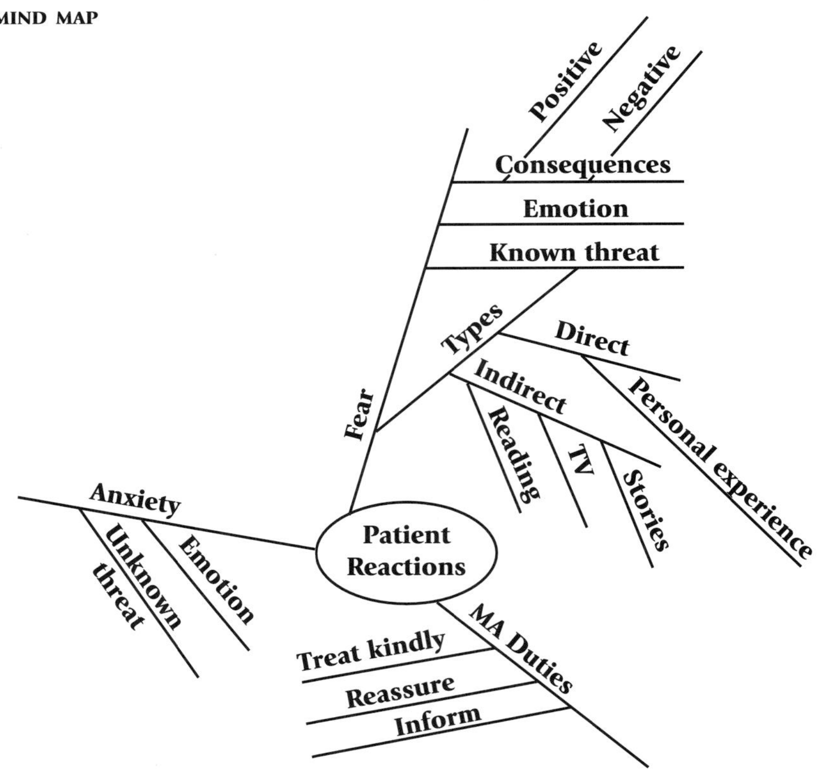

KEY WORDS

Fear and anxiety. Known & unknown threats
Positive & negative motivation
Pain & death
Direct & indirect experience
Exaggerated
Need understanding
Patient rapport
Face future fear

Note-Taking Guides

Some instructors distribute preprinted outlines to help students focus on the important points of their lectures. These can be very helpful but should be used with care. Do not go on automatic pilot during lectures and listen only for those points that are on the guide. You can miss other valuable information that you should write on your own notepaper if there is not enough space on the guide. Another habit students sometimes fall into is copying down exactly what the teacher says. This is appropriate for recording definitions, formulas, and rules. However, you increase your chances of learning if you use your own words to take notes.

To Tape or Not to Tape

There are conflicting opinions about the value of taping lectures. Some educators warn that students who tape their lectures pay less attention in class. Tapes do not include important nonverbal language and visual aids. Also, listening to tapes is time-consuming. On the other hand, taping can be useful if you find that listening is an effective way for you to review. It can also help students who have trouble understanding English. If you decide that taping is a good idea for you, be *sure* to obtain your instructor's permission. Some schools and/or individual instructors don't allow lectures to be taped. They believe that students must develop good listening skills in class.

PRESCRIPTION FOR SUCCESS 4–4

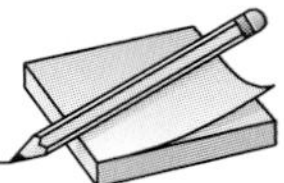

What Works for You?

1. Did you find a note-taking method that might work better than what you are doing now? Why?
2. If "yes," try it during the next class lecture you attend and report on how it works.

   Did it help you better follow or did it detract from the lecture? Explain. Would you use this method again? Why or why not?

MORE IDEAS FOR TAKING GREAT NOTES

1. Be there! Do your best to be present for both the beginning and end of lectures. Introductions and conclusions often contain valuable information about what the instructor considers to be most important. Conclusions may clarify points that seemed fuzzy or unrelated earlier in the lecture.
2. Leave some blank space between the major ideas or clusters of related information so that you can make additions when you edit and review. You may think of something you forgot to write down or find helpful explanations in your textbook or other sources. If you have trouble understanding the material or if you get lost and have gaps in your notes, leave a lot of space to fill in later.
3. Write out examples, definitions, formulas, and calculations.
4. Write on only one side of the paper so that you can lay the pages out to relate information and review. Some students use blank facing pages to create study notes (Fig. 4–3).

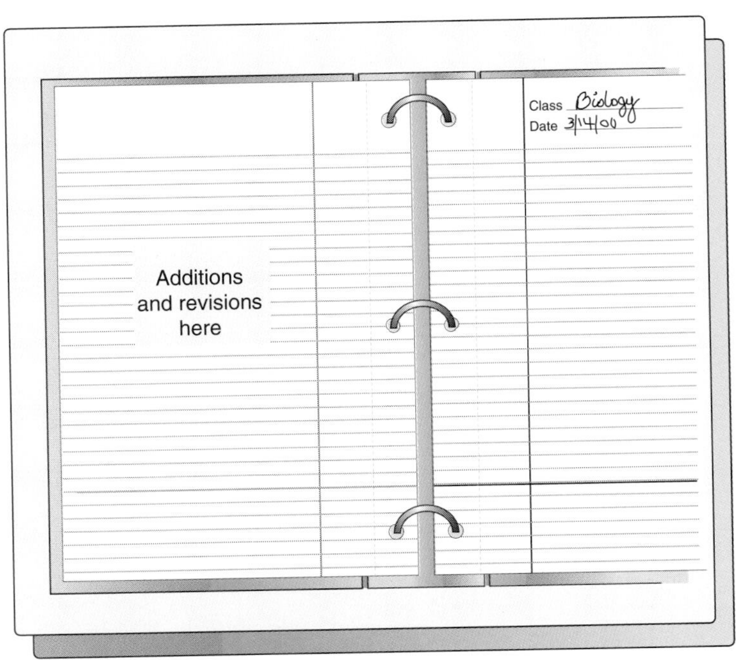

FIGURE 4–3 Use the facing page or reverse side of your note pages to write additions or revisions.

5. Do your best to write down words you do not know. Guess at the spelling and circle the words so that you can look up their meanings or ask the instructor.
6. Write as neatly as possible. Practice improving your handwriting if necessary. Try printing if it does not slow you down too much. Aim for a balance between speed and legibility. Recopying notes to make them neater takes time that you could use more productively. There are, however, a few circumstances in which rewriting, typing, or word processing notes is recommended. If you have strong keyboarding skills, you may find that this process serves as a good review of the lecture. If you are a kinesthetic learner, you may benefit from the activity of keyboarding. Finally, on those few occasions when your notes are a total disaster, it may be worth your time to clean them up. Keep in mind that good handwriting is important on the job because the quality of patient care depends on the ability of other health professionals to read your written documentation. Because many records are summoned to court, their legibility can be critical in defending the actions of health care personnel.
7. Erasable pens are good for note taking, although regular pens can be used if you make corrections neatly. Pencils can break or need sharpening, and the writing tends to fade and smudge over time.
8. Create a set of symbols to mark your notes as you take them. Here are some ideas:

   T = test item (instructor announced or hinted).
   ?? = got lost and need to fill in later.
   P = personal thoughts: your own ideas that you want to jot down before you forget. (Or you can bracket your own thoughts to distinguish them from what the instructor says.)
   J = important for job success, something employers look for.
9. Develop abbreviations to increase your recording speed. Use standard abbreviations or invent your own—or use a combination. See Table 4–1 for suggestions.

TABLE 4–1 ***Developing Abbreviations for Note Taking: Standard Abbreviations***

Word	Standard Abbreviation
and	&
and so forth	etc
equals, same as, means	=
for example	eg
less than	<
more than	>
negative	–
not the same as, does not equal	≠
number	#
of, per	/
positive	+
regarding	re
therefore	∴
times	×
to, toward, leads to, goes to	→
versus	vs
with	w/ or c̄
without	w/o or s̄

TABLE 4–1 ***Developing Abbreviations for Note Taking: Standard Abbreviations*** *(continued)*

Spell words as they sound, leaving out silent letters	
Examples	**Phonetic Spelling**
	(Finally, spelling just like its sound!)
although	altho
through	thru
Shorten words by leaving out the vowels	
Word	**Shortened Form**
blood	bld
book	bk
homework	hmwrk
learn	lrn
patient	pt
Develop your own short forms of common words	
Word	**Shortened Form**
anatomy	anat
appointment	appt
because	bec
determine	det
important	imp
information	info
introduction	intro
necessary	nec
procedure	proc
psychology	psych
venipuncture	venip
Learn common medical abbreviations	
Word	**Abbreviation**
cardiopulmonary resuscitation	CPR
electrocardiography	EKG
medical assistant	MA
occupational therapy	OT

If you create your own set of abbreviations, it is a good idea to make a directory that you keep with your notes in case you forget your coding system. Since you cannot anticipate all the words you might shorten during a lecture, write out potentially confusing abbreviations as soon as possible after class.

Here are the outline notes from our previous example. This is how a shorthand approach can help you take notes more quickly.

Pt emotions
  Fear = react to known threat
  Anx = react unkn threat
Fear
  Strng emot
    Pain & dth
  Both + & − types/fear
    Pos
      Motiv seek med care
    Neg
      Avoid care
      Destruc

Fear = result/exper
  Direct = hap to pers
    Touch stove
  Indir = hap to others
    Hear, read
      Stories
      TV
      Bks & mag
How MA helps
  Try to underst bas/fears
    Recog import to pt
    Treat kindly
    Give reassur
Results/MA's act
  + rapport w/ pts
  Help pt face fut fears

Abbreviations are used extensively in health care work, so learning to apply them is an important skill. The following is an example of notes on a patient history form.*

Chief complaint: Ⓛshoulder pain p̄ playing basketball this AM
Present illness: Soreness and immobility L shoulder × 8 hours; strained upon collision w/another player

PRESCRIPTION FOR SUCCESS 4–5

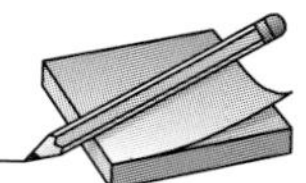

Create Your Own

Create a list of twenty abbreviations to use in your note taking.

MAKING YOUR NOTES WORK FOR YOU

It takes work to record good notes in class. Now let them work for you. Review them as soon as possible after class. Try not to wait more than twenty-four hours. The average person forgets more than half of what was said during a typical class lecture within that time. Why take notes if you are just going to let them sit and not serve you further? Even a brief review will help create memory pathways for new information. Here are ways to help you review and edit your notes productively:

I. Read them over and fill in any missing words or abbreviations with meanings you might forget.
II. Fill in ideas or reorganize as needed.
   A. Keyword notes: Fill in with additional information or details; create an outline or mind map and add supporting facts from recall; or write a sentence explaining each one.
   B. Write-it-all notes: These can be difficult to study from, especially if the lecture was disorganized or hard to follow. Create an outline, mind map, or other structure to organize the material so that it makes sense to you.
   C. If there are gaps where your mind wandered or you did not understand well enough to take clear notes, look in your textbook, ask a classmate, or plan to speak with the instructor.
   D. Consider rewriting notes that are extremely disorganized or if you think that a different format might help you. For example, if the topic emphasizes relationships and you wrote paragraphs, create a mind map. If the lecture was organized by classifications, design a chart that lays out the various categories.

* From Chester, 1998.

E. Mark anything that needs clarification or further explanation so that you can ask about it at the next class meeting.

III. Mark key words or phrases with a highlighter or colored pen to make reviewing easier.

IV. Consider organizing all or part of the material in a way that corresponds to your learning style. If you learn facts before understanding the big picture, list them and then write a summary that describes how they relate to each other and form concepts. If you see the big picture first, write out concepts and then create a list of supporting related details. Linear learners can look for **logical** patterns in the material. Holistic learners can create their own formats, such as mind maps, that show relationships. (If you decide to revise or add to your notes, be sure to leave the spaces on the left side and bottom of each page.)

V. Employ the Cornell system.
   A. Use the space in the left column on each page to write words or phrases to help you review and study your notes. You can do this in several ways:
      1. List key words or headings.
      2. Write phrases that state major points.
      3. Write brief summaries.
      4. Make up test questions about the content.

      If you find that you don't have enough room in the study space, use the back of the previous page (see Fig. 4–3).
   B. Use the space at the bottom of each page to write a summary, in your own words, of the material on the page. (If you have trouble writing a summary, this is a good indication that you do not fully understand the material.)

USING KEYWORDS	**LECTURE NOTES**
Fear vs Anxiety	Pt emotions Fear = react to known threat Anxiety = react unknown threat
Fear Positive Negative	Fear Strong emot Pain & death Both + & – types of fear Pos Motiv to seek med care Neg Avoid care Destruc
Experience Direct Indirect	Fear = result/exper Direct = happens to person Touch stove Indirect = happens to others Hear, read about Stories TV Bks & mag
MA responsibilities	How MA can help Try to underst basis/fears Recog import to pt Treat kindly Give reassur
How MA helps	Results of MA's actions Better rapport with patients Help patient face future fears

USING STUDY TEST QUESTIONS	LECTURE NOTES
What is the difference between fear & anxiety?	Pt emotions Fear = react to known threat Anxiety = react to unknown threat Fear Strong emot Pain & death Both + & – types of fear
How can fear be a positive motivator? When can fear be destructive?	Pos Motiv to seek med care Neg Avoid care Destruc
What influences the fear experienced by an individual?	Fear = result/exper Direct = happens to person Touch stove
What is the difference between direct & indirect fear? How can stories add to a person's fear? How can the MA help alleviate patient fears?	Indirect = happens to others Hear, read about Stories TV Bks & mag How MA can help Try to underst basis/fears Recog import to pt Treat kindly Give reassur Results of MA's actions
Why is it important to reduce patient fears?	Better rapport with patients Help patient face future fears

VI. Personalize your notes. Use color, drawings, arrows to show relationships, pictures from magazines, or anything else that helps you focus on and better understand the material. Consider taping your edited notes for a listening review.

VII. Think of ways to relate new material to your own experience or to something that you already know.

PRESCRIPTION FOR SUCCESS 4–6

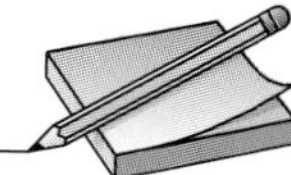

Give It a Try

Write a three-sentence summary of the lecture segment on fear and anxiety.

REVIEWING PRODUCTIVELY

I. The *most important* thing you can do with your notes is to *review them often,* at least twice a week. If your classes last for less than one month, review even more often. As we discussed in Chapter 3, the key to long-term memory is repetition over time. Your review sessions do not have to be long, but make them a regular part of your study schedule. Keep in mind that you are not simply learning to pass a test. You are accumulating knowledge to assist you in attaining future excellence as a health care professional.

II. Engage your mind actively when you review. Passively reading and rereading your notes will not store them in your mind. Use the review column to the left of your notes to prompt recall of the information. Cover the notes you took in class, and answer the questions or explain the headings or key words. This is the *most effective part* of the review because it forces you to think and helps transfer the content of your notes into your long-term memory.

III. Other review suggestions for various learning styles:
   A. Visual: picture the words and concepts in your mind as you review; label drawings from memory; draw sketches (rough ones are fine—no one is grading the art).
   B. Auditory: review out loud, even if you must speak in a soft voice. Have someone read your key words and questions and check your answers as you give them out loud. Listen to recordings of your notes.
   C. Kinesthetic: stand up, move around, re-create the lecture. Or teach someone else by explaining one-on-one. Use movement and gestures to emphasize important points. If the content concerns a procedure or something that involves movement, act it out or actually perform it as much as possible.
   D. Interactive: exchange notes with a study partner or group. Discuss and quiz each other. Make flash cards with questions on one side and answers on the back.

IV. Create practice tests based on your notes. They can be written out or taped. Do not take your "test" for at least three days. Suggestions for questions:
   A. What is the definition of ______?
   B. What is the meaning of ______?
   C. What are the steps in performing a ______?
   D. What is important to remember about ______?
   E. Why must you ______?
   F. What are the principal parts of ______?
   G. How does ______ function?
   H. What is the purpose of ______?

PRESCRIPTION FOR SUCCESS 4-7

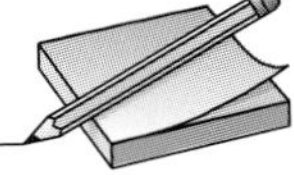

Note-Taking Practice

Set up a couple of pages using the Cornell format. Choose a recording method and take notes while someone reads you the lecture segment that appears on page 100 (don't look!). Write study questions in the review column, and write a brief summary at the bottom of the page.

Reading: Now and on the Job

Reading, along with listening and taking notes, is one of the principal ways you will acquire information as a student. And reading will continue to be an important skill in your professional life. It will allow you to increase your proficiency continually and keep up with the rapidly advancing field of health care.

READING TO LEARN

To read without reflecting is like eating without digesting.—Edmund Burke

Like effective listening, reading to learn requires that you pay attention and participate actively. It should be approached purposefully, and you must work at understanding, remembering, and applying new material. If you were reading instructions about how to perform a medical procedure, you would ask yourself, "Do I understand this? What, exactly, am I supposed to do?" and then read carefully to make sure that you got it right. Your goal in reading textbooks is also to comprehend and know what to do with your new knowledge. You will spend a great deal of time reading textbooks, so it makes sense to learn how to gain the most benefit from your efforts.

Earlier in this chapter, we discussed why you should take notes. You might wonder why you have to read *and* take notes. There are several reasons:

1. The more ways you take in information, the more likely you will be to remember it. Paths are worn over time by many walkers. If no one uses them, they disappear. Your memory pathways are also created and maintained by repeated use. Even if a subject is discussed in class, reading gives you one more encounter with it.
2. As we suggested in the section on taking notes, reading will give you background for class lectures. It also reinforces what you hear in class.
3. Textbooks provide a permanent means of saving information. You can refer back to them over and over as needed.
4. Books generally contain more supporting details, examples, graphics, and organizational aids than lectures.

Getting Ready to Read

There are several prereading activities that will make your reading easier and more beneficial.

1. Clear your mind of clutter. Reading requires concentration, and this is difficult when you have unfinished business on your mind. If something is bothering you that can be handled *quickly*, take care of it before you start studying. (But try not to let "urgencies" be an excuse to put off getting together with your books indefinitely.) If it will take more than a few minutes of your attention, write it down (the list notebook would be a good place) so that you can deal with it later.
2. Find a place that encourages reading rather than sleeping or daydreaming. Many people find that a straight-backed chair at a desk works best (you will be doing some writing as you read). Give your back good support, and make sure the light is adequate. An uncomfortable environment can tire you and cut your reading time short.
3. You need more than just your textbook to read actively, so gather your tools: notebook, pen or pencil, highlighter, and dictionary. Develop the habit of thinking ahead and gathering needed supplies. This is an important health care practice, too. You would not want to interrupt a patient procedure because you forgot to bring something from the supply room. Your study time is valuable, too, and should not be interrupted looking for the dictionary.

First Step to Effective Reading: Previewing

Advice worth repeating: Always work smarter, not harder.

Many methods have been developed to help students get maximum benefit from their reading assignments. Some have many steps and others just a few, but they *all* recommend that you **preview** before you start reading. Referring back to our medical procedure example, you would never perform a treatment on a patient without taking a few preliminary steps: identify the patient, introduce yourself, verify the procedure, gather necessary supplies, and put on gloves. Previewing in reading means that you look over the entire selection, learn any new vocabulary, and use clues in the text to anticipate and think about the content. These steps transform your reading from a passive activity to an active process in which learning takes place. Fortunately, most textbooks are set up to help you and contain many features to guide your previewing and reading.

When you start using a new textbook, take a few minutes to look it over carefully. Don't wait until the end of the course to discover something that could have made your life easier.

1. **Preface:** This is an introductory section at the beginning of the book. It typically contains a statement of the author's purpose and an overview of the book's content and structure. Some prefaces include information of special value to students, such as study tips and career ideas.
2. Table of contents: Some books supplement the usual list of chapter titles with a complete listing of chapter sections. This detailed format gives you a very good overall view of all the topics covered.
3. **Appendices:** These appear at the end of the text. Their contents are based on the book's subject and vary widely. Look these over early in your courses. You may discover valuable resources to help you understand both the textbook and the subject and learn about sources of career information. They can serve as reference guides. Examples from recent editions of health care textbooks include guidelines for infection control, important abbreviations, a metric conversion chart, Spanish translations of common health care phrases, laboratory test values, and a Celsius–Fahrenheit conversion scale.
4. Index: An alphabetical listing with corresponding page numbers of the book's contents. This is very useful when you need specific information or are reviewing.
5. Bibliography: A list of references used by the author or recommended readings if you want to learn more about the subject. Each chapter may have its own bibliography or there may be just one at the end of the book. Bibliographies provide sources of supplemental information whether you want to learn more or are having trouble understanding the assigned text. Remember the students discussed in Chapter 2 who identified specific career interests early in their studies? Bibliographies are excellent resources for expanding your knowledge of specific areas that can help you achieve your career goals.

PRESCRIPTION FOR SUCCESS 4–8

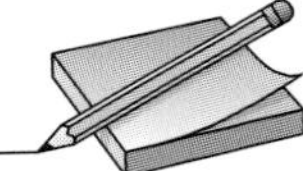

Book Report

Look over your current textbooks. Which of the following features do they contain?

____ Preface
____ Detailed table of contents
____ Appendices

____
____
____
____

____ Index
____ Bibliography(ies)
____ Other ____
____

Here are more potential gold mines you can use when previewing:

I. Vocabulary or key terms: These are often listed at the beginning of each chapter. Because reading is based on understanding words, learning new vocabulary before you begin to read is essential for comprehension. There are two ways to use vocabulary lists, depending on how a book is organized.
   A. If the definitions are included, take a few minutes to study them before you read the chapter. Mark the words you find most difficult.

B. If the definitions are not included, look them up in the **glossary,** an alphabetical list in the back of the book that is like a mini-dictionary. Most textbooks have a glossary. It yours does not, use a standard or medical dictionary and create your own word list: on a sheet of paper, written in the margins of your book, on your computer, or on flash cards. This will help you learn new vocabulary.
C. If your book defines the vocabulary or key terms as they appear in the text, you can use that feature to watch for the terms as you read instead of looking up the definitions as part of your preview. Once you become familiar with your books, you can choose the best method for learning new vocabulary.
D. Word lists contain clues about what the author considers to be most important. Key terms are like shortened forms of the important concepts.

II. **Objectives:** These are statements that tell you what you should learn or be able to do as a result of reading the chapter. Knowing the chapter objectives gives structure and purpose to your reading. Objectives are useful to check your understanding after reading the material. Go back to the beginning of the chapter and see if you have met them. Here are some examples:
A. Name six ways to display professionalism.
B. Recognize emergency situations in the reception area. (Chester, 1998)
C. List the possible causes of an increased or decreased red blood cell count.
D. Describe the purpose of rapid chemical tests. (Stepp and Woods, 1998)

III. Chapter introductions: In addition to giving an overview of chapter content, these often explain why the material is important and how it relates to your career.

IV. Headings: These words or phrases divide and label sections of text to give you an idea of the chapter's content. An important part of previewing is to go through the assigned selection page by page and read the headings. You will see they are organized like an outline, often with several levels of subheadings. Some books distinguish the levels with different colors and lettering styles. The following example of headings comes from a chapter entitled "Dealing with the Medical Patient" in Chester's *Modern Medical Assisting:*

Stress
  Flight, Fight, or Submit
  Defense Mechanisms
    Repression
    Regression
    Affiliation
    Deployment
    Control

Headings provide a logical structure to guide your reading. In the example, you learn several things before even reading the chapter: there are three responses to stress; defense mechanisms are related to stress; and there are at least five different defense mechanisms.

We know that one way to increase learning is to relate new information to what we already know. Based on what you find out about the content from reading the headings, take a few moments during the preview to think about what you already know about the topics.

You may be thinking that previewing is a waste of time and that it would be better to just jump into the reading and get it done. Not true! You are not "just reading." You are engaging in a learning activity and previewing adds greatly to your ability to comprehend and remember the information presented in your textbooks. Previewing is an excellent investment of your time.

Getting the Most from Your Reading

There are two activities that help you interact with your textbooks: asking and answering questions and marking or highlighting your book. They focus your attention and serve as comprehension checks as you proceed through the text. Here's how to use these techniques:

1. Convert each section heading into a question and then look for the answer as you read. When you find it, *stop* and answer the question aloud or quietly to yourself. This technique was developed almost sixty years ago when methods to increase the speed of learning were researched for World War II soldiers (Wahlstrom and Williams, 1997). It has proven to be one of *the* most effective ways to master written material developed to date. The following examples are questions based on a few of the headings from "Dealing with the Medical Patient":

   What is meant by "flight, fight, and submit"?
   What are "defense mechanisms"?
   How do they relate to health care?
   What is "repression"?
   What is an example of patient behavior that might be a sign of repression?

   There are no right or wrong questions. The only purpose of these questions is to help you learn. With practice, you will ask the questions that best help you benefit from your reading assignments.

   It is usually not necessary to write out the answers, although you may find it helpful with very difficult material. In that case, write both the questions and answers in your notebook so you can use them to review.

2. Mark your book *after* you finish reading each section. Highlight or underline the most important information. This transforms your book into a personal study aid. Busy students do not have time to reread entire textbooks before exams, and marking directs your attention to the major points. Try not to mark too little or too much. Too little and you miss important ideas that you need to know for testing and your future work. Too much and the whole page becomes a "must know" and you have not achieved your goal of identifying what is most important.

   In addition to marking, you can further increase your learning by writing in your book. This may take the form of key words, short summaries, questions, or responses. Develop symbols, like the ones you use when taking notes, that are logical and easy to remember:

   T = information instructor indicates will be on test
   ?? = I don't understand and need to ask about
   * = important
   ** = very important
   circled word = new term

   Many students like to use colored highlighters to mark their books. If this is your preference, avoid very bright colors that can cause eye strain. You can also use a pen or pencil to underline and make notes. A tool that combines the features of the highlighter and pen is a colored pen. When it is used to underline, the color draws your attention for easy review. Use the same pen to write in your book. Save time this way by not having to switch back and forth between a highlighter and a pen.

Additional Reading Tips

1. Look up unfamiliar words that were not included in the vocabulary. Use the book's glossary, a general dictionary, or a medical dictionary. You can write the definition in your book, in your own glossary that you keep in your notebook, and/or make flash cards.
2. Take advantage of illustrations, charts, lists, and boxed text. These are designed to work together to give you additional opportunities to master the material. Boxes often provide summaries of text content and serve as valuable aids to review.

3. Read through procedures carefully if they appear in your text. Do not assume that the instructor will explain everything you need to know. Find out what will be expected ahead of time. Pay special attention to the rationale. It is important that health care professionals understand the reasons behind their actions. Nothing in health care is routine. You must think through every action and know why you are performing it. Written instructions will be part of your professional reading, and learning to read and understand this format is an important health care skill.
4. Read in short sessions. Depending on the difficulty of the material, you may find that you are able to read and absorb for only twenty to thirty minutes without a short break. Experiment to see what works best for you. Just don't wander off too far or get involved with a two-hour movie on TV!
5. Don't worry about speed. Health care textbooks contain a lot of technical and detailed information. Your goal is not speed; it is comprehension. Read at a rate that keeps your attention and also allows you to comprehend the material. One way to prevent getting bogged down is to avoid saying each word, even if you are only doing this mentally. Try to read in phrases. When you drive a car, you see and act on many things at once. The same is true for reading, and with practice, you can see and process several words at a time.

Reviewing—the Final Step

As we discussed in the section on note taking, regular reviews started soon after your first exposure to new material is the key to ensuring that it becomes stored in your long-term memory. Review techniques for reading are similar to those suggested for reviewing notes:

I. Review *within twenty-four hours.* Start laying down memory pathways before you forget most of the information. What a waste to spend an entire evening reading an assignment, only to forget most of it by bedtime the next night! Even a quick review is effective.

II. Do more than look at the words. Passive rereading is not likely to increase your comprehension and retention significantly. Use the note-reviewing techniques discussed in the previous section. Use prompts such as questions, headings, and key words in the margin *without looking at the text.* This forces you to think and checks your understanding. If you have trouble remembering, review the section and try again. If you continue having trouble, this is a sign that you don't understand the material.

III. Use study techniques that fit your learning styles.
   A. Visual: Use text illustrations to prompt recall. Create scenarios around the illustrations to help anchor concepts in your mind. Attach significant concepts to people in a photograph. While looking at a picture of a piece of equipment, recall the name and function of each part, as well as how and for what purpose the equipment is used. Later you can call up the pictures in your mind as a trigger to remember facts and concepts. Cover the labels on drawings and say or write down the names.
   B. Auditory: Do "out-loud" activities. Explain the text in your own words. Create a dialogue to discuss the material. Have someone else ask you questions. Record important points about text or your questions and answers created from the headings.
   C. Kinesthetic: Stand up or move around while you review. Point to illustrations as you describe them. When appropriate, imagine how it feels. A lot of health care text describes processes and procedures. Go through them as realistically as possible in your mind or act them out. For example, open and close your hand as you read about how the heart pumps blood. Imagine yourself taking a file off the shelf, opening it to the correct section, and entering patient information.

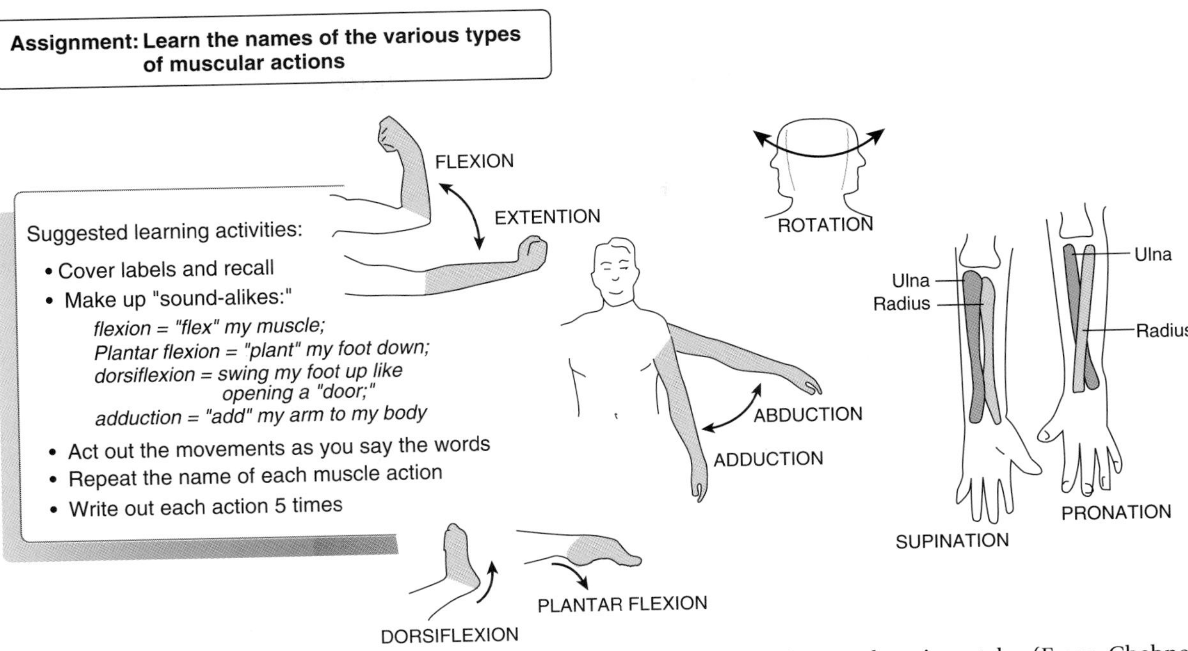

Assignment: Learn the names of the various types of muscular actions
Suggested learning activities:
• Cover labels and recall
• Make up "sound-alikes:"
flexion = "flex" my muscle;
Plantar flexion = "plant" my foot down;
dorsiflexion = swing my foot up like opening a "door;"
adduction = "add" my arm to my body
• Act out the movements as you say the words
• Repeat the name of each muscle action
• Write out each action 5 times
FLEXION
EXTENTION
ROTATION
ABDUCTION
ADDUCTION
Ulna
Radius
Ulna
Radius
SUPINATION
PRONATION
PLANTAR FLEXION
DORSIFLEXION

FIGURE 4–4 Create learning activities that match your learning style. (From Chabner, Davi-Ellen, *Language of Medicine,* 5th ed. Philadelphia: W.B. Saunders Company, 1996, p. 529, used with permission.)

D. Linear: Outlines may be especially helpful because they create a logical structure for new material. Use the headings as a guide. Charts that show relationships are also good. If the text does not include them, create your own.
E. Global: Create mind maps of the entire chapter or major sections.
F. Deductive: To be sure that you master the concepts along with the facts, try writing short summaries that state the principal ideas.
G. Inductive: List the important facts that support the major ideas. Make flash cards with facts on one side and explanations or details on the other (Fig. 4–4).

IV. Outline the chapter: This is optional—unless it is assigned by your instructor, of course. It can be helpful when reading material that is not well organized, lacks descriptive headings, or is very difficult. It can also help you determine how the information is related.

V. Learn all new vocabulary. Clear and effective communication in health care requires the correct use of both general and medical language. Learning new words as you encounter them helps you understand your reading and adds to your value as a future employee.

VI. Test yourself. Make up practice tests as suggested for learning from your class notes. Converting chapter objectives into questions is an excellent way to review. Here are a few examples:

Identify character traits that are desirable in a professional medical assistant.
What are the most important character traits in a professional medical assistant?

Assist patients in planning a daily menu in accordance with a physician's dietary guidelines utilizing the food pyramid and a calorie counter.

What is the food pyramid? How do you use a calorie counter? What are the elements of menu planning? What is the proper way to give patient instruction? (Chester, 1998.)

Handle insurance claims in the physician's office to minimize their rejection by insurance carriers.

What can you do to minimize the rejection of insurance claims? What are some reasons why insurance claims are rejected? (Fordney, 1997.)

VII. Work in a study group. Each student makes up several test questions and exchanges them with the others. Practice quizzing each other.

Some Final Remarks about Note Taking and Reading

You may think that the processes for note taking and reading are too long and unnecessary. Remember that repetition is essential for storing information in your long-term memory, the sign of true learning. And it is true learning that will help you achieve your goal of becoming a competent health care professional equipped with the knowledge to perform your job (Box 4–1). The suggestions given in this chapter can actually increase, not decrease, your learning efficiency.

Doing Research

Research is not limited to finding information about a paper you have to write. We do research all the time: when we investigate how to cook a turkey, remove a stain from the sofa, or buy a car. Research simply means finding sources of reliable information and getting what you need from those sources.

LIBRARY

Your school's library may be large and contain thousands of books and loads of other material, or it may be small and focused on the specialized items needed to support the programs offered at your school. You should get to know both your school library and your local public library. If there are other schools of higher education nearby, inquire whether they allow the public to use their libraries. Some even give checkout privileges for a yearly fee. Hospitals and clinics often have libraries for employees. It is possible that you will have access to these during your clinical experience.

The key to using any library effectively is to find out what is available and how to find it. See Table 4-2 for some of the most common items found in a library.

Some libraries offer database searching services. **Databases** are specialized collections of information that are transmitted over phone lines by computer. Huge amounts of information are organized by topic. There are databases on every subject imaginable, including health care topics. Databases are not the same as the Internet, and special librarians perform searches for the information that you request. Sometimes a fee is charged for the service.

Every library is different. Walk around and explore. Look for informational brochures and how-to guides and ask the librarian for help.

BOX 4–1. ON THE ROAD TO MASTERY: THE MANY WAYS TO LEARN NEW MATERIAL

Read	*Listen*	*Create*
Preview	Take notes	Mind maps
Highlight	Organize material	Outlines
Ask questions	Write questions	Charts
Review!	Review!	Drawings

TABLE 4–2 ***Library Materials—Know What's Available***

Item	Where to Find	How to Find/Use
General books	Open shelves	Library catalog. May be entered on 3 × 5" cards organized alphabetically in drawers; on microfiche, which must be read on a special machine; or on computer. However stored, all books will be listed alphabetically by title, author, and subject.
Reference books	Open shelves, usually placed separately from general books.	Library catalog. Many reference books have "How to Use" guides in the front.
Books in Print	With reference books or in computerized form.	Lists all books currently in publication. Will be listed separately by title, author, and subject.
Journals	Periodical section. Older issues may be stored separately from current issues. Information tends to be more current than that found in books.	*Index to Periodical Literature* lists articles, by subject, in general periodicals like *Newsweek, Ladies Home Journal,* and *Popular Mechanics.* There are specialty indexes that cover specific subjects. Some even contain abstracts—short summaries of each article. Useful indexes for health care students include *Nursing Abstracts, Psychological Abstracts, Medline, Biological Abstracts, Cumulative Index to Nursing and Allied Health Literature, Excerpta Medica,* and *Index Medicus.* Indexes are now computerized, in addition to being in print format. Some are also available on microfiche and on the Internet.
Looseleaf services: regularly updated materials kept in binders or on computer	Reference shelves, secured area, or on computer.	Content is kept current. There are services for a wide range of subjects, including health care.
Audiovisual materials: tapes, films, CDs, software, etc.	Secured area.	Ask librarian how to access.

PRESCRIPTION FOR SUCCESS 4–9

Check out the Library

If you did not visit your school library and list its resources for Prescription for Success 1-11, do it now.

INTERNET The **Internet,** with its ability to connect millions of computers throughout the world, is a valuable source for all kinds of information. Literally anyone or any organization can create a **web site** and get on the Internet for everyone to access. Here are just a few examples of what is available:

Articles from newspapers and magazines
Informative articles by researchers
Directories of all types
Dictionaries
Opportunities to communicate with experts
Job postings and applications
Information about diseases and injuries for both patients and health care professionals
Career advice from professional organizations
Photographs
Video-type presentations
"Stores" from which you can order almost any product or service imaginable

If you don't own or have access to a computer, check with your school to find out what is available. A discussion on how to search the Internet is outside the scope of this book. However, if you are unfamiliar with it, here are a few facts about its potential as a research tool:

I. The Internet is easy to access and takes no special computer knowledge.
II. You can find information in two ways:
    A. All sites have an address, just like houses. If you know the address, you simply type it in. Sample addresses:
    American Association of Medical Assistants
    http://www.aama-ntl.org/
    Profiles of major allied health employers
    http://www.healthopps.com/healthopps/health3.html
    Information about types and severity of burns
    http://www.alpha-tek.com/burn/type.htm
    B. If you do not know which sites have the information you are looking for, just type in key words and the search is on!
III. There are many companies that provide access to the Internet, perform searches, and organize information so that you can find it more easily.
IV. A word of caution—the Internet is not controlled by any organization or agency that checks on content or keeps the connections up to date. For serious research, be sure to check the credibility of the supplier of the information. Questions to ask about a web site include:
    A. Who is the sponsor? Universities, government agencies, professional organizations, research institutes, and established publishers are usually good sources.
    B. Who is the author? He or she should have education and/or experience in the subject matter.
    C. What is the purpose of the web site? Many sites are designed to sell products or persuade viewers to believe in a cause. The material provided may be not be well-researched.
    D. How are claims supported? Check for statistics and references to original sources of information.
V. This is new technology, and not all web pages are well organized or easy to follow.
VI. There are many directories, like the one listed in the bibliography at the end of this chapter, that list addresses to make it easier for you to go directly to the information you need. Keep in mind that sites close down, merge with others, or change address.

INTERVIEWING The informational interview, described in Chapter 1, is a form of research. Many important studies are based on interviews. Effective interviews require that you identify your purpose in advance and prepare good questions. You will use your note-taking skills to ensure that you record all the key points given by the interviewee. Examples of interviews that a student or health professional might conduct are the following:

- Request career advice from a graduate of your school to learn how you can make the most of your education.
- Ask a local specialist a series of questions about a health condition in which you have a special interest.
- Talk with personnel at community offices of organizations like the American Heart Association and American Cancer Society to learn what information and services they have available.

PRESCRIPTION FOR SUCCESS 4–10

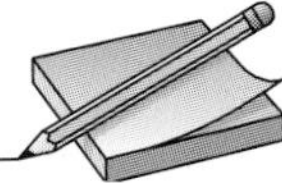

Go to the Source

Choose a topic in which you have an interest and locate five different sources of reliable information. Briefly describe each source and state why you believe it to be reliable.

1. ______________________
2. ______________________
3. ______________________
4. ______________________
5. ______________________

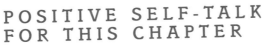

SUMMARY OF KEY IDEAS

1. Class notes can be powerful study aids.
2. Effective listening is one of the most valuable skills for a successful life.
3. Repetition is the key to long-term memory.
4. Reviewing the same material frequently is much more effective than one or two long review sessions just before the test.
5. Reading to learn is an active process that requires your participation.
6. There are many effective ways to learn. Find the ones that work best for you.
7. Research is an everyday activity that is not limited to library books.

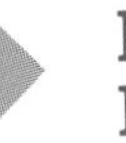

POSITIVE SELF-TALK FOR THIS CHAPTER

1. I am an active listener.
2. I take good notes in class.
3. My notes are good study tools, and I review them regularly.
4. I use techniques that I enjoy and that help me learn.
5. I learn from my reading assignments because I preview before I read and review afterward.
6. I use a variety of sources to conduct research.

BIBLIOGRAPHY

Chester, Gail A. *Modern Medical Assisting.* Philadelphia: W.B. Saunders Company, 1998.

Fordney, Marilyn. *Insurance Handbook for the Medical Office,* 5th ed. Philadelphia: W.B. Saunders Company, 1997.

Griffin, Attrices Dean. *Directory of Internet Sources for Health Professionals.* Albany, NY: Delmar Publishers, 1998.

Pauk, Walter. *How to Succeed in College,* 6th ed. New York: Houghton Mifflin Company, 1997.

Stepp, Craig and MaryAnn Woods. *Laboratory Procedures for Medical Office Personnel.* Philadelphia: W.B. Saunders Company, 1998.

Wahlstrom, Carl and Brian K. Williams. *The Commuter Student: Being Your Best at College and Life.* Belmont, CA: Wadsworth Publishing Company, 1997.

"Lecture Segment" for Prescription for Success 4-7 Autoclaving*

The autoclave is an instrument that works like a pressure cooker in the home. It sterilizes by steam under pressure. Steam under pressure increases the effectiveness of boiling.

Boiling kills most organisms. However, boiling does not destroy spores. Autoclaving kills all spores. Spores are a protective mechanism for some bacteria, and the reproductive stage for some fungi. The spore-forming bacteria convert to the spore form when conditions are not ideal for growth.

Spores have a terrific survival rate. For example, the bacillus causing anthrax, a disease of cattle that may infect and kill humans, can survive for hundreds of years as a spore. Once the conditions are good for growth of the bacteria, the spore converts to the bacterial form to reproduce. The spore is not a reproductive form for bacteria.

The autoclaving process requires specific conditions for sterilization. The most effective sterilization process is maintaining 121 degrees C for 15 minutes with 15 pounds per square inch pressure. If these conditions are not met, the process of sterilization is not complete. To be effective, the steam must come into contact with the entire item being sterilized.

* From Chester, 1998, p. 490.

5

Developing Your Paper Skills II: Output of Information

OBJECTIVES

THE INFORMATION AND ACTIVITIES IN THIS CHAPTER CAN HELP YOU TO:

- Understand why it is important for health care professionals to have good writing skills.
- Evaluate your own writing skills and, if necessary, devise a plan to improve them.
- Know how to locate and use writing tools to help you write more effectively.
- Plan and organize various types of writing projects.
- Understand how tests are part of the daily life of a health care professional.
- Use tests as incentives to learn rather than as instruments of torture.
- Apply effective techniques to maximize your performance on classroom tests.

KEY TERMS

Audit, auditors: To check an organization to see if it is following certain laws and regulations. It also refers to reviews by professional organizations to ensure that their standards are being met.

Bibliography: A list of the information sources for any type of writing assignment. It can have a variety of sources including books, journal articles, websites, movies, and interviews.

Consonant: All the letters in the alphabet *except* A, E, I, O, and U.

Credibility: Believability and integrity. The degree to which people have confidence in and trust you is your credibility.

Criteria: Established standards used to measure performance.

Documentation: Written records. In health care, it refers to detailed recordings of facts about and observations of patients and their care. In the computer world it also refers to the written instructions that explain how to use equipment and software.

Draft: The first version of a piece of writing. Its purpose is to get ideas and preliminary organizational ideas on paper. Drafts are revised and sometimes even completely rewritten before the work is released to readers.

Essay: A short piece of nonfiction (true—not made up by the writer) that is meant to inform, persuade, or entertain the reader. Essay questions on tests require you to write at least several paragraphs and include facts to support your answer.

Fraud: Dishonesty or trickery, especially in business. Accepting payments from the government for health services that were not provided is a serious form of fraud.

Freewrite: Recording ideas as they come to you without worrying about perfect organization, grammar, and spelling.

Grammar: A system of rules for putting words together that is meaningful to speakers and writers of a language. The rules differ among the world's languages. For example, in Spanish subjects are indicated by verb endings and adjectives follow nouns: "Vivo en una casa blanca" translates as "I live in a white house." Note: vivo = I live, casa = house, blanca = white.

Protocols: Established ways of performing procedures. They refer to the specific steps required for carrying out various tasks. Protocols are developed by health care facilities to ensure safety and quality control.

Reimbursement: Payments from a third party for services given. For example, insurance companies pay physicians on behalf of patients who purchase insurance plans.

Suffix: A syllable attached to the end of a word such as "ing" and "ly". Suffixes are used extensively in medical terminology to add to and change the meaning of medical words.

Syllable: The shortest part of a word that can be pronounced as a unit. Examples: immunization has five syllables: im-mu-ni-za-tion. Oxygen has three syllables: ox-y-gen.

Text: Written material as contrasted with illustrations, drawings, graphs, and so on.

Vowel: Any of the following letters: A, E, I, O, and U.

Your Writing Ability: A Key to Professional Success

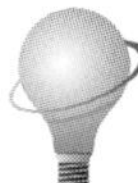

Take a Moment to Think

Which statement best describes how you feel about writing?

____ I love to write!
____ I am a good writer and enjoy writing.
____ My writing skills are okay, but I don't really like to do it.
____ I don't mind writing, but I'm not very good at it.
____ I don't like to write, and I avoid it whenever possible.
____ Other ________________________

Clear communication is critical for the delivery of quality health care. Notes on patient charts, letters to insurance companies, and printed instructions for patients must be written clearly and accurately. Consistency of care, proper billing and **reimbursement** for services, and good relations between health facilities and the public they serve depend on the quality of written documents. You may believe that you will not do much writing in your future work. Not true! Almost every job in health care today involves paperwork and some writing tasks.

Your writing is a personal advertisement. When you are speaking, you can revise and correct yourself. Writing, however, has a permanent form. It influences the opinions of other people about you and your work. Even if you have excellent technical skills, you can appear incompetent if you make grammatical and spelling errors or organize information poorly because most patients notice these problems. How well you write also represents your employer and the health care facility where you work. It is an important skill to master.

E-mail, in which you correspond electronically over the computer, is replacing a lot of the communication that until recently was conducted over the telephone. While e-mail messages tend to be informal and often use phrases instead of complete sentences, they must be expressed clearly and in an organized fashion in order to be useful to the receiver. Technology is actually increasing, rather than decreasing, the need for you to develop your writing skills.

Many students find writing difficult and dread assignments in which they have to write more than a few words. Maybe this applies to you. Perhaps you thought your English classes were boring or you were never required to do much writing. Or maybe English is not your first language. Whatever the reason, it is not too late to upgrade your skills. This chapter discusses some of the basics of good writing and includes suggestions to help you write more effectively. However, a complete writing course is beyond the scope of this book. The main goal here is to encourage you to care about your writing skills and motivate you to improve them, if necessary.

In Chapter 4 we discussed how you can use writing to increase your learning. For example, taking notes in class, preparing outlines, writing summaries, and jotting down key words and questions in the margins of your books force you to think about what you hear and read. The act of writing down new information, in any format, increases the chances that it will be stored in your long-term memory. Some educators suggest that you do a lot of writing that no one else sees by regularly writing summaries of what you are learning. This is an excellent investment of your time, because you receive the double benefit of practicing a critical basic skill as you increase your learning of other subjects (Campbell, 1997).

There is no denying that learning to write well takes practice and self-discipline, but it is an important part of becoming a professional. Starting now to work on improving your writing skills will significantly affect your future success and provide positive payoffs throughout your life.

Write On! Developing Good Writing Skills

Writing requires a variety of skills which we will divide into two categories: content and form. Content refers to *what* you write about: the information and ideas. Form is *how* you present it: grammar, spelling, and formatting. You must pay attention to both aspects in order for your reader to receive your intended message.

CONTENT: DETERMINING WHAT TO WRITE

When journalists write articles, they ask themselves a series of questions. You can use questioning to help you select and organize your content. The first step when starting to write is to think about what you want to accomplish. Your purpose determines what you say and how you say it, so it is important that it is clear in your own mind. The following examples illustrate the writing goals that are common for students and health care professionals.

1. *Demonstrate your knowledge.* This is the reason instructors ask you to write research papers (also called "term papers" or "reports") and answer essay test questions. They use these assignments to assess what you know about a subject. To do well on papers and tests, it is important that you know about your subject, state information clearly, and give accurate facts to support what you write. When your purpose is to show what you know, it is important not to pad your writing with repetition or statements that add nothing meaningful to the content. A common mistake of students is to use many words to make it look as if they've said a lot when they really have said very little.

2. *Persuade your reader.* A common classroom assignment in school is to write a paper about a controversial topic in which you must convince the reader to accept your point of view. Outside of class, you may write with the goal of influencing the reader to take certain actions. For example, you will write application letters to include with your resume when you are looking for employment. You want to convince prospective employers to interview you. Persuasive writing can be used on the job to present your ideas about how the facility might run more smoothly, or to

request a promotion or a pay raise. Supervisors often ask that you submit these ideas and requests in writing, so it is important that you know how to write convincingly.

There are various ways to persuade readers. One is to present facts that support your arguments. In the case of the letter to a prospective employer, you could list the ways you can be of benefit. Another method is to appeal to readers' emotions. For example, if you want to convince them to take action against cigarette advertising aimed at children, you could point out the need for adults to express their love for vulnerable children by protecting them from potential health hazards. Sometimes it is effective to use both methods so that they support each other and strengthen your case. In the argument against cigarette advertising, you could cite the number and ages of children who start smoking each year, along with statistics about diseases and deaths caused by smoking.

3. *Provide an explanation.* Some school assignments, such as exercises in workbooks, ask you to explain the steps in a procedure or explain why something is done a certain way. Test questions that require short answers are often requests for explanations. On the job, you may write instructions for patients or directions for coworkers. Explanatory writing that takes the form of instructions may includes lists of steps. It is important that this type of writing be very clear and organized in a logical order. Including information about why something should be done or why it should be done in a specific way is known as the rationale. People tend to be more willing and able to follow instructions when they know the purpose of their actions.

4. *Narrate a story or event.* If you take an English or writing class, creating a story may be one of your assignments. While stories are not commonly used in workplace writing, they can add interest and provide examples in persuasive or explanatory works. The principal considerations in narration are to use your imagination to create interesting stories and to write good descriptions.

5. *Make a request.* This is related to persuasive writing, but it is usually more direct and has the goal of initiating a definite response. While writing a request is not a common school assignment, you might use this form for tasks at school outside of class. For example, some schools require that you submit a written request if you need a leave of absence. Or you may want to request information about your student loan. During your job search, you may wish to submit requests to health care facilities for information about their hiring requirements. Once on the job, you may submit requests to vendors for information about their products, compose letters to physicians asking them to send you patient records, or write to insurance companies requesting action on unpaid claims.

Many times there will be more than one purpose for your writing. It is more effective if you combine your purposes so that they reinforce each other. For example, when preparing instruction sheets for patients, they can be more effective if you include persuasive language that encourages the patients to follow their special diet or perform their exercises every day.

PRESCRIPTION FOR SUCCESS 5-1

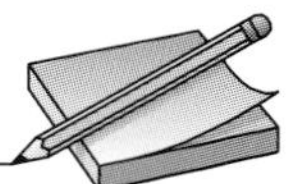

What's the Purpose?

What do you think would be the major purpose of each of the following writing projects?

1. A three-page report about a skin disease that includes the causes, methods of diagnosis, and treatment.
2. An instruction sheet explaining how patients with leg casts can take a shower without getting the cast wet.

PRESCRIPTION FOR SUCCESS 5-1 (*continued*)

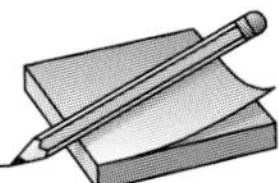

3. An **essay** in which you tell why quitting smoking can improve the quality and increase the length of a person's life.
4. A letter asking for a transfer to a job at your facility which requires more experience than you currently have but for which you feel you are qualified.
5. A letter of recommendation for a coworker who is moving to another state.
6. A letter to your local newspaper in which you express your ideas about the lack of affordable medical care for the poor.
7. Directions for using the office copy and facsimile (fax) machines.

What Do I Know about This Topic?

One reason students have trouble with writing is that they don't know enough about their topic. A related problem is that they can't think of anything to write about when told to choose a topic. Writing sometimes requires research and always requires thought. This may sound obvious, but many people simply start writing without any preparation or in-depth thinking. The result is a collection of words and sentences that don't say much.

1. *Assess what you know.* One of the purposes of research and term papers is to help you learn about a topic. Instructors often specify the kind and number of resources you must use in preparing your report. Start out by writing down what you already know in the format you find most useful: lists of key ideas and facts, a mind map, or an outline. Or you can put ideas on 3 × 5 cards that you use later to organize your content.

2. *Identify what you need to find out.* If the instructor assigned a topic about which you know very little, develop a list of questions to help guide your research. For example, if you are to write about infectious diseases, your questions might include:

What are the major infectious diseases?
What are the symptoms?
What causes these diseases?
How are they spread?
How are they treated?
How widespread are these diseases? How many people are affected each year?

3. *Choose topics wisely.* If part of your assignment is to select the topic, it is tempting to put this off until just a few days before the finished product is due. Don't wait! Start early and give yourself a chance to benefit from the paper by choosing something that is related to the kind of work you will be doing in the future. (If you have a mentor who works in your field, ask him or her for recommendations.)

4. *Locate resources.* If you know almost nothing about the topic, start your research with nontechnical resources that provide definitions and general information. These resources include encyclopedia and journal articles, textbooks, or books on the subject whose purpose is to inform the general reader. Once you have an overall view of the topic, you can focus your research on specific aspects of interest. Review the section on research in Chapter 3 to get ideas for resources. (Note: Your instructor may require you to consult certain types and numbers of resources beyond your textbook. He or she may also have good suggestions for finding out more about your topic.)

5. *Take notes.* As you consult each source of information, take notes in which you list important facts and ideas. Many people like to use note cards. Start a new card for each separate topic or subtopic. If you need more than one card for each topic, number or mark them in some way to keep them organized. You also need a system to keep track of your resources so that you can cite them appropriately when

you begin to write. Another method is to take notes on sheets of paper (one side only), organizing by resource rather than topic. There may be several pages for each source. When it's time to organize, you can either cut the paper up and create piles of related information, or you can color-code them or write key words in the margins to identify various topics to refer to when you write.

6. When taking notes from books and journals, be sure to write down all the information you will need for your **bibliography.** This includes the name of the book or journal and article; the author's name; the publisher; and the place and date of publication. Even if your project does not require a bibliography, it is a good idea to write down your sources so that you can find them later if you need them. One way to keep track of your sources is to create a numbered list and then write the corresponding number on each note card or page when you take notes. Remember that information sources are not limited to books and journals but may also include ideas from interviews, information from pamphlets, and printouts from Internet searches. Details about these sources should also be recorded for your bibliography.

7. *Skip steps 2 through 5.* Yes, you read that correctly. If you are answering essay test questions, obviously you will not do any outside research. However, take a little time to assess what you know before you start writing. It might help to write major ideas and brief outlines in the margins of your test paper to help you review mentally and get organized.

Who Are My Readers?

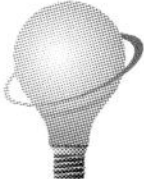

Take a Moment to Think

In what ways would instructions you write for a coworker differ from those you write for a patient? What factors are helpful in determining how to direct your writing?

Effective writers consider the needs of their readers. This is especially important in health care, where safe and consistent care depends on how well health care professionals communicate with patients and with each other. The National Health Care Skill Standards, introduced in Chapter 1, include many references to both verbal and written communication skills. Here are several standards that emphasize the need to understand the needs of patients:

- Assess others' ability to understand.
- Adapt communication to individual needs.
- Use language appropriate to the situation.
- Be sensitive to multicultural and multilingual needs.

The same principles apply whether you are addressing patients, coworkers, supervisors, or the general public. Whenever you write, consider what you know about the readers' ages, cultural backgrounds, knowledge of health issues, and purpose for reading the material. Remember that you will not usually be present to clarify information, answer questions, or see from their facial expressions that they do not understand or agree with what you have written. This is why it is so important to write clearly and organize your **text** so that readers can follow it easily. If you are addressing a mixed audience, plan your writing for the readers who will have the most difficulty understanding. When writing class assignments and tests, your instructor is the audience. He or she wants you to demonstrate what you know about a subject and how well you express yourself. There may also be specific requirements about the form that you should follow (Box 5-1).

BOX 5–1. ANTICIPATING YOUR READERS' NEEDS

- Relationship to you: patient, supervisor, coworker, or instructor
- Their purpose in reading: learn from you, receive instructions, evaluate you
- Educational and reading levels
- Knowledge of English
- Knowledge of health care
- Age
- Cultural background

Getting Started

Since it is not possible to think about everything all at once, most experienced writers handle a piece of writing in stages.—Diana Hacker

When you are assigned a research paper or have a report to prepare for work, one of the hardest parts is deciding how to organize the information you have collected from your research and your own experience. Some instructors require students to prepare an outline as the first step in writing. If you find it difficult to think in outline form (you're just not linear) or you just don't know where to start, outlining can be as intimidating as writing the paper itself. Don't despair. There are other ways to tackle the problem of getting things in order and getting started.

1. *Mind maps.* These are good if you don't have a clear idea of the order you want for your material. You don't have to worry about running out of room under a heading if you think of more ideas later. Mind maps also help you think about how ideas relate to and support each other. If you have several major ideas, you can make a series of maps.

2. *Idea sheets.* As you think of major ideas, write each one at the top of a separate sheet of paper. Then list all related and supporting ideas on the pages. To organize, lay the sheets out and move them around until the order makes sense to you.

3. *Note cards.* Dave Ellis, writer of popular student success books, recommends the use of note cards for generating creativity and organization (Ellis, 1998). Think about all of your ideas, both major and supporting, and list each on a 3×5 card. Sort the cards by topics or categories and then arrange them in logical order. You can lay them out on a flat surface or pin them to a wall or large bulletin board.

4. *Brain dump.* Get out some paper and just start writing. Narrow the topic as best you can, and write everything you can think of. This is not always the most efficient method because you can end up with a jumble that has to be unsnarled, but it can get started if you find yourself in a state of organizational paralysis. Many people use the brain dump to promote creativity and the free flow of ideas, because they are not confined to any particular structure. Use this method when you have trouble identifying the major topics. Write quickly, and get as much on paper as possible. Then go back through your writing and look for ideas and themes that you can pull out and put into some kind of logical order.

5. *Questions.* Think of questions you would like answered about the main topic and subtopics. Then organize your information as you research and find the answer to each question.

PRESCRIPTION FOR SUCCESS 5–2

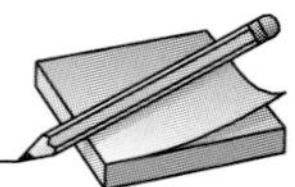

What Works for You?

1. Which of the organizational techniques presented best fits your learning style?
2. Explain why.
3. Have you used any other techniques that worked well for you?
4. If yes, explain.

Organizing Content for Your Readers

Everyone prefers to read material that is easy to follow. Good writers achieve this by organizing material logically, and you can do it too. Here are suggestions for organizing different types of documents that you might write at school and on the job.

Letters, research papers, and long essay answers are easier for the reader to follow if they are divided into sections:

1. Introduction: Present your major points. Tell what you are writing about. State your purpose.
2. Middle or body: Develop, support, and explain your ideas. You may have several sections, one for each topic or idea.
3. Conclusion: Show how everything you have said pulls together. Give your "final word" on the subject. Summarize your points. State what you have attempted to prove with your information. Tell the readers what action you hope they will take as a result of your writing.

Instructions and directions within the piece can be organized into lists or other clumps of related information:

1. Lists: steps or activities in the order in which they should be performed or in order from most to least important.
2. Rationale: include just before or after the step or action to which it relates.

Short answers to test questions and brief letters and notes require tight organization to cover all necessary material in a small space:

1. Give your answer or state your purpose or main point in the first sentence.
2. Give supporting details in one or two paragraphs.
3. Limit your conclusion to one or two sentences.

See Figure 5–1.

Do Not Aim for Perfection

Not on your first **draft,** anyway. Writing is not easy for anyone, not even professional writers. Many people find a piece of blank paper very intimidating. A good way to beat the blank-paper monster is to *just start writing.* Begin with a rough draft, and don't worry about how rough it is. There are several purposes for writing a rough draft: to overcome the fear of writing, stop procrastinating, and start the flow of creativity (Fig. 5–2).

Writing creatively and writing perfectly and correctly require different intellectual skills that can actually cancel each other out. Peter Elbow, a professor who wrote a very helpful book about how to write, says that trying to write perfectly the first time is "dangerous writing" because you can't generate good ideas and be critical of your work at the same time (Elbow, 1981). He recommends that you spend half of the time on a project **freewriting** the rough draft and the other half revising (a good argument for starting your writing assignments well in advance of the due date!).

When freewriting, don't worry about starting with your introduction. Starting with the introduction puts unnecessary pressure on you to start out "just right" and think of good opening sentences. You may not be completely clear at this point

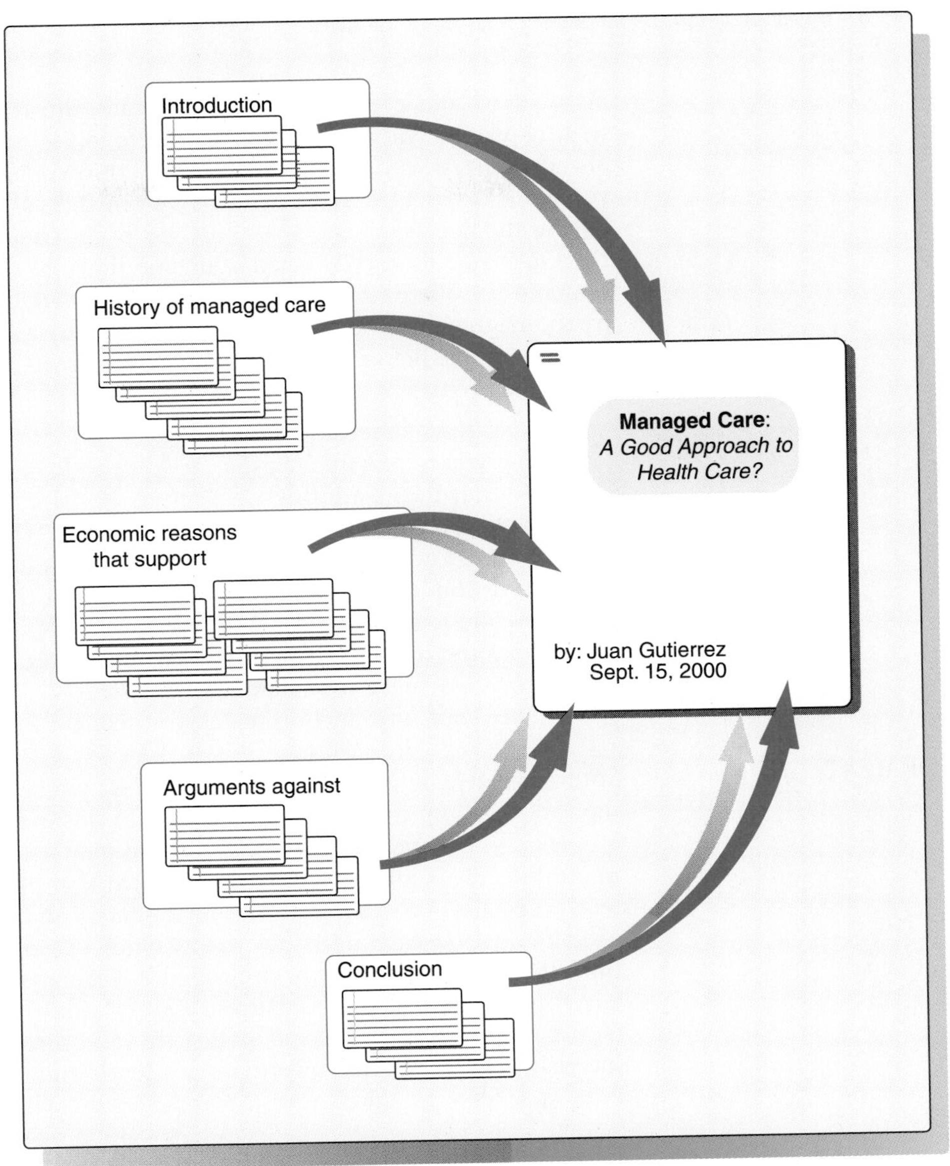

FIGURE 5–1 Organize your material *before* writing the final draft of the research paper.

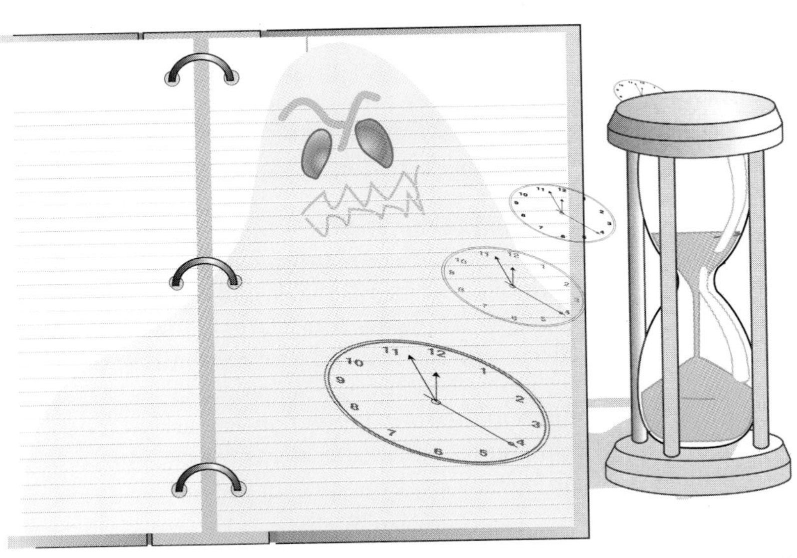

FIGURE 5–2 "Come on. I dare you to write something!"

about how your piece will turn out because ideas are developed throughout the writing process and you may add or delete topics or even change your purpose. Go ahead and start with the middle section if this works for you. (An exception is when you write answers to essay questions on timed tests, when it is best to state your answer at the beginning and spend the rest of the time supporting it.)

Once you have completed your first draft, let it rest for a couple of days (or hours, if the due date is directly ahead). Then assume the role of your readers and try to imagine that you are reading the piece for the first time. Read it aloud to hear how it sounds. Better yet, have someone else read it so that you can listen for the following points:*

- Does it make sense?
- Can you follow the ideas?
- Do they flow smoothly?
- Have you supported your ideas?
- Is there enough information about each topic or idea?
- Have you included unnecessary details that should be left out?
- Do you repeat yourself unnecessarily?
- Does the conclusion summarize your information?
- Do you achieve your stated purpose?
- Does your introduction match your conclusion?

FORM: ATTENDING TO THE DETAILS

Your content may be important, interesting, and well organized, but poor **grammar** and spelling can cause your readers to misunderstand what you have written and even to question your **credibility.** You may believe that worrying about grammatical details is unimportant. However, work in health care demands that you attend to details every day. Performing accurately and following exact procedures are valuable health care skills. In many types of written health care **documentation,** the contents are strictly controlled by federal and state law as well as by nongovernmental regulatory agencies. For example, California law requires that reports prepared to document patient home care visits be written on the day of the visit, contain specific information, use certain abbreviations, make corrections in a specific way, and show the time of the visit using the twenty-four-hour system.

Written documentation is often the only proof to show that patients have received appropriate care. It is recognized in court and by **auditors** who perform compliance reviews of medical institutions. A standard rule in health care is "If it was not documented, it was not done." We might add "If it's written poorly, it's not documented properly." Most patients are covered by some type of insurance, and payment to the health care provider depends on clear and accurate claims submitted by health care facilities. Even if your job does not include preparing insurance claims, your notes may provide the information on which the claim is based. Learning to write correctly and developing the habit of paying attention to details are skills worthwhile developing.

First Aid for Grammar

All languages are organized into systems of rules that determine how sentences are organized. Correct grammar is especially important in writing. Mistakes may be overlooked when we speak. But writing is permanently recorded on paper for the reader to see again and again. Using proper grammar will result in writing that reflects competence and professionalism.

Tables 5–1 through 5–3 are designed to help you review rules you may have forgotten. If they don't look familiar, ask your instructor how to find resources that can help you learn to write in a way that represents you well. The time you spend now will be well worth it later on the job.

* Adapted from Palau and Meltzer, 1996.

TABLE 5–1 ***Common Sentence Ailments***

Ailment	Example	Corrected
No subject	Said his tooth hurts.	He said that his tooth hurts.
Run-on (no punctuation or connecting word)	He needed an x-ray the radiologist was called.	He needed an x-ray, so the radiologist was called.
No pronoun agreement	Every patient should take their prescription to the pharmacy.	Every patient should take his or her prescription to the pharmacy. OR All patients should take their prescriptions to the pharmacy.
No subject-verb agreement	Both the nurse and the physician sees the fracture on the x-ray. An ECG machine, cables, and limb and chest electrodes are the equipment needed to perform the ECG.	Both the nurse and the physician see the fracture on the x-ray. An ECG machine, cables, and limb and chest electrodes is the equipment needed to perform the ECG.
Incorrect pronoun	Me and Jamie are going to the same dental office. Give your urine sample to the doctor or myself. The AARC has a special newsletter for we respiratory therapists.	Jamie and I are going to the same dental office. Give your urine sample to the doctor or me. The AARC has a special newsletter for us respiratory therapists.
Incorrect verb form	The patient already drunk the glass of water. Mr. Daley has broke the same leg twice.	The patient already drank the glass of water. Mr. Daley has broken the same leg twice.
Unclear references	When he hit his arm against the window, it broke.	When he hit his arm against the window, his arm broke. OR He broke his arm when he hit it against the window.

TABLE 5–2 ***Cures for Capitalization Problems***

When to Use	Examples
First word of a sentence	The test for strep throat was negative.
Proper nouns and adjectives: names of people, places, organizations, institutions, religions	Diane is working as a nurse in Kenya on a United Nations project in a Catholic hospital.
Professional titles when used with the person's name	I understand that Dr. Nguyen is a leading oncologist. (BUT: I understand that the doctor is a leading oncologist.) They are here to see Nurse Edmonds. (BUT: They are here to see the nurse.)
The major words in the titles of books, articles, movies, software programs, etc.	Two popular software programs for use in the medical office are Medical Manager and Medi-Soft. *The Language of Medicine* is a popular medical terminology textbook.
The first word of a quotation	The physical therapist told the patient, "It is critical that you do these exercises every morning and evening."
Days, months, and holidays	I think Christmas was on Friday last year.
Trade names of products and drugs	The physician recommended Sudafed for the patient's nasal congestion. The lab technician used Acetest to confirm the presence of sugar in the patient's urine.
Abbreviations	AIDS (acquired immune deficiency syndrome) CPR (cardiopulmonary resuscitation) EKG (electrocardiograph) RDA (registered dental assistant)

TABLE 5–3 ***Punctuation Remedies***

Mark	When to Use	Examples
Comma ,	Connect two sentences (independent clauses) into one with a connecting word (and, but, or, nor, yet, for, so)	The surgeon performed the knee replacement surgery, and the physical therapist directed the patient's rehabilitation program. The patient was very nervous about the procedure, so the physician ordered a sedative.
	Separate items in a series	Encephalitis, epilepsy, meningitis, and multiple sclerosis are disorders of the nervous system.
	After introductory phrases	While the patient filled out the necessary forms, the dental hygienist gathered her supplies. When the EMT couldn't detect a pulse, he quickly began to perform CPR.
	Around optional information (Nonrestrictive clause)	Mrs. Washington, who has been seeing Dr. Gonzalez for several years, is doing well on her new medication.
	After transitions (however, therefore, for example, in other words)	She is doing well with her diet; however, she needs to walk at least a mile each day. Alternative medicine is gaining popularity in the United States; for example, many patients have found pain relief with acupuncture.
	After the closing in letters	Sincerely, Very truly yours,
	With dates, addresses, titles, and numbers with more than four digits	The surgery is scheduled for August 12, 1999, at Grand General Hospital. Dr. Sally Halloway, M.D., will perform the surgery. There were 86,000 procedures performed in the United States last year.
Semicolon ;	Connect two sentences (independent clauses) not joined with a connecting word	Occupational therapists help patients regain as much normal function as possible after a serious injury; they also help patients adjust psychologically to their disabilities.
	Connect two independent clauses joined by a transitional expression (examples: however, also, therefore, furthermore, meanwhile, as a result, in conclusion)	I believe that medical care should be available to everyone in the United States; furthermore, it should be affordable.
Colon :	After an independent clause that is followed by a list	There are several habits that contribute to heart disease: smoking, a high-fat diet, lack of exercise, and psychological stress.
	After the salutation in a formal business letter	Dear Dr. Chang:
	With hours and minutes	Your appointment is at 4:15 p.m.
	With proportions	The ratio of medication to water should be 2:1.
Apostrophe '	Show possession	The patient's cast needs to be changed today. Please get John Bergen's file out for the dentist.
	Substitute for missing letters in contractions	Let's see if we can find better prices for these supplies. You're doing well with your therapy. It's a good method for sterilizing instruments.
Quotation Marks "/"	Around direct speech	"You should eat at least five servings of fruits and vegetables each day," said the dietitian.
	Around titles of articles, poems, short stories, songs, TV programs	"The Rising Costs of Health Care" that appeared in today's paper was an interesting article. "Nova" had a good review of current AIDS research on public television last night.
NOTE: Put periods and commas inside quotation marks. Put colons and semicolons outside quotation marks.		
Dash —	Give emphasis	Diseases that were thought to be conquered—tuberculosis, measles, and hepatitis—have once again become public health concerns.
	Show change of thought	Mrs. Crawford—who reminds me of my grandmother—comes in every Wednesday for chemotherapy treatment.

PRESCRIPTION FOR SUCCESS 5–3

How's Your Grammar?

1. How would you rate your knowledge of English grammar?

   ____ Excellent ____ Very Good ____ Good ____ Fair ____ Poor

2. If you scored yourself as "fair" or "poor," what can you do to improve?

   ____ Take classes at school
   ____ Use special services at school, such as a computer lab or tutoring program
   ____ Study on my own
      ____ Workbooks
      ____ Software
      ____ Videos
      ____ Other

First Aid for Spelling

Spelling English words is not easy. English is a combination of many languages and contains silent letters, different ways of pronouncing the same letter, different ways of spelling the same sound, and other irregularities. There are a few rules, but the spelling of many words must simply be memorized. Use the memory techniques suggested in Chapter 3. Spelling can be a family activity, something you can do with your children in which everyone benefits. Or you can work on spelling in a study group. Have contests, give small prizes, and make learning fun. Start your own dictionary and spelling list to keep in your notebook. If you use a computer, you can keep your lists alphabetized and up-to-date.

Learning medical language is an important part of your education. Accurate spelling of medical terms is critical. Some words look alike and can be confused. Errors can negatively affect patient care. Developing a good learning system for spelling now will be a valuable study skill when you learn medical language. Begin to practice good spelling habits by learning everyday English words. Tables 5–4 through 5–6 contain spelling rules, as well as commonly misspelled and commonly confused words. Use them as a study guide and add your own problem words. If the suggestions for learning commonly confused words don't make sense to you or seem silly, you can create your own hints for remembering.

PRESCRIPTION FOR SUCCESS 5–4

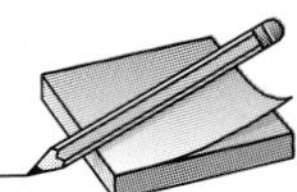

Spelling Test

1. How's your spelling? Quiz yourself by having someone read the words in the tables for you to spell.
2. After correcting your quiz, separate out any words that you missed. (Didn't miss any? Congratulations! Skip the rest of the assignment and consider volunteering to help classmates who have trouble with spelling.)

continued

PRESCRIPTION FOR SUCCESS 5-4 *(Continued)*

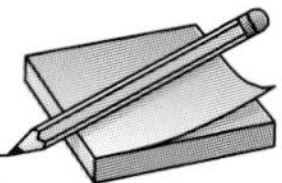

3. For those of you who missed a few words, make a commitment to learn them in the next few weeks. Devise your own plan. Here are a few suggestions.

   Set a goal to learn a certain number of words each week.

   Use techniques that complement the way you like to learn: use flashcards. Spell aloud. Visualize in your mind. Think of hints and associations. Put the cards where you will see them often, such as the bathroom mirror. Imagine them printed in large colored letters on a movie screen that you flash in your mind. Practice writing them over and over again. Use colored pens. Write larger than you usually do. Pay attention to what you are writing; don't just go on automatic pilot.

   Reward yourself when you reach your goals.

TABLE 5-4 ***Spelling Prescriptions***

Rules	**Examples**	**Exceptions**
I before E except after C and when the word sounds like AY, as in SAY	relieve receive neighbor weigh	either foreign height seizure
Drop final silent E when adding a **suffix** that begins with a **vowel**	achieve—achieving care—caring	change—changeable
Keep final silent E when adding a suffix that begins with a **consonant**	achieve—achievement care—careful	argue—argument judge—judgment true—truly
When adding -ING to a word that ends in IE, replace the IE with Y	die—dying tie—tying	
Double the final consonant of a one-**syllable** word when adding a suffix that begins with a vowel *unless* there are two vowels or another consonant before the final consonant	trim—trimming look—looking test—testing	
Plurals		
Add S to most words	disease—diseases wound—wounds	
Words that end in a consonant + Y: change the Y to an I and add ES	laboratory—laboratories pregnancy—pregnancies	
Words that end in S, SH, CH, and X: add ES	crutch—crutches	
Words that end in SIS: change to SES	diagnosis—diagnoses urinalysis—urinalyses	
Words that end in a vowel + O: add S	radio—radios	
Words that end in a consonant + O: add ES	echo—echoes	

TABLE 5–5 ***Commonly Misspelled Words***

absence	disease	leisure	receive
absorption	efficiency	license	recognize
accessible	eighth	loneliness	recommend
accidentally	eligible	magazine	reference
accommodate	eliminate	maintenance	resuscitate
accumulate	embarrass	management	rhythm
achievement	emphasize	maneuver	safety
acknowledge	encourage	marriage	satisfactory
acquire	enthusiastic	miscellaneous	schedule
address	entirely	necessary	scissors
affiliated	environment	negligible, negligence	secretary
aggravate	equipped	neighbor	seize, seizure
analyze	equivalent	noticeable	sensible
appropriate	especially	obstacle	separate
assistant	exaggerate	occasion, occasionally	several
association	exercise	occur, occurrence	severely
athlete	exhausted	often	significance
beginning	experience	original	similar
behavior	extremely	pamphlet	sincerely
belief	fascinate	parallel	strategy
beneficial	fatigue	particular	strictly
bureau	February	patience	substantial
business, businesses	fluctuation	perform	succeed
cafeteria	foreign	persistent	success
caffeine	forty	physically	surprise
calendar	fourth	physician	sympathy
cancel, canceled	fragile	pneumonia	technique
column	friend	possession	temperature
coming	government	practical	thorough
committee	harass, harassment	precede	though
commitment, committed	height	preference	tongue
communicate	hygiene	prejudice	transferred
comparative	impatient	privilege	typical
competition	indefinitely	probably	until
cooperate	infinite	proceed	urgent
correspond	intelligence	prominent	useful
criticism, criticize	interesting	psychiatry	usually
decision	jewelry	psychology	vacuum
definitely	judgment	qualified	vague
describe	knowledge	quantity	vegetable
despair	knowledgeable	questionnaire	view
develop	label	quiet	Wednesday
discipline	laboratory	quite	weight
	legitimate	receipt	writing

TABLE 5–6 ***Commonly Confused Words***

Word	Meaning	Sample Hints for Learning
accept	to take or receive	take—accept
except	excluding, all but	exclude—except
access	way of entering	
excess	too much	extra—excess
adapt	adjust	adjust—adapt
adopt	to take as one's own	own—adopt
advice	helpful suggestions	
advise	to give advice	
affect	to influence	
effect	result; to bring about	
allowed	permitted	
aloud	capable of being heard	loud sound
already	before now, so soon	
all ready	completely prepared	It's all done.
capital	official seat of government; form of wealth	
capitol	building in which members of government meet	
choose	to select	
chose	selected (past tense of "choose")	
coarse	rough	The dog has a rough coat.
course	class; path or track	Our class is on track.
conscience	part of the mind that determines right and wrong	
conscious	awake; aware	
council	governing body	
counsel	advice; to give advice	
defer	delay	
differ	to be different; to disagree	differ—different
desert	dry land area	1 rain shower in the desert.
dessert	eaten at the end of a meal	2 cups of sugar in dessert
it's	contraction of "it is"	The apostrophe replaces a word
its	possessive form of "it"	
later	after the usual time	
latter	the second of two	2 Ts = 2nd of 2
lay	put or place something (past = laid)	
lie	rest on a surface (past = lay!! - confusing!!)	
lead	type of metal; to guide; connecting wire	
led	guided (past tense of "lead")	
loose	not tight	Bigger word, like a shirt, is looser
lose	to be unable to find	I lost one O.
maybe	perhaps	
may be	possible, permissible	
miner	mine worker	
minor	younger than the legal age	
overdo	to do too much	
overdue	late or past due	
patience	quality of being uncomplaining, unhurried	
patients	people under medical care	

(*continued*)

TABLE 5–6 ***Commonly Confused Words*** *(Continued)*

Word	Meaning	Sample Hints for Learning
passed	went by, earned a satisfactory grade	
past	before now, ended	
personal	private	
personnel	employees	
principal	head of a school, main or most important	The principal is your pal.
principle	general truth or rule	
stationary	not moving	Stay in one place
stationery	paper for writing letters	Letters are written on stationery
than	compared to	
then	at that time	
their	possessive of they	
there	in that place	
they're	contraction of "they are"	Apostrophe stands for "a"
to	toward, for the purpose of	
too	also, very, more than enough	
two	2	
weather	climate conditions	Weather can be wet and windy
whether	introduces alternatives	
who's	contraction of "who is"	Apostrophe stands for "is"
whose	possessive of "who"	
you're	contraction of "you are"	Apostrophe stands for "a"
your	possessive of you	Our is possessive; so is your

Tests: Part of School, Part of Life

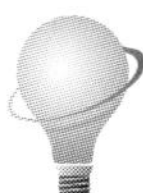

Take a Moment to Think

What are some similarities between classroom tests and working on the job as a health care professional?

Taking tests is not limited to your life as a student. As a health care professional, much of what you do every day is a kind of test. Let's compare some typical classroom test questions with the performance of a procedure on a patient.

PAPER AND PENCIL TEST IN CLASS	PERFORMANCE OF PATIENT PROCEDURE
Supply definitions	Recall procedure you are instructed to perform
List items needed to perform procedures	Gather equipment and supplies for procedure
Recall information	Create mental checklist of steps
Write explanations	Provide patient with clear explanation and instructions
	Perform procedure correctly
Supply short answers	Write results accurately on patient chart

TAKING THE TERROR OUT OF TESTS

Classroom tests and work on the job both involve sets of instructions (questions and job tasks), time limits (class session and appointment schedules), standards (instructor **criteria** and facility **protocols**), and indicators for level of performance (grades, patient satisfaction, evaluations, and raises). In reality, performing on the job is more serious in terms of requirements and consequences than any classroom quiz or final exam. Students can repeat a test—or a course, if necessary—but winning back an unhappy patient or reversing the poor opinion of your supervisor is more difficult. At the extreme is the possible damage done by an incorrect procedure or inaccurate medication dosage.

The intention here is not to terrorize the future health care professional but to put the subject of tests in perspective. They are a fact of life, and if approached with the right attitude, classroom tests can provide you with opportunities to increase your learning.

1. Tests encourage students to study. Most of us perform best when there is a consequence for our actions. In Chapter 3 we discussed how "good stress" can stimulate us physically and mentally to be alert and take appropriate actions. In the same way, you can harness the anxiety of future tests to energize yourself and focus your efforts on applying effective learning techniques. Use tests to mark your progress toward achieving your long-term goal of becoming a competent health care professional—which is, after all, the ultimate reason for learning.

2. Tests teach students to work under pressure, a daily reality for health care professionals. You can never take your tasks for granted. Classroom tests can help you practice working calmly and efficiently when it counts. Planning and preparing ahead, thinking about what you are doing, and performing to the best of your ability are habits that apply to both test-taking and work.

3. Test results help students improve, advance their learning, and make progress toward becoming health care professionals. Answer sheets and scores are not for the exclusive use of your instructors. And contrary to what you may believe, the only purpose of tests is not to assign you a grade. Take advantage of them to help *you* as a student. Use tests for *your own* benefit to find out what you know and don't know. Review your answers to identify the material you haven't mastered. What did you not understand? What do you need to ask the instructor? What should you review again? (If your instructor collects and keeps the answer sheets after reviewing them with the class, take notes quickly during the review.) Fill the gaps in your knowledge now, while you are still in school. Don't brush off wrong answers and hope that the knowledge all comes together on the job. Remember why you are in school: to learn the basics of your profession. Sometimes you will make mistakes, a fundamental student right. *Learning* from your mistakes is a fundamental student responsibility.

WHAT TESTS ARE—AND ARE NOT

Think of a test as a challenge instead of a threat.—Walter Pauk

Tests can turn otherwise sensible individuals into quivering masses of anxiety. For many students, the grades earned on tests influence their feeling of self-worth. As an adult student, you may be concerned about appearing stupid and worry that you don't have the ability to learn. Or you may feel insecure about your test-taking skills. In reality, the life experiences accumulated by adult learners are often helpful in dealing with tests and other stressful situations. While there is no denying that tests are used as indicators of progress by both instructors and students, understanding more about tests and their purpose can help you control *them* rather than letting them control *you*.

Well-prepared tests can measure your knowledge and ability in certain specific areas. They can also measure how much you have packed into temporary memory as a result of last night's cram session. Therefore, they may or may not indicate the extent of true learning (how long you will retain what you know today) or your ability to perform effectively on the job. And remember that tests are *never* a measure of your value as a person. You can be an "A" in life even if you do not receive straight As in the classroom. Here are some realities about tests:

1. Tests only ask for samples of what you are expected to know. Many students express disappointment when everything they studied does not appear on the test.

They believe they have wasted their time and should have been told just what was going to be on the test. The truth is, health care professionals must master a great deal of information. If instructors included everything on tests that students should know, there would only be time for testing and none left for learning! Samples are reliable indicators of overall knowledge. For example, if you are expected to learn 1000 medical terms, the instructor may randomly select 50 for a test. The percentage of those 50 that you know is a good indication of how many of the 1000 you know. (Another example: If you know the steps to follow in eleven procedures, you may be asked to give the steps for three.) Remember, you are learning for the future. Knowing more than what is on the test is a *requirement* for job success, *not* a waste of your time.

2. Classroom tests provide instructors with feedback about their teaching. Tests help them adjust their classroom strategies to ensure that students have every opportunity to master the subject and skills. If many students do poorly on all or part of a test, it means that the information was not presented effectively. Instructors want and need this feedback.

3. Poorly prepared tests do exist. Test writing is a skill, and good test questions are not easy to create. Even instructors with good intentions write questions that are unclear and confusing. They may teach more than one class and forget exactly which material was—and was not—presented in each section. They may ask questions that are different from those they announced would be on the test. This does happen, and the best strategy is to ask the instructor *politely* to review the information (especially if it appears to be important information that you will need on the job). If the problem continues, meet with the instructor privately to discuss the situation.

PRESCRIPTION FOR SUCCESS 5-5

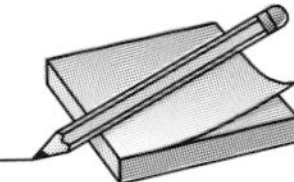

Make Tests Work for You

Describe five ways you can use tests to your advantage as you prepare for a career in health care.

PREPARING EFFECTIVELY FOR TESTS

The *best* way to prepare for tests is the same way you will prepare yourself for career success: *Start preparing early and study to learn.* Being prepared for tests means *mastering the content of your courses.* We discussed some of the ways to do this in Chapters 3 and 4:

1. Manage your time so that studying is a priority.
2. Identify and apply techniques that correspond with your learning styles to make the best use of your study time.
3. Use learning techniques that help move information into long-term memory.
4. Take good notes in class and review them often.
5. Read textbooks actively and review them regularly.
6. Seek help early if you are having trouble.

In addition to developing and practicing study habits that work for you, be proactive and create a study plan to ensure that you are prepared as well as possible. Even if you have been studying consistently, you need at least a week to prepare for a major test such as a final exam. The following steps can help you develop an effective plan:

I. Find out as much as possible about the test. Gather any notes or handouts about it that the instructor has distributed. Ask the instructor for suggestions on how to prepare.

II. Quickly review your notes, textbook, handouts, and any other class materials to check your comprehension. Is there anything you don't understand or can't remember, even after reviewing? Write a list of questions to ask in class. (This is why you start your review early, *not* the night before the exam!)

III. Make a schedule, and divide what you have to review over the time you have available so that you don't run out of time before you have had a chance to review everything (another good reason to start reviewing a few days *before* the test).

IV. Use the study tools you developed when you reviewed throughout the class—or create some now!
   A. Keywords or questions to prompt recall of notes and text.
   B. Mind maps, charts, or outlines to help you organize the material meaningfully.
   C. Flashcards to practice recall. Put aside the ones that you know well and concentrate on the ones you have the most difficulty remembering. Your goal is to move all cards into the "know-these" pile.
   D. Create practice tests with the types of questions you think might be on the test.
   E. Say aloud or write answers to your prompts and practice questions. It is important that you are actively involved in creating the answers, not passively reading the material and thinking you know the answers.
   F. Set a time limit, and practice writing short answers and essays. Many students find it difficult to collect and organize their thoughts quickly to respond to essay questions. You wouldn't do a procedure on the job that you hadn't practiced many times. Test-taking is a skill, too. Give yourself the same advantage by doing a few practice runs.

V. Identify and concentrate on the material you find most difficult and have the most trouble remembering. Don't keep restudying material that you know. (Except when you are deliberately overlearning, as discussed in Chapter 3.)

THE ANXIETY MONSTER

You have studied throughout the course, you have reviewed for the test, and you feel pretty secure about your knowledge of the material, but you are panic-stricken by the prospect of your final exam. You just know you'll freeze up and won't be able to remember a thing. You may feel physically ill when you enter the classroom on test days, and there doesn't seem to be any way around it—you just can't take tests. This is a real problem for many students, and solving it is an important step toward achieving your professional goals. Here are some suggestions to help you manage test anxiety:

1. Evaluate your study habits and test-review methods. Can you improve them? Are you really using you study time efficiently? For example, some students spend a lot of time reading notes over and over but never actually quizzing themselves on the information. They think they know it, but without their notes they can't remember very much.

2. Think about your actual test preparation. It may *seem* that you are spending a lot of time reviewing because you feel worn out by it. In reality, if you engage in a marathon review session the last two days before the test, you may feel as if you studied a lot but are too tired to remember much of the material.

3. Be honest with yourself. Do you have trouble understanding in your classes but don't ask for help because you are embarrassed? Remember that instructors are there to help you, and asking for help is not nearly as embarrassing as failing a test or finding that you lack information needed to perform your job. Do you lack the time after class to stay for extra help? Is there another reason? If you are serious about achieving your career goals, you must decide to make school a priority and organize your life so that you can study when and as much as needed.

4. Don't let your classmates freak you out. If you worry about competing with them, such as finishing the test first or earning a higher grade, you can get distracted from focusing on your own performance. Your education is not a race with winners and losers; the goal of a health care program is for everyone to win by graduating as a competent professional. Although the awarding of grades tends to set up a competitive environment, modern health care is delivered by teams of individuals who must work cooperatively, not competitively.

Some classmates are even more anxious about tests than you. These people often express their nervousness by talking a lot and predicting total gloom and doom. Be upbeat with them rather than letting their negative talk increase your own anxiety. Avoid participating in "ain't it awful" conversations around test time.

5. Join forces with positive students. Organize a small group to review, share ideas, quiz each other, and cheer each other on. Have each person make up a few test questions and quiz the others. Seek out classmates who are dependable and will contribute to the group. Keep the number small (between three and five) so that everyone can make a contribution. If the group is too large, organizing meetings to accommodate everyone's schedule can be very difficult.

6. Use visualizations and positive self-talk that promote learning and good test performance.

7. Practice good health habits and the stress management techniques described in Chapter 3. Remember that vigorous physical exercise releases endorphins, the body's natural tranquilizers. Do your best to get enough sleep before major tests so that you're not exhausted and more subject to anxiety. Finally, the relaxation exercise described in Chapter 3 is effective just before taking a test. Take deep breaths to help quiet the mind. Help your body work for instead of against you.

If you review thoroughly and try the suggestions for relieving anxiety, and *still* find yourself freezing up during exams and feeling as if even dynamite couldn't blast facts out of your brain, you can try a technique called "desensitization." This is a treatment developed for people who have anxieties that interfere with their daily lives. It consists of providing exposure to small doses of whatever they are afraid of and then gradually increasing the size and number of exposures (Fry, 1996). Develop a plan to increase your exposure to tests. Have a friend or family member make up and give you tests, starting with short quizzes. Make them as realistic as possible. For example, set and stay within a time limit. Ask your instructor to give you outdated or practice tests. Find out if you can take these in a classroom under conditions as close to those of a real test as possible. This may seem like a lot of work and even a little embarrassing, but if test anxiety is running your future career off track, desensitization is worth trying.

TRIPPING YOURSELF UP

Some students procrastinate in preparing for tests because of a fear of failure. The fear instills a kind of paralysis that prevents them from taking positive steps to prepare. For others, not studying creates an excuse for failure. After all, if they try their best and *still* fail an exam, this might mean that they lack ability.

Another problem is feeling overwhelmed—there is just so much to learn that they can't figure out how to get started and give up without really trying. If you believe that one of these situations may be your problem, make a deal with yourself to try something new. *Study throughout the course,* use the suggestions in this chapter on preparing for tests, ask for help, and work with a study group. The chances are very good that you will experience success, and that can be habit-forming!

TEST DAY: PREPARE TO SHOW WHAT YOU KNOW

Okay, it's the day of the test and you feel reasonably prepared. You certainly don't want to perform poorly because you fail to follow some commonsense test-taking guidelines. Following are some important things to do that apply to any test situation.

1. You deserve a good start, so plan to arrive early. Don't stress yourself out by rushing in late, scrambling to find a seat, or missing the introductory instructions.

2. Bring your supplies, including books, notes, and a calculator if these are allowed. An erasable pen works well because the instructor can read your answers and you can make corrections neatly.

3. Listen to all instructions. Ask for clarification of anything you don't understand. This is not the time to be shy. You have a right to know exactly what is expected. Asking for clarification is also an important career skill. You must be able to ask your supervisor questions about any aspect of your work that you don't understand.

4. Review the *entire* test before starting. Read *all* directions on *every* page. This is another health care skill because you must be able to read and follow directions. If you have questions and the test has begun, go to the instructor and ask them quietly.

5. If there are different types of questions, note which ones will take longest to answer and/or are worth the most points. Then quickly plan how to divide your time among the different parts of the test.

(Important note: If the test is longer or more difficult than you expected, do *not* panic. Take a deep breath, follow the guidelines, and work systematically through the test. Keeping your cool now is good practice for days on the job when you must handle a series of demanding tasks.)

6. Give yourself a boost by answering the easiest questions first. When there are different types of questions, it is usually best to move from the shortest to the longest answers: true/false, multiple-choice, matching, fill-in, short essay, long essay. This is like giving yourself a warm-up. Also, the questions that have the answers provided for you to choose may give you ideas for questions in which you must supply the answers from recall.

7. Limit the time you spend on difficult questions. Mark them and return later after you complete the rest.

8. Proofread your answers before you turn in your test. Did you answer all the questions? Mark the correct boxes on the answer sheet? Follow all directions correctly? Check for spelling errors, words left out, and other careless errors? Checking your work is another health care skill that ensures safety and accuracy. For example, a medication is never given to a patient until the label identifying it has been checked *at least three times.*

9. Use all the time allowed if you need it. You don't earn extra points by finishing early, and hurrying may cost you a few correct answers.

SPECIFIC TEST-TAKING TECHNIQUES

A message that has been repeated throughout this book is the importance of mastering the knowledge and skills presented in your classes in order to become a competent health care professional. Patient well-being depends on what and how well you learn. We have pointed out that high grades are not final goals but signs that you are on your way to a new career. The purpose of studying, then, is to learn for the future, not simply to pass tests. Tests may measure the effectiveness of your study efforts, but they are not the reason for them.

While the best way to prepare for tests is to know your material well (Pauk, 1997), learning about the different question formats can help you be more effective in showing what you know. Students who are unfamiliar with question formats can use up time and energy figuring them out. Test-taking techniques, however, do *not* substitute for knowledge. For example, if you hear that the longest multiple-choice answer is often the correct one, don't let *that* steer you away from what you believe to be the right answer! The suggestions given in this section are based on the experience of many students. However, they are only guidelines and should be used mainly as backup when you are stumped by a question.

Keep in mind that some of the techniques suggested for answering test questions would be downright dangerous if applied to work in health care. For example, most study skills books recommend that if there is no penalty for incorrect answers, go ahead and guess. With true/false questions, you have a 50-50 chance; with most multiple-choice questions, the chance is 25%. But there is no room in health care for a 50-50 chance of correct performance. Some activities, such as administering medications, must be 100% correct. There is no guesswork allowed here!

True/False Questions

Purpose: to test your recognition of correct facts, statements, and cause-and-effect relationships, as well as your ability to distinguish fact from opinion.

Examples: *Read each of the following statements. If the statement is true, circle the T. If it is false, circle the F.*

T F 1. Classroom tests are always good indicators of how well students understand a subject.

T F 2. Test performance can be improved by cramming as much as possible the day before the test is given.

T F 3. Reviewing material regularly throughout the course is the best way to do well on tests.

Suggested Techniques for Answering

1. Be sure that every part of the answer is correct. If any part of it is false, the entire answer is false.
2. Watch out for words like "always" and "never." Think about it: how many things are so final? Statements with these words are often false. (But not always. For example, there are safety rules in health care that must *always* be followed and legal rules, such as those concerning release of patient records, that can *never* be violated.)
3. Answers with middle-of-the-road words like "usually," "sometimes," and "often" tend to be true (*except* as noted previously).
4. Some wording makes it difficult to understand the statement. For example, double negatives are confusing. Read these questions carefully and try canceling out the two negatives to interpret their meaning correctly.
5. Guess *only* as a last resort (and *only if* there is no penalty).

Multiple-Choice Questions

Purpose: to test your knowledge of terminology, specific facts, principles, methods, and procedures.

Examples: *Circle the letter to the left of the response that* best *answers each question.*

1. Which is the *best* reason for learning to spell correctly?
   A. Patients are impressed by correct spelling.
   B. Patient care can be negatively affected if words are misspelled on medical documentation.
   C. Students who spell correctly get better grades in school.
   D. It increases the chances of receiving a promotion at work.
2. The Cornell note-taking system has proven helpful to students because it
   A. Prevents them from having to review notes after class.
   B. Helps them record everything the instructor says.
   C. Provides a format that encourages review.
   D. Teaches specific active listening techniques.

Suggested Techniques for Answering

1. Read the instructions and questions carefully. If the question asks you to identify the "best" answer, it is possible that more than one is correct.
2. Read through *all* the answers before selecting one.

3. If the instruction says to select the correct answer (as opposed to the "best," "most complete," etc.), consider each statement separately and ask yourself if it is true or false.
4. If the answer requires a math calculation, do the problem yourself *before* you look at the answers.
5. Match each answer to the question rather than comparing the answers to each other.
6. If you are guessing, choose an answer that has information you recognize.
7. You can sometimes eliminate choices by using logic. For example, if two answers say basically the same thing, they must both be incorrect. As with true/false answers, if any part of a statement is wrong, the entire answer must be wrong. If the answer is silly or farfetched (instructors sometimes like to have a little fun), eliminate it immediately.
8. If you are allowed to write on the test, circle or underline key words in the question to focus your attention when you read the answers.

Matching Questions

Purpose: to recognize correct facts based on simple associations.
Examples: *On the line to the left of each number in Column A, write the letter from Column B that explains one of its uses.*

COLUMN A	COLUMN B
____ 1. Comma	A. Substitute for letters that are dropped when contractions are formed
____ 2. Semicolon	B. Indicate a change of thought within a sentence
____ 3. Colon	C. Connect two sentences into one long sentence when a connective word is used
____ 4. Apostrophe	D. Follow the greeting in a formal business letter
____ 5. Dash	E. Connect two sentences into one long sentence without the use of a connective word
	F. Place at the end of a sentence

Suggested Techniques for Answering

1. Read the instructions carefully. Note whether any item can be used more than once.
2. Quickly count each column to see if both columns have the same number of items.
3. Read through both columns before you write in any answers.
4. Do the ones you know first.
5. Some students find it easier to read the longer answers first (usually placed in the right-hand column) and then look for the shorter match. See which method works best for you.
6. Mark or cross out each item as you use it.

Fill-in-the-Blank Questions

Purpose: to test your ability to recall terminology, facts, and procedures and to interpret information.
Examples: *Fill in each blank with a word or phrase that correctly completes the sentence.*

1. The huge group of interconnecting computers located around the world is called the ______.
2. Learners who are both visual and global sometimes find that ______ is a useful note-taking technique to record information in a way that clearly shows relationships.
3. An explanation of why a procedure is performed in a certain way is called the ______.

Suggested Techniques for Answering

1. Read the entire statement before attempting to fill in the blank or blanks.
2. Write answers that fit the form and content of the words around them.

3. It sometimes helps to convert the phrase into a question in which the answer is the correct fill-in.
4. The length of the space *may* be a clue to the answer, but there is a chance that whoever typed the test didn't even know the answers and randomly chose the lengths. This is not a reliable way to select an answer.

Short-Answer Questions

Purpose: to recall facts and definitions or supply brief explanations that demonstrate your understanding.
Examples: *Write a short answer to each of the following questions using the spaces provided. Some questions have several parts. Your answers do not need to be complete sentences.*

1. List three reasons why a three-ring binder is recommended by most educators for keeping your notes and class materials.
2. Explain why previewing is a critical part of the reading process.
3. Describe four ways of starting to write a paper when you are having trouble determining exactly what to write and/or how to organize it.

Suggested Techniques for Answering

1. Read the instructions to find key words that tell you exactly what is expected in the answer. Are you asked to explain? Give two examples? List five reasons? Define? Give the steps?
2. If you are asked to write several sentences, answer the question as directly and completely as possible without padding with unnecessary information.

Essay Questions

Purpose: to demonstrate ability to select, organize, relate, evaluate, and present ideas. These questions provide an opportunity to show what you know about the topic.
Example: *Write a well-organized essay at least one page long explaining the meaning of this statement: "Study skills are career skills." Support your answer with examples and references to SCANS and the National Health Care Skill Standards. You will be graded on how well you demonstrate understanding of the concept, as well as on spelling and grammar.*

Suggestions for Answering

1. As with the short-answer questions, read the instructions to see what you are supposed to include in your answer. Provide evidence for your response? Give examples to illustrate? Give the sequence? Explain reasons and purposes? Defend your answer? Compare and contrast?
2. Don't be too skimpy with your answers. Even if the question does not specifically ask for examples or evidence, you will be expected to fully explain or defend your answer.
3. Don't spend time beating around the bush with introductions that lack substance. Answer questions directly.
4. If you have trouble organizing an answer in your head, quickly jot down a few key ideas, an outline, or a mind map.
5. Follow the rule that journalists use when they write a newspaper article: state the most important information first by answering the question as quickly as possible. Use the rest of the time to develop your answer, write examples, provide evidence, and so on. This way, if you run out of time, you know you have covered the most important information.
6. Include the principal ideas of the course, as appropriate, especially ones that the instructor emphasized.
7. Use the principles of good writing discussed in this chapter.

POSTTEST STRATEGIES

Much as you'd like to forget about the test you just took, *don't*. Just like athletes who analyze each game to learn which plays worked and which didn't, you can use de-

TABLE 5–7 ***Common Test Problems***

The Problem	What to Do
You didn't study at all or waited until the last minute and crammed.	You *know* what to do!
You studied but couldn't remember the information.	Check your understanding. Information that you don't comprehend well is very difficult to remember. Did you use prompts to study or did you simply reread your notes and textbook? Passive review is not effective for most people.
You were extremely anxious during the test and froze.	Review the section on anxiety and seek additional help if needed.
You made careless errors.	Allocate time to proofread your test before turning it in.
You didn't understand what the question meant.	If there were certain vocabulary words you didn't know, were these part of the subject and should they have been studied along with the content? If English is your second language, see your instructor for help.
The questions were different from what you expected. For example, you memorized a lot of facts and definitions, but the test required you to apply information to new situations.	Review your notes or other information about the test to see if you misunderstood. If you did not take notes (or attend the class in which the test was explained), make it a point to attend all classes, especially around test time. If you believe that the instructor was unclear about the format of the test, speak with the instructor privately about his or her expectations.

briefing to your advantage. As soon as possible after finishing the test, review your notes and books to find the answers to the questions you were unsure about or just didn't know.

When the test is returned in class, try not to react emotionally. If you earned a top score, give yourself credit. If you did poorly, don't lose heart. Listen to any review of the test. If you have to return it to the instructor, take notes on a separate sheet of paper. Pay special attention to the questions you missed and write the correct answers. If the instructor reexplains points, be sure to take notes. Ask questions. (If your instructor does not discuss tests with the class and you did poorly, make an appointment to discuss it privately.)

At your earliest opportunity, review your notes and the marks you made in your books. Did you miss some of the major points? Study the wrong material? Not really understand it? What can you do to improve your performance next time? See Table 5–7 for suggestions on dealing with test problems commonly encountered by students.

SOME FRANK TALK ABOUT CHEATING

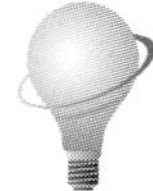

Take a Moment to Think

1. Do you believe that cheating in school is justified if that is the only way you can pass?
2. What are some possible future effects on the job for students who passed their courses by cheating instead of studying?

Working in health care demands high ethical standards. Quality patient care and safety depend on them, and there is no room for cheating in any form. Furthermore, governmental regulations have increased, and **audits** of health care facilities are common. The consequences for **fraud**, taking shortcuts, and even trying to just "get by" are severe, including fines and closures of health care facilities.

You may believe that cheating on tests in school isn't as serious as cheating on the job, but this is not true. Health care graduates who have substituted cheating for the acquisition of knowledge are likely to be dangerous practitioners. You are in the process of becoming a professional, and what you do now is setting the groundwork for your future actions. Integrity is an essential characteristic of the health care professional, and cheating undermines that integrity. Cheating is an unsatisfactory and potentially destructive way of approaching your education. It converts the opportunities offered by tests to learn course content and develop positive study habits into unacceptable behaviors.

Even if you do not cheat yourself, helping others to do so promotes incompetence in the health care system. Would you or one of your family members want to be treated by "professionals" who cheated to pass their classes? Do you want to carry the load at work for a coworker who is used to taking the easy way out? Helping friends cheat enables them to avoid taking responsibility for themselves. This can lead to the habit of dependence and unsatisfactory performance.

A Word about Professional Exams

Many health care professions have exams that you must pass in order to work in the field. Their purpose is to promote high standards for practitioners by testing for competence. They may be administered by a governmental agency or a professional organization. Passing these exams entitles the professional to use one of several special designations such as "licensed," "certified," or "registered." Most exams require a fee. Your school may have included this cost in your tuition or fees. The school may also assist you in applying to take the exam. Some exams are given year round, others only on certain dates. As we discussed in Chapter 2, find out whether you must take a professional exam and, if so, learn as much as possible about it while you are still in school.

Some professions do not require testing for graduates to work. However, voluntary testing is available and recommended for many careers. For example, there are no formal approvals required of medical assistants in any state. However, many physicians prefer to hire only certified or registered medical assistants. These designations must be earned by passing professional exams administered by the American Association of Medical Assistants and the American Medical Technologists, respectively.

Here are some suggestions for increasing your chances of passing professional exams the first time you take them:

1. Start preparing early (note that the word is "prepare," *not* "worry"). This suggestion is not intended to add further stress to your already busy class and study schedule. It is a reminder that if you prepare over a period of time, you will be better prepared and less stressed when the time comes to actually take the test.
2. Keep your notes, handouts, and textbooks organized so that you can use them for review before the exam.
3. Pay attention to any clues that your instructor gives you about the content of professional exams.
4. Some textbooks refer to specific exams and professional organizational requirements, and the authors design their content and review questions to help students prepare throughout their courses. Take advantage of these features.
5. Find out if there are any review books available in your school library or for purchase that direct you what to focus on in your classes.

6. Practice tests are available for many professional exams. Check with your professional organization.
7. Find out if review workshops are available in your area.
8. Plan to take the exam as soon as possible after you are eligible (usually on graduation from your program). You are less likely to forget information and lose your confidence.
9. Think of the timed tests you take in school as opportunities to practice taking an important exam under pressure.

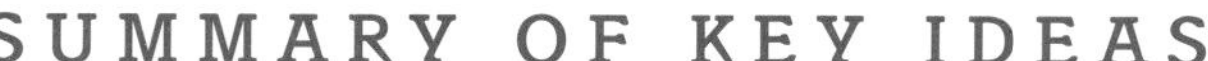

SUMMARY OF KEY IDEAS

1. Your competence is often judged by how you write.
2. Writing correctly takes effort and practice.
3. It's not too late to improve your spelling and grammar skills.
4. Tests are part of life.
5. Test anxiety can be conquered.
6. The best preparation for a test is to know the material.

POSITIVE SELF-TALK FOR THIS CHAPTER

1. I write clearly and effectively.
2. I spell and use grammar correctly.
3. I use the act of writing to help me learn new material.
4. I use tests to motivate me to do my best in school.
5. I prepare in advance for all my tests.
6. I manage test anxiety effectively.

REFERENCES

Campbell, William E. *The Power to Learn: Helping Yourself to College Success,* 2nd ed. Belmont, CA: Wadsworth Publishing Company, 1997.

Chester, Gail A. *Modern Medical Assisting.* Philadelphia: W.B. Saunders Company, 1998.

Elbow, Peter. *Writing with Power: Techniques for Mastering the Writing Process.* Oxford: Oxford University Press, 1981.

Ellis, Dave. *Becoming a Master Student,* 8th ed. New York: Houghton Mifflin Company, 1998.

Fry, Ron. *How to Study,* 4th ed. Franklin Lakes, NJ: Career Press, 1996.

Hacker, Diana. *A Writer's Reference,* 4th ed. Boston: Bedord/St. Martin's, 1998.

Palau, Susan Marcus and Marilyn Meltzer. *Learning Strategies for Allied Health Students.* Philadelphia: W.B. Saunders Company, 1996.

Pauk, Walter. *How to Succeed in College,* 6th ed. New York: Houghton Mifflin Company, 1997.

6

Developing Your Practical Skills

OBJECTIVES

THE INFORMATION AND ACTIVITIES IN THIS CHAPTER CAN HELP YOU TO:

- Apply strategies to help you get the most out of laboratory sessions and master hands-on skills.
- Explain the importance of knowing how to apply math skills in health care.
- Approach the learning of math with a positive attitude and, if necessary, apply techniques to overcome math anxiety.
- Evaluate your own math skills and, if needed, devise a plan to improve them.
- List the purposes and benefits of the educational clinical experience.
- Describe how to maximize learning and gain the most benefits from clinical experience.
- Develop skill in using a problem-solving process to make good decisions in both your personal and professional lives.
- Plan and start putting together a personal reference guide that will help you in school, during your job search, and on the job.

KEY TERMS

Aptitude: The ability to learn and apply new knowledge. Our level of aptitude varies among subjects; some are easier for us to learn than others.

Contaminate: To make impure or infect by introducing organisms, such as bacteria, that can cause disease.

Dosage: The amount of medication to be administered.

Evaluate: To judge or determine the worth or condition of something. For example, when you are deciding whether to buy a certain car, you evaluate it to determine if it is worth the selling price. When treating patients, the first step is to evaluate their current condition.

Math anxiety: The fear of math. People with math anxiety believe that they don't have the ability to learn math. This belief is generally based more on negative past experiences and emotions than on their actual ability to learn.

Metric system: A system of measurement used throughout the world that is based on meters (length), grams (weight), and liters (volume).

Nursing process: An orderly approach to patient care that nurses use to identify and resolve patients' health problems.

Protective equipment: Special clothing and accessories worn by health care workers to protect themselves against body fluids that may be infectious. These include goggles, face shields, and clothing that prevents the passage of liquids. They are also referred to as "personal protective equipment" (PPE).

Role play: A way of practicing interpersonal exchanges in which students play the parts of health care professionals, patients, supervisors, and coworkers. Specific situations may be assigned for students to act out and resolve.

Standard precautions: Practices used to avoid the transmission of infection via body fluids.

Theory: Ideas and knowledge as seen in the mind. Also refers to systematic statements of principles. Theories are usually explained in words during class lectures before related procedures are practiced in the lab.

The Importance of Practical Skills

Health care work involves a lot of hands-on activity, and the level of your performance is critical to your success on the job. Learning to apply the theory you learn in class to practical situations is an important component of your education. You must learn to think through problems and select appropriate alternatives for action. Some students don't consider the practical portion of their training to be as important as the classroom-based courses. This is a serious mistake because hands-on practice builds a bridge between school and the world of work. There is a big difference between knowing *about* a procedure and being able to actually *do* it well. Performing a blood draw is much different from hearing about it. Practice sessions provide you with opportunities to take risks in a safe, monitored environment where you can learn from your experience—and from your mistakes.

Learning in Lab

Labs and practice sessions give you opportunities to participate actively and apply the **theories** you learn in class. Lab sessions include opportunities to practice procedures, **role play,** do computer exercises, and complete pencil-and-paper activities such as filling out insurance forms. You may solve problems, perform procedures, conduct tests, or do calculations. Future health care professionals must learn a variety of skills that range from filling out forms accurately to performing a urinalysis to taking an x-ray (Fig. 6–1).

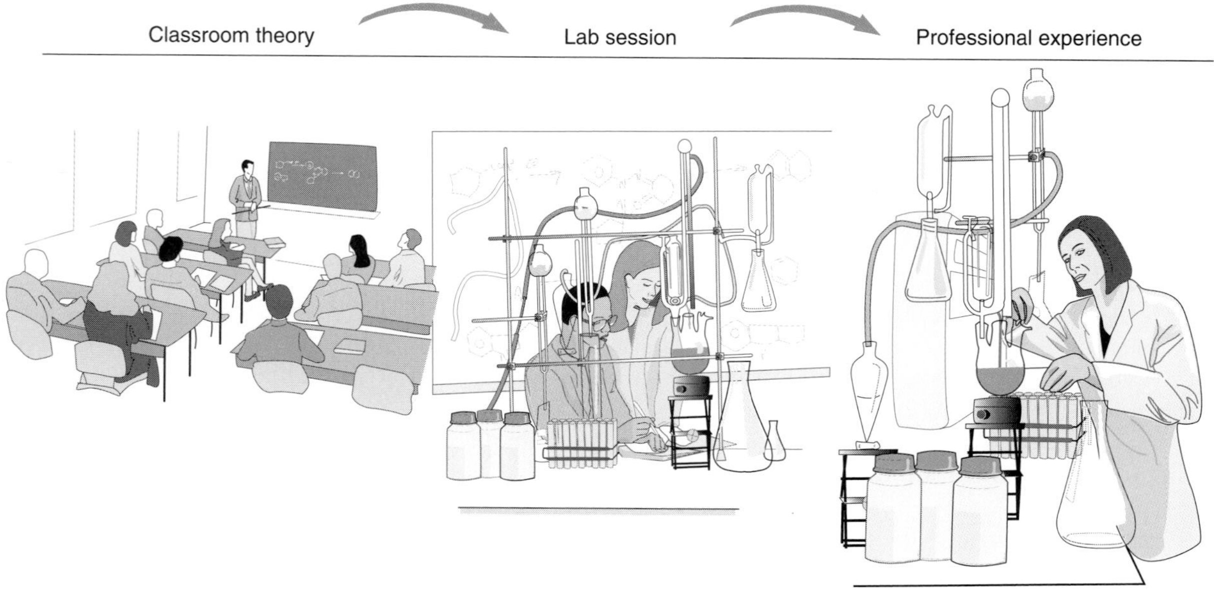

FIGURE 6–1 Laboratory work and clinical practice build a bridge between class theory and real work.

BEING PREPARED

Advance preparation will help you benefit fully from lab sessions. Lab time is often limited, and the instructor will expect you to proceed with the assigned activities without delay. The following suggestions will help you increase both how much you learn and the quality of your performance:

1. Read your textbook. Don't depend on your instructor's explanations or on being able to "figure it out." Reading gives you time to think through the steps and, as we discussed in Chapter 4, gives you a framework for lectures and demonstrations. Many health care textbooks present procedures in recipe or how-to formats. Read through each step. Pay special attention to the hints and cautions, which contain important safety information for you and the patient. Rationales may also be included. These explain the reasons for performing a step. Understanding the "why" can make it easier to remember the "how."

2. Study the illustrations in the text. Are the health care professionals wearing gloves? How are they positioned in relation to the patients and equipment? What do the equipment and instruments look like? How are they held? In which direction should movements be made? For example, in disinfecting a surgical site on the skin, it is important that cleansing be done in a circular motion, moving from the center toward the outside edges to avoid **contaminating** areas already disinfected. The effectiveness of a procedure is often based on details like these.

3. When your instructor explains or demonstrates, follow along. Be sure to sit where you can see and hear clearly. Focus on what the instructor is doing. Take notes only if it doesn't prevent you from watching and listening. If action is involved, mirror the instructor as closely as possible. For example, when watching a demonstration of the proper way to hold a syringe, use your highlighter or pen to copy the motion at your desk. Developing the ability to observe carefully is a valuable health care skill.

4. Ask questions about any point you don't understand. Gain as complete an understanding as possible before going to the lab in order to minimize mistakes and avoid wasting practice time.

5. Pay special attention to learning and practicing safety rules. You may be operating expensive and potentially dangerous equipment and handling chemical and biological hazards. The human immunodeficiency virus (HIV) and the hepatitis B virus can be spread through the mishandling of blood and certain body fluids. Proper disposal of contaminated items is regulated by law. Be sure to learn and follow the **standard precautions** developed by the U.S. Public Health Service's Centers for Disease Control (Fig. 6–2).

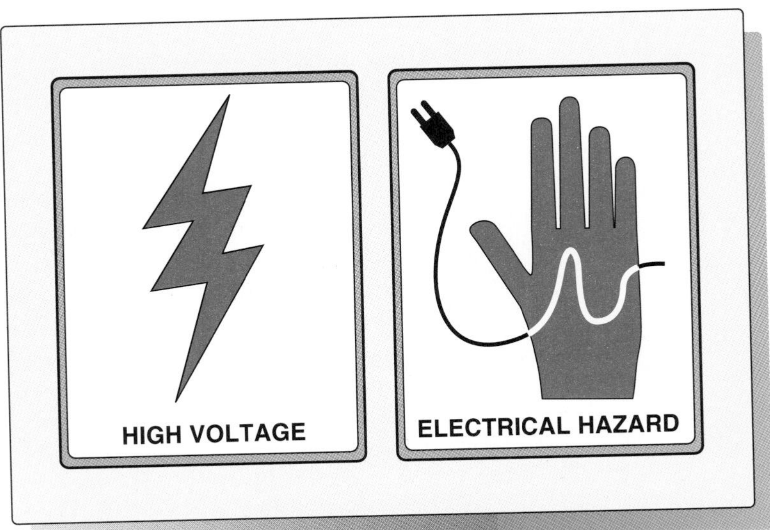

FIGURE 6–2 Pay special attention to all warnings and safety rules when working in the lab. (From Stepp, C.A. *Woods' Laboratory Procedures for Medical Office Personnel*. Philadelphia: W.B. Saunders Company, 1998, p. 10, with permission.)

6. Learn the theory and background information that support the procedures you will practice in the lab. For example, giving injections requires that you understand the principles of infection control. Insurance coding requires a knowledge of basic human anatomy terminology and medical diagnoses.

7. Rehearse the steps for each procedure in your mind. Act them out. Develop mental checklists of the steps. Some students find it helpful to use memory tricks to help recall them. For example, the mnemonic RICE is a popular way to remember the immediate first aid treatment for bone breaks and sprains:

R = rest
I = ice
C = compression
E = elevation

8. Take any study materials, reference books, supplies, or **protective equipment** needed to participate in the lab activities. Set them out the evening before if you have an early start the day of the lab.

GETTING THE MOST FROM LAB SESSIONS

1. Participate fully. Take advantage of the time allotted to practice. Don't put off the scheduled activities. Some students, especially if the class is large, fade into the woodwork and don't use lab time effectively to practice. Remember that you learn and remember best when you review and repeat activities over time. You will miss this opportunity if you waste time and do only enough at the last minute to get by. Give yourself a chance to master every procedure and enjoy your experiences in the lab.

2. Keep up on the laboratory portion of course requirements. Many health care courses feature "check-off" sheets which the instructor uses to observe the student's performance of each required procedure. As each skill is completed satisfactorily, it is checked off on the sheet. Plan to complete these sheets in a timely way as you progress through each course (Fig. 6–3).

3. Take lab sessions seriously. Never think of them as a "relief" from class lectures. Most health care careers require many hands-on activities. Lab sessions give you opportunities to perform actual work activities. This is your chance to develop and refine the skills you will use with real patients during your clinical experience.

4. Respect your instructor's time but ask questions as needed. If the instructor is busy observing or assisting other students, write down your questions so that you don't forget them.

5. Strive for accuracy. All health care tasks depend on accuracy to ensure safe, high-level patient care and adherence to various laws and regulations. In many procedures, "almost correct" is not good enough. *Only perfection is acceptable.* For example, a sterile field is a germ-free area prepared to prevent infection during procedures such as minor surgeries. It is either sterile or it is not. Brushing an ungloved hand against an object in the field may seem like a minor error, but the field is no longer sterile.

Accuracy is also critical in the administration of medications. The label on a medication package must be checked at least three times before the medication is given to a patient. Always follow this practice in the lab. Never skip a step because this is "just practice" and these are not "real surgeries" and "real medications." You are establishing habits, and it is important that everything you do in the lab be as realistic as possible.

6. Treat the students you work with as if they were real patients. Demonstrate the same courtesy and concern that you would on the job. Think and act like a professional. (Remember, "your career starts now.") If you are entering patient data on

EVALUATION OF COMPETENCY

Procedure 2—1: Measuring Body Temperature—Electronic Thermometer

Name: ________________ Date: ________________

Evaluated by: ________________ Score: ________________

Performance Objective

OUTCOME: Measure oral body temperature.
CONDITIONS: Given an electronic thermometer and oral probe.
Given an oral probe cover.
STANDARDS: Time: 5 minutes
Accuracy:
1. The temperature recording must be identical to the reading displayed on the digital display screen.
2. Satisfactory score on the Performance Evaluation Checklist.

Performance Evaluation Checklist

Yes	*No*	*Performance Standards*
____	____	Washed hands.
____	____	Assembled equipment.
____	____	Attached oral temperature probe to thermometer unit.
____	____	Inserted probe into the face of thermometer.
____	____	Removed thermometer unit from its rechargeable base.
____	____	Grasped probe by the collar and removed it from the face of thermometer.
____	____	Is able to state what occurs when probe is removed from the face of thermometer.
____	____	Attached disposable probe cover to probe.
____	____	Is able to state the purpose of probe cover.
____	____	Identified patient and explained procedure.
____	____	Correctly inserted the oral probe in patient's mouth.
____	____	Held probe in place until the audible tone was heard.
____	____	Noted patient's temperature reading on the digital display screen.
____	____	Removed probe from patient's mouth.
____	____	Discarded probe cover in an appropriate receptacle.
____	____	Did not allow fingers to come into contact with cover.
____	____	Returned probe to its stored position in the thermometer unit.
____	____	Is able to state what occurs when probe is returned to the face of the thermometer.
____	____	Washed hands.
____	____	Charted the results correctly.
____	____	The temperature recording was identical to the reading on the display screen.
____	____	Stored thermometer unit in its base.
____	____	Is able to state why thermometer unit must be stored in its base.
____	____	Completed the procedure within 5 minutes.

FIGURE 6–3 Use check-off sheets to monitor your progress. (From Bonewit-West, Kathy. *Student Mastery Manual for Clinical Procedures for Medical Assistants.* Philadelphia: W.B. Saunders Company, 2000, p. 65, used with permission.)

the computer or practicing patient scheduling, work as if the students in the exercises are real people who are depending on your ability to maintain accurate and efficient records and schedules.

7. Think about what you are doing as you work. Nothing can be taken for granted in health care. When you are working with real patients, you will have the added pressure of time restrictions and potentially serious consequences if you make a mistake. Each patient encounter presents a different set of circumstances that you will have to **evaluate.** Procedures sometimes need to be altered in order to accommodate patient needs. You cannot assume that automatically following the steps you learn in class will prepare you adequately for work in the field.

8. Concentrate on completely mastering each technique. Keep in mind that your long-term goal is to serve patients well, not simply to master the class performance requirements.

9. Understand that there may be more than one way to perform a task. For example, your instructors may each have a different way of performing a venipuncture. While certain rules must be followed for safety and effectiveness, there may not necessarily be only one correct way for every procedure. The important thing is that your technique is effective and safe for both you and your patients.

LAB FOLLOW-UP

As with any learning situation, follow-up and review are as important as the original activity. This is your opportunity to reinforce what you have learned and ensure that it enters your long-term memory.

1. Join or organize a study group to practice procedures and quiz each other on the rationale, safety concerns, and supporting theory.
2. Write out the steps of each procedure from memory. Include any safety concerns or rationale.
3. Make flashcards to help you remember important facts: rules and regulations, normal values (blood cell counts, body temperature), purpose of various lab tests, and so on.
4. Make charts, using color and illustrations to highlight important points about each procedure.
5. Review each procedure periodically. Just as with lecture notes and textbooks, regular reviews will help shift what you have practiced into your long-term memory. Maintain a list of all procedures, adding to it throughout your program.

Use the list as a checklist for review.

PRESCRIPTION FOR SUCCESS 6-1

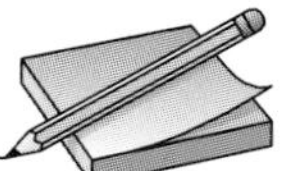

Making the Most of Labs

1. Describe any previous experience you have had with lab courses. How well do you learn from practical sessions?
2. Which study and learning techniques do you think will work best for you?
3. Describe how you think working with patients on the job will differ from the practice sessions in labs, in which you work with and on other students.

Math Skills

Math is necessary for performing many health care tasks. Examples include measuring a child's height, calculating the correct amount of medication to give a patient, conducting tests, and determining how much to bill an insurance company. It is not necessary to be a math genius, but there are a few basics you must understand in order to safely carry out the responsibilities of your job.

Many students find math difficult and dread the idea of having to deal with it in any form. You may be in this category, but the truth is that with practice, almost everyone can master the fundamentals. Here are some common reasons why students have trouble with math in their health care courses:

1. They either didn't learn or they forgot how to perform basic operations, especially those involving fractions, decimals, percentages, ratios, proportions, and simple equations.
2. They don't understand the metric system. Many Americans don't know what metric measurements refer to—how big, how much, or how long—because they don't generally use them in daily life.
3. The signs and symbols, called "notations," look strange. Students know they mean something—but what?
4. Numbers are abstract, so students have trouble visualizing math operations in their minds.
5. They memorize formulas without really understanding and knowing when to apply them to solve problems.
6. They avoid taking math classes. When this is impossible, they may skip class or neglect the homework. While this is a natural reaction to avoid difficult situations, this behavior limits their opportunities to learn, making the subject seem even more difficult.

PRESCRIPTION FOR SUCCESS 6–2

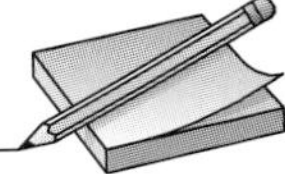

Math Check

1. How would you rate your current feelings about math?

 ____I really like it and find it interesting.

 ____I appreciate it as a handy tool to solve everyday problems and figure things out.

 ____It's okay. I sort of get by.

 ____Ugh! Don't even mention it!

2. Describe your previous experiences with math classes. Were they positive or negative?
3. Are you able to use math in your everyday life? For example, do you understand how interest on loans is calculated? Do you balance your checkbook each month? Can you double a recipe or calculate how much paint to buy for a home-improvement project?

SOME TRUTHS ABOUT MATH

Knowing the truth about something can be helpful. For example, if you are told that "math is really easy" and you find it difficult, you might wonder what is wrong with you and worry that you are not smart enough to understand it. It would be better to hear that while it may not always be easy, it can be mastered with persistence and practice. So, here are a few truths about math:

1. It is not always easy or fun. Learning math is like learning to use a computer. The strange symbols and unfamiliar language make it seem difficult, but once students learn to use it, it helps them perform many tasks quickly and efficiently.
2. Accuracy in performing math calculations is critical to patient safety. According to Chester (1998, p. 578), "medication errors and mishaps rank second only to improper diagnosis as a source of malpractice lawsuits."

3. Math knowledge builds on itself. You must master each principle and skill before moving on to the next. Walter Pauk (1997), a noted expert on study skills, believes that the reason students have difficulty with math is almost always because they didn't understand an earlier principle or process.
4. Getting behind in class can really trip you up. Failure to understand one concept leads to failure in the next. The self-fulfilling prophecy can occur: you get behind and don't understand what's going on, so you avoid the subject because you don't understand it. This leads to failure, and you "prove to yourself" that you can't do it.
5. Memorization is helpful, but understanding is essential. In order for math to be useful on the job, you must be able to apply it to new situations. You can do this only if you understand how concepts and formulas work.

RELIEVING MATH ANXIETY

While many students cringe at the thought of having to deal with numbers, others become downright panicky. They may do very well in other academic subjects but feel completely helpless and stupid when faced with math. These feelings have been labeled **math anxiety.** Stanley Kogelman and Joseph Warren (1978) developed a series of workshops to help people of all ages approach math with confidence. They firmly believe that math problems are more emotional than intellectual. The following suggestions are adapted from their book *Mind Over Math:*

1. Accept your feelings of anxiety and realize that many students experience the same feelings.
2. Don't run away from your emotional reactions. Be aware and allow yourself to experience them.
3. As an adult student, you have life experience to draw on, and once you overcome math anxiety, you can learn arithmetic in a relatively short time.
4. Know that your feelings and imagination can be just as important in math as reasoning and logic. Trust yourself to make estimates and to know when an answer just doesn't "feel right."
5. Accept that there is usually more than one way to think through and solve a math problem. Your way may be just as correct as the next person's.
6. Have confidence in yourself. Self-confidence is one of the most important factors in developing math ability.
7. Realize that no one—not even most mathematicians—works all problems quickly or "in his head."
8. Understand that it is almost impossible to concentrate and focus, which are essential to learning math, when you are anxious and nervous. In other words, math anxiety itself, not your lack of ability, can be the cause of your problems.
9. Read and work through math texts and problems slowly and carefully. Don't worry about speed.
10. Don't listen to anyone who puts you down about your math skills—especially your own negative voice!
11. Avoid saying "I can't do math." This prevents you from trying and doesn't allow you to identify what you don't know so that you can learn it. Negative self-talk defeats you before you even start.
12. Take breaks when you feel stuck. Your unconscious will continue to work, and you may find that the "impossible" problem you left is not so difficult after all.
13. Don't avoid math and procrastinate on studying and assignments. Putting time pressure on yourself will only add to your anxiety and make things worse.
14. Don't worry if you have to go over a concept many times before you get it. *That's okay!*

15. Look at the challenge of overcoming math anxiety as an opportunity to increase your overall self-confidence and ability to take control of other areas of your life.
16. Think of ways that overcoming math anxiety will help you better understand and control your personal life, such as your finances.

SUGGESTED LEARNING STRATEGIES

The following activities address the various learning styles. Try the ones that look most helpful.

1. Make flashcards for learning "math facts," such as the multiplication tables, formulas, and common conversions.
2. Draw pictures of concepts to help you understand.
3. Use paper plates, clay, blocks, and other materials to make shapes and help you see how parts relate to the whole in fractions and decimals.
4. Do a lot of practice problems. Persistence and repetition pay off when you are learning math.
5. Look for examples of math applications in everyday life: shopping, bills, bank statements, recipes, weights, measurements, taxes, and interest on loans.
6. Read math explanations aloud. Be sure that you understand each word or idea before moving on.
7. Reread materials as many times as necessary.
8. Mark your book with questions or your own explanations.
9. Study, work all examples, and practice problems in your book or study materials. Explanations often don't make sense until you've actually worked with the problems yourself.
10. If you don't understand the explanations in your own books or materials, look for others in the library or bookstore or ask your instructor for resources. Sometimes a different approach helps.
11. Be proactive. Ask questions about anything you don't understand.
12. Write down any calculations that the instructor does in class. Be sure to include each step so that you can review it later.
13. Join or form a math study group. Members should provide each other with support and learn different ways to approach the problems.
14. Take problems apart to see if you understand how they work.
15. Learn how to check your work for correctness. For example, use multiplication to check division problems.
16. Explain concepts out loud to yourself or try teaching someone else. By having to say it, you may clarify and understand it better.
17. Explain concepts and processes in writing. Pretend you are writing a letter to a friend in which you describe what you are learning in class.
18. When studying math, plan to concentrate fully. Remove as many distractions as possible, and try to spend at least thirty minutes of focused time before taking a break.

FIRST AID FOR MATH

This section contains a review of the math concepts you are most likely to encounter in health care work. If it contains skills you think you have never learned or if you need more extensive help, see your instructor for help. Working on your math skills now will help prepare you for the math portions of your health care courses.

The Language of Math

Most of the fundamental ideas of science are essentially simple, and may be, as a rule, expressed in a language comprehensive to everyone.—Albert Einstein

Math has its own special language. The various parts of calculations and notations have names that make it easier to explain math operations. Knowing this vocabulary can help you better understand your teachers and textbooks. See Table 6–1 for a list of common math terms.

TABLE 6–1 ***The Language of Math***

Word or Phrase	What It Means	Examples
Digit	Any of the numerals 0–9.	The number 834 has three digits: 8, 3, and 4.
Factors	The numbers being multiplied in a multiplication problem.	8 × 10 = 80 8 and 10 are the factors
Product	The answer to a multiplication problem.	8 × 10 = 80 80 is the product
Fraction	Used to represent equal parts of a whole. Always written as two numbers, one on top of the other.	1/2 represents 1 of the 2 equal parts into which a whole of something has been divided. 5/12 represents 5 of the 12 equal parts into which a whole has been divided.
Numerator	The top number in a fraction. It tells you how many pieces of the whole you have.	In the fraction 1/2, 1 is the numerator. In 5/12, 5 is the numerator.
Denominator	The bottom number in a fraction. It tells you into how many equal pieces a whole has been divided. The larger the number, the smaller the pieces.	In 1/2, 2 is the denominator. In 5/12, 12 is the denominator.
Proper Fraction	A fraction in which the numerator is smaller than the denominator.	3/4 3 is smaller than 4
Improper Fraction	A fraction in which the numerator is larger than the denominator.	4/3 4 is larger than 3. This represents a whole number and a fraction: 1 1/3. (There are 3 thirds in a whole, which equals 1. 1/3 represents the additional—or 4th—third.)
Lowest Common Denominator	The smallest number that can be evenly divided (no remainder) by all the denominators in a series of fractions. It is necessary to find this number when you want to add or subtract fractions.	The lowest common denominator for 1/6, 3/4, and 5/8 is 24. 24 divided by 6 = 4 24 divided by 4 = 6 24 divided by 8 = 3
Simplest Form	A fraction in which the numerator and denominator cannot be evenly divided by the same number.	1/2 is the simplest form for the following fractions: 2/4, 3/6, 4/8, 5/10, 25/50
Decimal	Special fractions. They are written with decimal points, the same symbol as a period. When decimals are written as fractions, they always have denominators written in units of 10 (10, 100, 1000, 10,000, etc.).	0.3 = 3/10. Both represent 3 of the 10 equal parts of a whole.
Whole Number	A number that has no fraction or decimal.	5, 67, and 1893 are whole numbers.
Mixed Number	A number that has two parts: a whole number and a fraction.	1 1/3, 4 1/2, 17 2/5
Percentage	A fraction with a denominator of 100 which is expressed as a whole number with a percent sign.	37% represents 37 of the 100 parts of a whole. It is the same as 37/100 and 0.37 (see Fig 6–4).
Cubic Measurement	Measure of volume, or the amount of space that something takes up. Medications are sometimes measured in cubic centimeters. (See Table 6–3 for an explanation of the centimeter.)	To calculate the volume of a box, multiply the height times the width times the length. A box that is 3 feet long, 2 feet high, and 5 feet wide = 3 × 2 × 5 = 30 cubic feet (see Fig 6–5).
Dividend	In a division problem, the number to be divided.	8⟌64 ← dividend

TABLE 6–1 *The Lanuage of Math (Continued)*

Word or Phrase	What It Means	Examples	
Divisor	The number by which the dividend is divided in a division problem.	8⟌64 divisor	
Ratio	Expresses the relationship of 2 numbers. They can be written several ways.	The relationship between 1 and 2 can be written as 1 to 2, 1:2, or 1/2.	
Proportion	Statement that 2 ratios are equal.	1:2 = 5:10 1/2 = 5/10 (1 is to 2 as 5 is to 10)	
Equation	Statement which says that 2 quantities are equal. This equality is represented by an "equals" sign. Equations are used to help you find values for unknown quantities by using the information you do know. The unknown quantities are commonly represented by letters.	x + 12 = 18 6x − 4 = 30 + 26	
Place Value Chart	A chart that shows the unit values of the places that follow the decimal point.	Tenths Hundredths Thousandths Ten thousandths Hundred thousandths	0.1 0.01 0.001 0.0001 0.00001

Performing Basic Operations

Table 6–2 contains a brief review of some of the operations commonly used in health care—and commonly forgotten by students! Its purpose is to help you recall math skills you have already learned, not to teach new material. The explanations given here and the way the problems are set up may be different from the way you learned them. Remember that there is no one right way to work a problem. For example, division problems are not set up the same way in every country.

Try working the examples. The explanations may not make much sense until you look at some real numbers.

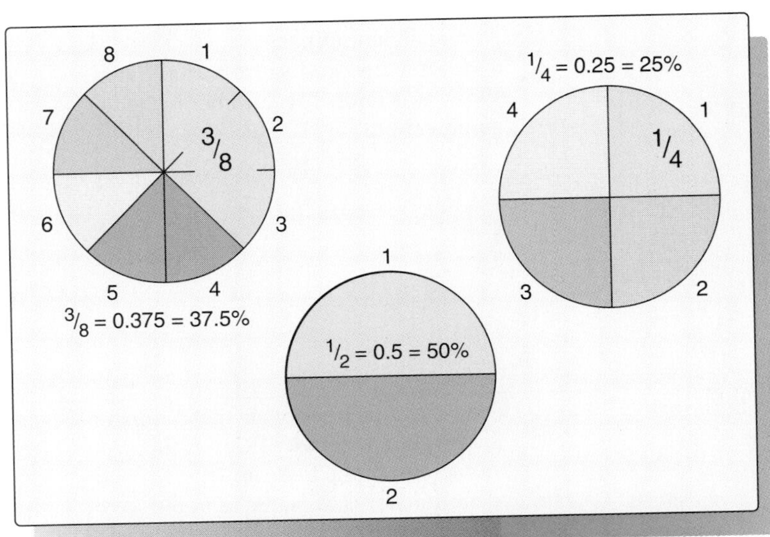

FIGURE 6–4 Relationship of fractions, decimals, and percentages.

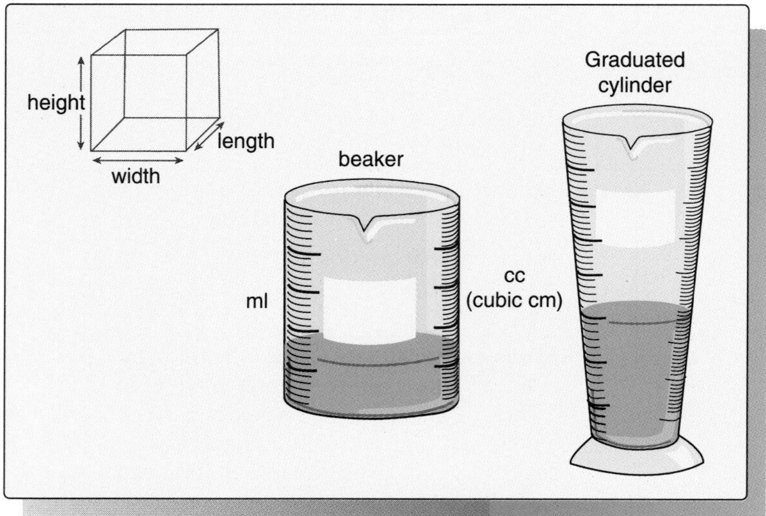

FIGURE 6–5 Volume measures space.

TABLE 6–2 ***Basic Operations***

Operation	What to Do	Examples
	Fractions	
Reducing fractions	Find a number that divides evenly into both the numerator and the denominator. You may have to do this more than once if you want it to be at its lowest terms (meaning that there are no other numbers by which both can be evenly divided).	18/30 Both 18 and 30 can be divided evenly by 2, resulting in 9/15 Both 9 and 15 can be divided evenly by 3, resulting in 3/5 (This can also be done in one step by dividing 18 and 30 by 6 = 3/5.)
Changing fractions so that they share the lowest common denominator	1. Find the smallest number that can be evenly divided by all the denominators in a series of fractions. This is the new denominator. 2. Divide the new denominator by the original denominator. 3. Multiply the product from step 2 times the numerator. This number is the new numerator.	By trial and error, we discover that the lowest common denominator for 1/6, 3/4, and 5/8 is 24. To convert 1/6, divide 24 by 6. The answer is 4. Multiply 4 times the numerator, 1. The new fraction is 4/24. To convert 3/4: 24 divided by 4 = 6 6 × 3 = 18 New fraction is 18/24 To convert 5/8: 24 divided by 8 = 3 3 × 5 = 15 New fraction is 15/24
Simplifying improper fractions	Divide the numerator by the denominator. If there is a remainder (R), it is the numerator of the fraction. The denominator is the same as in the improper fraction. Reduce the fraction, if necessary.	10/4 is improper because the numerator is larger than the denominator. 10 divided by 4 = 2 R 2 2 2/4 = 2 1/2

TABLE 6–2 ***Basic Operations (Continued)***

Operation	What to Do	Examples
	Fractions	
Adding and subtracting	1. If the fractions do not have the same denominator, find the lowest common denominator. 2. Add or subtract the numerators. 3. Use the common denominator in the answer. 4. Simplify the result if it is an improper fraction. *Caution:* When subtracting mixed numbers, it is best to change them to improper fractions before subtracting the numerators.	1/6 + 3/4 + 5/8 = ? 24 is the lowest common denominator. 4/24 + 18/24 + 15/24 = 37/24. 37/24 is an improper fraction, so divide 37 by 24 = 1 R 13. 37/24 = 1 13/24 5/8 − 1/4 = ? 8 is the lowest common denominator. 5/8 − 2/8 = 3/8
Multiplying fractions	1. Multiply the numerators and then the denominators. 2. Reduce the fraction, if necessary.	1/2 × 3/4 = ? 1 × 3 = 3 2 × 4 = 8
Dividing fractions (everyone's big fear!)	1. Invert (switch) the numerator and the denominator of the divisor. 2. Multiply the numerators and the denominators. (That's right—you don't actually divide as we know it. This is what makes an otherwise simple operation seem confusing and hard to remember.) 3. If necessary, simplify to a proper fraction.	3/4 divided by 1/2 = ? Invert: 1/2 becomes 2/1 3 × 2 = 6 4 × 1 = 4 6/4 is an improper fraction. 6 divided by 4 = 1 R 2 = 1 2/4 = 1 1/2
	Decimals	
Adding and subtracting decimals	1. Line up the numbers so that the decimal points are aligned. 2. Use zeros to fill in the spaces to the right of the decimal point. 3. Add or subtract as you would any numbers. 4. Place the decimal point in the answer directly under the points in the numbers you added or subtracted.	To add 3.96, 4.229 and 6.1: 3.960 4.229 6.100 14.289 To subtract 18.453 from 72.5: 72.500 −18.453 54.047
Multiplying decimals	1. Multiply as you would whole numbers. 2. Count and total the digits to the right of the decimal point in each factor. 3. Place the decimal point in the answer that total number of spaces from the right. 4. Insert zeros as needed for placement of the decimal point.	16.953 × 3.502 59.369406
Dividing decimals	1. Set up the problem like any division problem. 2. If the divisor is a decimal, move the decimal point to the right and place it immediately following the last digit in the number. Then move the decimal point in the dividend to the right the same number of spaces. Add zeros if necessary.	2.5/10 2.5⟌10.0 4.0 25⟌100.0

Table continued on following page

TABLE 6-2 ***Basic Operations (Continued)***

Operation	What to Do	Examples
	Decimals	
	3. Divide the numbers. 4. Place the decimal point in the answer directly above the decimal point in the dividend.	
	Decimals and Fractions	
Changing decimals to fractions	1. Write the numbers in the decimal as the numerator. 2. Write the unit of the decimal as the denominator. (tenths, hundredths, thousandths, etc; see Placement Value Chart in Table 6–1). 3. Reduce the fraction, if necessary.	0.25 = ? Numerator is 25 0.25 has two places; therefore, use 100 for the denominator. 0.25 = 25/100 Both 25 and 100 can be evenly divided by 25: 25 divided by 25 = 1 100 divided by 25 = 4 0.25 = 1/4
Changing fractions to decimals	1. Set up a division problem in which the numerator is divided by the denominator. 2. Before dividing, check to see if the numerator is smaller than the denominator. If it is, write a decimal point and one or more zeros, as needed.	2/3 = ? 3⟌2 3⟌2.00 add decimal point and zeros .66 3⟌2.00 18× 20
	Percentages	
Changing percentages to decimals	1. Start counting from the decimal point and move it 2 places to the left. Fill in with zeros as needed. (Note: If the whole number does not have a decimal point written in, it is understood to be located at the far right side of the number.) 2. Drop the percent sign.	To change 41% to a decimal: The decimal point is understood to be to the right of the 1 41% = 41.0% Move the decimal point 2 places to the left: 0.41 41% = 0.41 To change 3% to a decimal: The decimal point is understood to be to the right of the 3. 3% = 3.0% Move the decimal point 2 places to the left: 0.03 3% = 0.03
Calculating amounts represented by percentages	1. Change the percent to a decimal. 2. Multiply the whole number by the decimal. 3. Count and total the digits to the right of the decimal point in the multiplier. 4. Place the decimal point in the answer that total number of spaces from the right. (Extra zeros on the far right may be dropped.)	To find 65% of 730: 65% = 0.65 730 × 0.65 474.50 65% of 730 = 474.5

TABLE 6-2 ***Basic Operations (Continued)***

Operation	What to Do	Examples
Equations		
Solving simple equations	1. Your goal is to find the value of an unknown quantity (x). You do this by reorganizing the equation so the unknown is by itself on one side of the equals sign. 2. Isolate x by adding, subtracting, multiplying, or dividing *both* sides of the equation in the same way. (You must always treat both sides of an equation the same way.) 3. You may have to do more than one calculation to isolate x completely. *Note:* Positive and negative numbers cancel each other out.	5 + x = 12 You want x by itself, so you need to eliminate the 5. Subtract 5 from both sides of the equation. 5 + x − 5 = 12 − 5 x = 7 6x − 3 = 15 Add 3 to each side: 6x − 3 + 3 = 15 + 3 6x = 18 Divide each side by 6: 6x/6 = 18/6 x = 3
Proportions		
Finding an unknown quantity in a proportion	1. Substitute x for the unknown quantity. 2. Write each of the 2 ratios as fractions. 3. Multiply the denominators by the opposite numerators. 4. Solve for x. 5. Write out the completed proportion.	1:2 = 10:x 1/2 = 10/x 1 × x = 2 × 10 x = 20 Therefore, 1:2 = 10:20 8:x = 14:91 8/x = 14/91 8 × 91 = 14 × x 728 = 14x 728/14 = 14x/14 x = 52 Therefore, 8:52 = 14:91
	Note: Another common way to discuss proportions is in terms of the "means" and the "extremes." In the example 1:2 = 10:x, 1 and x are the extremes and 2 and 10 are the means. The product of the means equals the product of the extremes. This is the same operation as cross-multiplying the fractions.	①:2 = 10:ⓧ mean extreme Multiply the means and extremes: 1 × x = 2 × 10 x = 20 Therefore, 1:2 = 10:20 8:x = 14:91 Multiply the means and extremes: 8 × 91 = x × 14 14x = 728 Isolate x: 14x/14 = 728/14 x = 52 Therefore, 8:52 = 14:91

The Multiplication Chart

Knowing the products of all possible combinations of the numbers 1 through 12 is a great time saver. This is *not* a substitute for learning how to multiply but a way to increase your efficiency. It is also a good study aid for learning the multiplication tables. To use the chart in Box 6–1, find the intersection of the two numbers you wish to multiply, one from the row across the top and the other from the far left column. For example, to multiply 3 times 4, find the 3 in the top row and the 4 in the first column. Move down from the 3 and across from the 4 until the lines meet at 12. This is the answer. Study from the table or make flashcards for any combinations you need to memorize. You can also use graph paper to set up blank tables to fill in to review and quiz yourself.

BOX 6–1. MULTIPLICATION CHART

	1	2	3	4	5	6	7	8	9	10	11	12
1	1	2	3	4	5	6	7	8	9	10	11	12
2	2	4	6	8	10	12	14	16	18	20	22	24
3	3	6	9	12	15	18	21	24	27	30	33	36
4	4	8	12	16	20	24	28	32	36	40	44	48
5	5	10	15	20	25	30	35	40	45	50	55	60
6	6	12	18	24	30	36	42	48	54	60	66	72
7	7	14	21	28	35	42	49	56	63	70	77	84
8	8	16	24	32	40	48	56	64	72	80	88	96
9	9	18	27	36	45	54	63	72	81	90	99	108
10	10	20	30	40	50	60	70	80	90	100	110	120
11	11	22	33	44	55	66	77	88	99	110	121	132
12	12	24	36	48	60	72	84	96	108	120	132	144

The multiplication table can also be used as a tool to reduce fractions if the numerator and denominator appear in the same column. For example, for 12/96, follow both 12 and 96 to the far left column: 12 becomes 1 and 96 becomes 8; 12/96 = 1/8. The fraction may need to be reduced further. For example, 24/48 = 2/4; 2/4 can be further reduced to 1/2.

PRESCRIPTION FOR SUCCESS 6–3

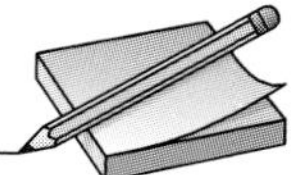

What's Your Math Status?

1. Based on your understanding of the preceding review, how would you rate your knowledge of math?

    ____Excellent ____ Very Good ____ Good ____ Fair ____ Poor
2. What math skills are required in your future profession?
3. If you don't know what math skills you will need, where can you find out?
4. If you rated yourself as "fair" or "poor," what plans do you have for improving?

    ____ Take classes at school
    ____ Use special services at school, such as computer lab or tutoring
    ____ Study on my own
    ____ Workbooks
    ____ Software
    ____ Videos
    ____ Other

Making Sense of the Metric System

The **metric system** is an obstacle for many students. It is actually a very logical system that is based on multiples of ten. Used in most countries of the world, it also serves as the measuring system for science and health care. People who come to the United States find it difficult to learn *our* units of measurement, because it is difficult to relate them to each other. Our units have names that don't follow any pattern: "inch," "foot," "yard," "pound," "mile," and so on. To make things even more confusing, some of these words—"foot," "yard," and "pound"—have other meanings as well.

Many Americans find the metric system difficult because we don't use it often in our daily lives. We know about how far a mile is, but we are lost if someone asks us if we'd like go on a five-kilometer walk. The first step in learning the metric system is to learn the names of the various weights and measures and get a feel for what each one represents. The second step involves doing conversions between the two systems, and this requires some math (see Figs. 6–6 and 6–7).

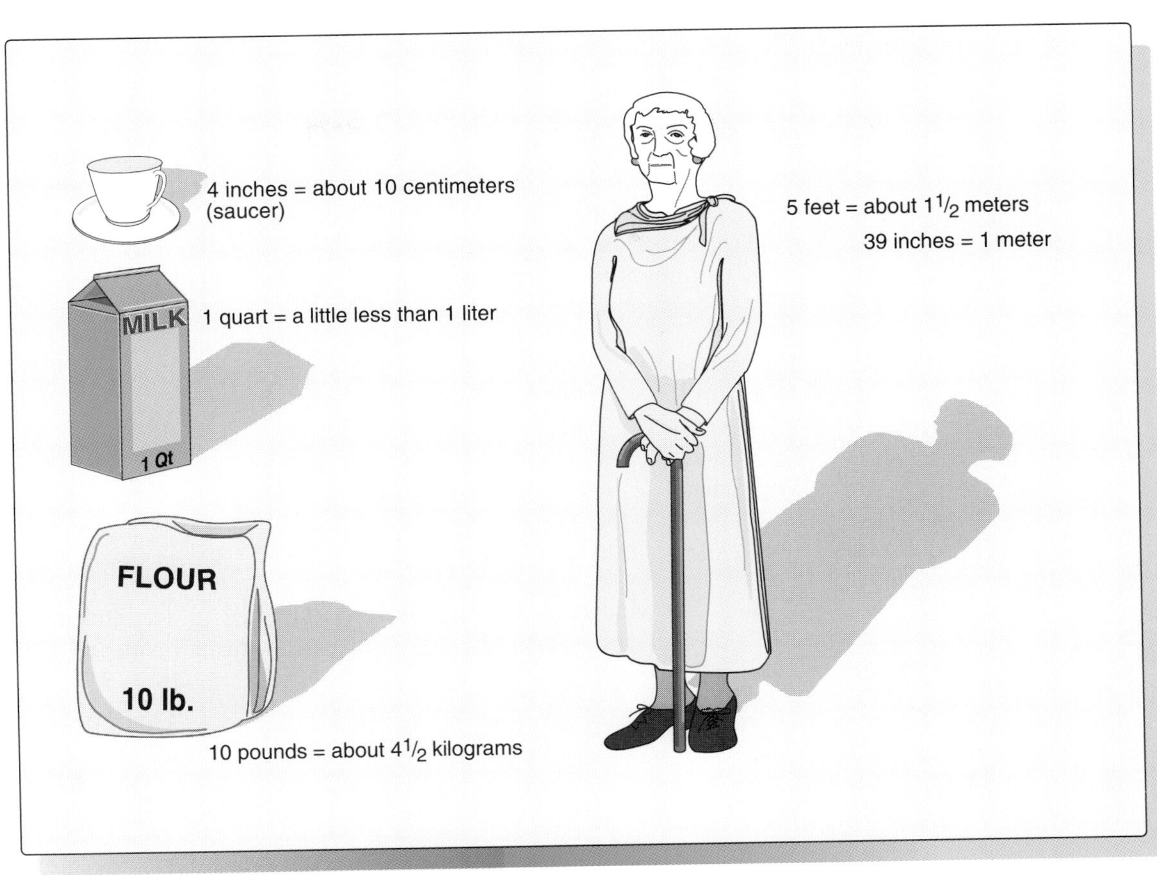

FIGURE 6–6 Some metric equivalents of U.S. units.

Nutrition Facts

Serving Size 1 cup (228g)
Servings Per Container 2

Amount Per Serving

Calories 90 Calories from Fat 30

	% Daily Value
Total Fat 3g	**5%**
Saturated Fat 3g	**0%**
Cholesterol 0 mg	**0%**
Sodium 300 mg	**13%**
Total Carbohydrate 13 g	**4%**
Dietary Fiber 3g	**12%**
Sugars 3g	
Protein 3 g	

Vitamin A 80%	Vitamin C 60%
Calcium 4%	Iron 4%

* Percent Daily Values are based on a 2,000 calorie diet. Your daily values may be higher or lower depending on your calorie needs:

	Calories	2,000	3,000
Total Fat	Less Than	65g	80g
Sat Fat	Less Than	20g	25g
Cholesterol	Less Than	300mg	300mg
Sodium	Less Than	2,400mg	2,400mg
Total Carbohydrate		300g	370g
Dietary Fiber		25g	30g

Calories per gram
Fat 9 • Carbohydrate 4 • Protein 4

FIGURE 6–7 Metric units are reported on food labels. (Adapted from *Understanding Food Labels*. Copyright © 1997 The American Dietetic Association. Used with permission.)

Facts about the Metric System

1. It is the universal system of measurement for science and technical fields.
2. It is more precise than the U.S. system.
3. It works on a base of 10. This means that units of measurement are created by multiplying to make larger units and dividing to make smaller units by powers of 10 (10, 100, 1000, 10,000, etc.).
4. Prefixes that designate multiples of 10 are added to the basic units of measurement to make them larger or smaller. The same prefixes are used for all the basic units, so you have to remember only one set.

micro	0.00001
milli	0.001
centi	0.01
deci	0.1
deka	10
hecto	100
kilo	1000

5. A knowledge of decimals is important for understanding metric units of measurement: See Table 6–3 for explanations of metric units of measurements.

TABLE 6–3 ***How the Metric System Works***

Type of Measurement	Units of Measurement	How It Compares with the U.S. System
Length or Distance	*meter* (m) = basic unit	A little more than 1 yard (1 yard = 36 inches and 1 meter = 39.37 inches)
	millimeter (mm) = 0.001 meter	About the size of the width of a pinhead. There are just over 25 millimeters in 1 inch.
	centimeter (cm) = 0.01 meter	About 2/5 (or 0.4) of an inch, the width of a child's little finger. There are about 2 1/2 centimeters in an inch.
	decimeter (dm) = 0.1 meter	About 4 inches
	dekameter (dam) = 10 meters	A little more than 10 yards
	hectometer (hm) = 100 meters	A little more than 100 yards
	kilometer (km) = 1000 meters	About 3/5 (or 0.62) of a mile
Liquids or Volume	*liter* (L) = basic unit	Approximately 1 quart (2 liters is now a popular-sized soft drink bottle; that's about 1/2 gallon because there are 4 quarts in a gallon)
	*milliliter** (mL) = 0.001 liter	*Very* small drop (commonly used in medicine)
	centiliter (cL) = 0.01 liter	About 2 teaspoons
	deciliter (dL) = 0.1 liter	Between 1/3 and 1/2 cup
	dekaliter (daL) = 10 liters	About 10 quarts or 2 1/2 gallons
	hectoliter (hL) = 100 liters	About 25 gallons
	kiloliter (kL) = 1000 liters	About 250 gallons

TABLE 6–3 ***How the Metric System Works (Continued)***

Type of Measurement	Units of Measurement	How It Compares with the U.S. System
Weight or Mass of Solids	*gram* (Gm, g) = basic unit	Approximately 1/28 of an ounce. About the weight of a paperclip.
	microgram (mcg) = 0.000001 gram	An incredibly small amount (1 millionth of 1/400 of a pound!!) Don't be fooled, however. This can be a significant amount in health care. The body depends on *very* small quantities of certain substances to function properly. It can also be harmed by minute amounts of the wrong substances.
	milligram (mg) = 0.001 gram centigram (cg) = 0.01 gram decigram (dg) = 0.1 gram	Also very small amounts, although they are many times heavier than a microgram.
	dekagram (dag) = 10 grams hectogram (hg) = 100 grams *kilogram* (kg) = 1000 grams	5/14 of an ounce About 3 1/2 ounces 2.2 pounds
Temperature	*Celsius* (commonly called centigrade) 0°C = freezing point of water 100°C = boiling point of water Celsius thermometers are marked in one-tenth intervals. Water freezes: 0°C Normal body temperature: 37°C Water boils: 100°C Sterilization occurs: 121°C To convert between the 2 systems: Fahrenheit to Celsius: 1. Subtract 32 from the F temperature 2. Multiply by 5/9 Celsius to Fahrenheit: (see Fig. 6-8) 1. Multiply the C temperature by 9/5 2. Add 32	Fahrenheit is the system commonly used in the United States. In this system, 32°F is freezing and 95°F is a sunny day at the beach. 1°C = 1.8 times 1°F 32°F 98.6°F 212°F 250°F 98.6°F 98.6 − 32 = 66.6 5/9 × 66.6 = 5/9 × 66.6/1.0 = 37 37 × 9/5 = 37/1 × 9/5 = 333/5 = 66.6 66.6 + 32 = 98.6

*A milliliter is the same amount as a cubic centimeter (cc). This is important to know in health care because these terms are sometimes used interchangeably.

PRESCRIPTION FOR SUCCESS 6–4

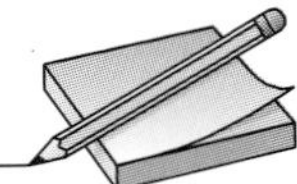

Learn with Practice

Practice learning the metric system by using it at home. It you don't have a yardstick or ruler that is marked in centimeters and millimeters, buy an inexpensive one. Measure and make labels for common items. For example, the height of a doorknob is about one meter from the floor.

MATH ON THE JOB Many health care applications require you to calculate metric units and to convert between metric and other systems of measurement. A goal of this chapter is to help you understand the metric system and realize that it is not mysterious and difficult.

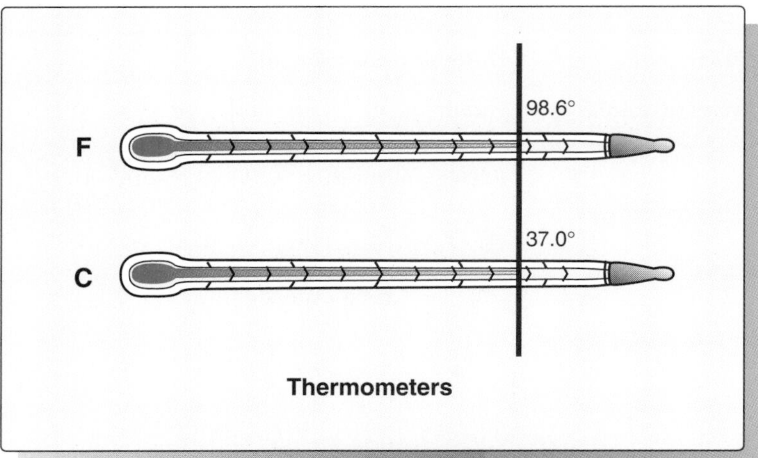

FIGURE 6–8 You may encounter both Fahrenheit and Celsius measurement systems in health care work.

Spend some time becoming familiar with the quantities represented by the basic metric units.

You don't have to become a math whiz to be a competent health care professional. But you should be motivated to overcome math anxiety, identify and work on areas you haven't mastered, and develop confidence in your ability to apply your knowledge. Here are some examples of how health care professionals use math:

1. *Calculating amounts of medication to administer.* This is one of the most important applications of math in health care occupations because of the critical need for accuracy to ensure patient safety. Medications are often ordered by the physician using a different system or **dosage** (amount) than those used by suppliers. It is often necessary to convert from one system to another and to calculate the proper quantity to administer. These calculations require that you understand the various systems of measurement, as well as how to use proportions and solve equations.

2. *Counting white blood cells manually.* White blood cells are counted to determine the number per cubic millimeter to see if the count falls within the normal range. Counts above and below normal can be indications of infection or leukemia. To perform the count, a blood sample is placed on a special slide, called a "hemocytometer," that is marked off in squares. With the use of a microscope, the white blood cells are counted in several designated squares. Various calculations are then carried out to determine the number of cells per cubic centimeter. These calculations include finding the average of several numbers, calculating 10% of the average, and performing addition and multiplication.

3. *Billing for services.* Patient bills must be calculated accurately and recorded properly to ensure proper payment from insurance companies.

4. *Taking vital signs.* The metric system is sometimes used when recording patient weight, height, and temperature. Blood pressure is expressed in millimeters.

Clinical Experience

Your clinical experience, whether it is called an "externship," "internship," "fieldwork experience," "practicum," or some other name, can be one of the most valuable parts of your education. It provides the final link between your education and your future career. Experienced professionals or clinical instructors will guide your work in a real occupational setting. This phase of your education provides you with opportunities to:

1. Apply the skills learned in class.
2. Gain confidence in performing these skills.
3. Learn firsthand about the expectations of employers.

4. Practice working with patients.
5. Think and problem-solve in real-life situations.
6. Demonstrate your abilities to a potential employer. (Students are sometimes hired to work at their clinical site after graduation.)

A successful clinical experience requires your full attention and effort. Some students make the mistake of thinking that this part of their education is less important than their academic classes, especially if they are graded on a pass-fail basis. Nothing could be further from the truth. The clinical experience really counts in the sense that you now have an impact on real people and real problems. It is also during the clinical experience that you begin to establish your professional reputation.

As in every area of our lives, not every clinical experience will be ideal. Things will not always go just as you expected or hoped. At these times, it may be necessary for you to adjust your attitude. Act as a professional and focus on doing your best to learn and achieve your career goals. Even difficult situations offer opportunities to practice getting along with others, adapt to a work environment, and solve problems. Start thinking now about how you can prepare to benefit fully from your clinical experience.

Here are some guidelines for maximizing your clinical experience:

1. Take advantage of the assistance and advice offered by your school. The staff has experience in setting up clinical experiences so that students have the best chance to succeed.
2. Strive to have excellent attendance. If you must be absent, *call the site* and let them know. Most schools require you to notify them, too.
3. Learn the policies and procedures at the facility. Ask for a copy of any that apply to the work you will be doing.
4. Be sure you understand what you will be expected and allowed to do. Some facilities have students start with relatively easy tasks before giving them more complex assignments. Others have students jump right in with a full set of duties.
5. Follow all rules and dress codes, even if others do not seem to be doing so.
6. Ask questions about anything you don't understand or want to learn more about. Try to determine the answers for yourself first, but don't hesitate if you are unsure. This is especially important regarding procedures that have safety consequences for you or the patient.
7. Ask an appropriate person to check your work if you are unsure about its accuracy.
8. Be courteous with everyone. These are your future professional colleagues.
9. Learn as much as possible from the staff. Observe them at work and get to know them as people. Do be careful, though, *not* to get involved in gossip sessions.
10. Become a contributing member of the health care team. Offer to help without being asked.
11. Find out how you will be evaluated. Be sure that you understand the performance expectations.
12. Set goals for yourself. Think about why you are there and what you want to learn.
13. Take advantage of any resources that are available at the facility. Find out if there is a technical library you can use. Does the facility have reference materials about topics in which you have a special interest? Are there additional opportunities for you to observe and talk with people about their work?

Take full advantage of your clinical experience to learn, make a good impression, and launch your new life as a health care professional.

PRESCRIPTION FOR SUCCESS 6–5

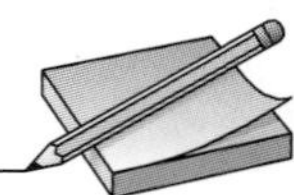

Having What It Takes

1. Which of your personal characteristics do you believe will most help you have a successful clinical experience?
2. Which personal characteristics do you think you might need to work on now to improve the benefit you receive from your experience (for example, shyness, impatience, or difficulty being on time)?

Problem Solving and Decision Making

Every day we are confronted with situations that require us to make decisions and solve problems, both large and small. The quality of your life depends to a great extent on your ability to make good decisions. On the job, this ability also affects the lives of your patients and coworkers.

Being able to problem-solve is an essential health care skill and is included in the National Health Care Skill Standards introduced in Chapter 1:

- Use analytical skills to solve problems and make decisions.
- Adapt to changing situations.

The nursing profession has developed a structured approach to patient care that is based on a problem-solving perspective. Known as the **nursing process,** it consists of five steps:

1. *Assessment:* Systematically collecting data about the patient.
2. *Nursing diagnosis:* Describing actual and potential health problems based on the data collected.
3. *Planning:* Setting goals for the patient and establishing a nursing care plan to achieve these goals.
4. *Implementation or nursing interaction:* Carrying out actions to assist the patient to promote, maintain, and restore health.
5. *Evaluation:* Measuring the patient's progress toward achieving the goals set in step 2. Determining ways to assist patients who do not reach their goals. Setting new goals for patients who are progressing as planned. (Adapted from Miller-Keane, 1997.)

Having a methodical way to approach problems and make decisions in your personal and professional lives helps you develop effective solutions and improves the quality of your decisions. Many helpful models have been developed. Like the nursing process, they consist of a series of steps that give structure to the process and help you sort out complex issues. The one presented in this chapter is organized into the following six steps:

1. Define the problem.
2. Gather information.
3. Brainstorm alternative solutions.
4. Consider possible results and consequences.
5. Choose a solution and act on it.
6. Evaluate the results and revise as needed.

STEP ONE: DEFINE THE PROBLEM

A problem well stated is a problem half solved.—Charles F. Kettering

The problem you are addressing may *seem* obvious, but sometimes what we believe to be the problem is only a symptom of a deeper underlying problem. For example, suppose that Kathy, a nursing student, is earning Ds and Fs in her pharmacology class. She may define the problem as "getting low grades in class." Grades, however, are only a symptom of the problem, not the problem itself. Asking questions can help her to identify the real problem.

- Do I understand the textbook? The lectures?
- Do I have good study habits?
- Do I put off studying for this class because I don't like it?
- Do I avoid attending this class?
- Does the teacher present the material in a disorganized manner?
- Does the subject require background knowledge that I don't have?
- Am I having trouble understanding what is asked for in test questions?
- Do I complete all homework assignments and projects?
- Do I have the math knowledge and skills needed to understand and perform the necessary calculations?

It's not always easy or comfortable to uncover real problems. We tend to avoid tough issues by ignoring them, or we blame circumstances or other people for our difficulties. If we fail to recognize our part in causing problems, we also give away our power to find solutions. For example, if we blame our poor grades on the teacher or the school, we become powerless to raise them. By accepting responsibility for ourselves, we also empower ourselves to direct our own lives.

Continuing with our example, suppose that Kathy identifies the problem as a weakness in math. She makes many mistakes when calculating dosages, converting between systems of measurement, and computing proportions.

STEP TWO: GATHER INFORMATION

We need up-to-date information to solve problems and make decisions. We don't benefit from opinions based on false facts or a limited number of facts. Even well-trained experts conduct research when confronted with new problems. When physicians begin working with patients who have unresolved heath problems, they gather as much information as possible. They observe the patient, ask questions, and run diagnostic tests. They call upon their own knowledge. They may discuss their findings with colleagues and consult reference books and recent technical articles. In summary, they gather as much information as possible from a wide variety of sources.

It is a sign of strength, not weakness, to admit that you don't know the answer. Our world is complex, and there is no way we can keep up in every field, even our own areas of expertise. The willingness to continue learning and seeking to find the best answers is the sign of a true professional.

Gathering facts helps avoid emotional and nonproductive reactions to life's problems. If Kathy's response to receiving low grades in pharmacology class is "I'm just dumb and I'll never get this," she will be discouraged from seeking an effective solution. If she passed the admissions requirements for her school and is receiving passing grades in her other classes, the evidence does not support the statement that she is dumb. Insisting that she is "just dumb" becomes a way to escape being responsible for seeking solutions to the problem. It avoids the work of going through the problem-solving process and making needed changes.

Relying on faulty opinions and emotional responses can also negatively influence the health care professional's work with patients. For example, if you assume that you know what patients are thinking or feeling, believe that you know what is best, or react emotionally, you may fail to ask appropriate questions and collect the information necessary to help them resolve their health problems.

There are many sources of information for help in addressing problems:

- Your own knowledge and observations. Review what you know that relates to the problem.
- The knowledge and opinions of others, especially those who will be affected by your actions. We often make assumptions without exploring the feelings and opinions of others. What we think is best for someone else may in fact be what is worst. Consult with friends, family members, instructors, and experts. Listen to what they say without arguing or judging. At this point, you are gathering information without screening the contents.

- Books, journals, and the Internet. There are many reader-friendly books about handling personal and professional problems.
- Classes, workshops, and conferences.

The number of resources you consult depends on the size, complexity, and importance of the problem. Some situations require only your current knowledge and a quick observation. Others require extensive research. (It may help to review the section on research in Chapter 4 for more specific sources and methods.)

A good professional practice is to keep up-to-date in your field by reading and pursuing continuing education opportunities. This will give you the background needed for making sound decisions. It will also enable you to judge the quality of the information you gather more effectively. Not all published information or material from the Internet is based on thorough research. It can have errors or be biased by the opinions of the writer. Up-to-date knowledge of the fundamentals of your area will help you distinguish fact from opinion.

Potential sources of information for Kathy's problem:

- Her math or pharmacology instructor
- Math tests that diagnose weak areas of knowledge
- Books, articles, and workshops about math anxiety
- Basic math textbooks
- Measurement and dosage practice problems

STEP THREE: BRAINSTORM ALTERNATIVE SOLUTIONS

There may be several effective solutions for a given problem. Brainstorm as many ideas as possible, even silly or impractical ones. Write down as many possible solutions as you can. Work quickly and don't discard anything. Even a foolish idea might lead to one that works.

Here are the results of Kathy's brainstorming session:

- Drop the class and hope she becomes smarter over time.
- Drop out of school. What's the use?
- Stay in the class, keep trying, and repeat the class if she doesn't pass.
- Drop the class and take it later. Use the extra time to work on her math skills.
- Stay in the class and spend extra time developing her math skills.
- Ideas to improve her skills
  - Work through a basic math textbook.
  - Use learning software.
  - Work with a tutor.
  - Form or join a study group.
  - Ask the instructor to work with her after class several times a week.
  - Ask a friend or relative who is good at math to help her.
- Go to a hypnotist who specializes in helping people overcome anxiety problems.
- Use positive self-talk and visualizations.
- Borrow her children's math books.
- Ask her children for help.
- Go to a learning supply store and buy math games and toys.

PRESCRIPTION FOR SUCCESS 6-6

Brainstorm five more examples of possible solutions for Kathy's problem.

STEP FOUR: REVIEW POSSIBLE RESULTS AND CONSEQUENCES

Now is the time to evaluate the brainstorming results. Review each idea and ask yourself, "What would happen if I took this action?" You may find that you need to ask more questions and gather more information. Look for ideas that can be combined or that suggest other workable solutions. Let's review a few of Kathy's ideas from step three.

Drop out of school. What's the use? This is an emotional response that's perfectly natural when a person feels frustrated and discouraged. Possible results and consequences:

- Disappointment at not reaching her goal of a career in health care.
- Missed opportunity to help others.
- Feelings of failure and depression.
- Student loans to repay and no job to help her financially.
- A feeling of relief. This just wasn't for her.

New questions to ask:

- How can she find out if she is really capable of learning the necessary math?
- How did she do in past math classes?
- Did she learn these skills at one time and just needs to review, or did she never learn them at all?
- Are review materials, tutors, friends, and family members available to help?
- What other career possibilities are open to her? Does she really want to change directions now?
- How much has her education cost so far? What would her student loan payments be each month?
- What other jobs is she qualified to start immediately? How much would they pay?

Stay in class and spend extra time developing her math skills. Possible results and consequences:

- She masters the math skills and does well in the class.
- She understands just enough to get by and passes the class.
- She tries but just never gets it and fails the class.
- She neglects her other classes when she spends extra time working on math skills.
- She passes all her classes, including math.

New questions to ask:

- How much review does she expect to need? Has she mastered at least the most fundamental math skills (for example, multiplication and division of whole numbers)?
- What resources are available to help her learn the necessary math skills?
- How much extra time can she devote to learning math? (Does she work, have a family to take care of, etc.?)

Go to a hypnotist to cure her math anxiety. Possible results and consequences:

- It works! She looks forward to working with numbers.
- It doesn't work. She still suffers from mental paralysis when faced with a problem that involves numbers.
- She still doesn't love math, but she can get through it to accomplish what needs to be done in her classes and on the job.

New questions to ask:

- Does she think that math anxiety is the problem, or has she just forgotten or never learned the necessary skills?
- Does she believe in hypnosis?
- Is she comfortable trying it?

- Is there a good hypnotist in the area?
- How much does it cost? Can she afford it?

While Kathy decides not to see a hypnotist, just considering this idea helps her realize that math anxiety may be a real problem for her. She decides to seek help from the school counselor and read a book about conquering math anxiety.

STEP FIVE: CHOOSE THE BEST SOLUTION AND ACT ON IT

It is common sense to take a method and try it. If it fails, admit it frankly and try another. But above all, try something.—Franklin Roosevelt

After weighing the various alternatives, select the one that best fits in with your mission and goals. It is easy to spend a lot of time thinking and then be afraid to take action. Think positively, make a plan, and do your best to implement the solution you have chosen. You may decide to combine several alternatives and attack the problem from several directions to increase your chance of success. Kathy decides to stay in the math class. She finds a math tutor and asks her sister to watch her children two afternoons a week to give her the extra time needed for meeting with the tutor and studying. She also decides to use positive self-talk to eliminate her negative feelings about math.

STEP SIX: EVALUATE THE RESULTS AND REVISE AS NEEDED

Did you achieve the desired results? Were there unknown facts or circumstances that resulted in unexpected consequences? How can you revise your plan to get the results you want?

After working with the tutor for three weeks, Kathy realized that this person, though well-meaning, was unable to explain the concepts so that she understood them. She decided to work on her own and bought a computer software program that the math instructor recommended. She also joined a study group in order to share ideas and gain support from other students. The results of her revised plan were positive. She learned the skills she needed, gained self-confidence, and passed her pharmacology class.

MAKING DECISIONS ON THE JOB

Work in health care involves problem solving and decision making. Some of this will be done quickly on the spot. Even in these cases it is important to think through situations, no matter how simple they seem. Health care work should never be performed automatically without thinking of the consequences of your actions.

PRESCRIPTION FOR SUCCESS 6-7

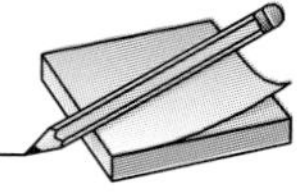

Try Something!

Choose an actual problem from your own experience and go through the six-step process to find and test a solution.

1. Define the problem.

____
____
____

2. Gather information.

   A. Sources

____
____
____

PRESCRIPTION FOR SUCCESS 6–7 (*continued*)

B. Facts, ideas, opinions

____

____

____

____

3. Brainstorm alternative solutions.

____

____

____

4. Consider possible results and consequences.

Results/Consequences	*Additional Questions/Information Needed*
______________	______________
______________	______________
______________	______________

5. Describe the solution you chose and the action you took.

____

____

____

6. Describe and evaluate the results.

____

____

____

Describe any needed revisions.

____

____

Creating a Personal Reference Guide

After graduation you may continue to use your textbooks, lecture notes, and completed assignments as resources. Creating your own reference guide adds even more value to your education by storing useful information that might otherwise be lost. Design the guide to be an organized, easy-to-access source of information that is helpful while you are in school and later in the job search and on the job.

The contents of your guide will vary according to your career area and personal preferences. Here are some suggestions:

- Names, phone numbers, and addresses of instructors and classmates with whom you want to keep in touch.
- Spelling words from the list in Chapter 5 and other words you find difficult to remember.
- New vocabulary words and their definitions.
- Important health care abbreviations. (When you become employed, your facility will have its own set of abbreviations that should be added to your guide.)
- Useful Internet addresses.
- Names, titles, organizations, phone numbers, and addresses of professional contacts. Make a few notes about each person to refresh your memory later.
- Titles of interesting books and journals. Also, titles of reference books that might be useful on the job. Many occupations have pocket-sized guides that contain frequently used measurements, formulas, summaries of common procedures, and so on.

- Inspiring and helpful quotations.
- Names and addresses of professional organizations.
- Sources of equipment and supplies that were used in your school. (This may be of use on the job if you are asked to make recommendations for purchases.)
- Summaries of the procedures you have learned. If check-off sheets are used in your classes, they might serve this purpose.
- Fact sheets that list measurement systems, test values, and so on. Your textbooks may include these within the body of the book or at the end in the form of appendices.
- Potential employers who you learn about from your instructors, graduates, guest speakers, job fairs, newspaper articles, and so on.
- Prescriptions for Success 1-4 and 1-5. These were the self-assessment exercises you completed in Chapter 1. Review them periodically to assess your progress in achieving workplace habits that help ensure on-the-job success.
- A page for each of the resume contents described in Chapter 2:
    1. Career objective
    2. Education
    3. Professional skills and knowledge
    4. Work experience
    5. Licenses and certifications
    6. Honors and awards
    7. Special skills
    8. Community service and volunteer work
    9. Memberships in professional and civic organizations
    10. Languages spoken
    11. References

Review the "To Do Now" suggestions in Chapter 2 for each part of your resume. Continue to add to your resume as you progress through your program. When it is time to actually write your resume, you'll have all the information you need in one place.

Collecting information is not useful if you can't find it when you need it. It can make life more difficult, rather than help, if it becomes simply another pile of stuff that gets in your way. Select a medium-sized or large three-ring binder and buy a package of index dividers. Start with a few categories and add to them as you proceed through your program. A table of contents will help you see what you have at a glance.

Incorporate the building of your guide with your study sessions. For example, writing new vocabulary lists can be part of your review for a terminology quiz. You can do the same thing when learning abbreviations, the steps in procedures, and other facts. You are applying the art of effective time management by accomplishing two things at the same time: creating a useful reference guide and reviewing to ensure maximum learning and retention.

PRESCRIPTION FOR SUCCESS 6–8

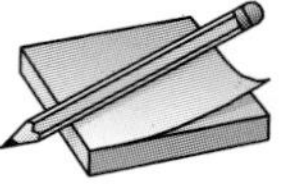

Create a Guide That Works

1. What type of information do you think might be helpful in your personal reference guide?
2. How would you organize a guide to be most helpful to you?

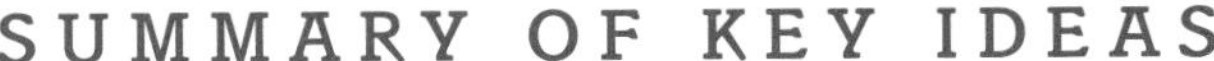

SUMMARY OF KEY IDEAS

1. Practicing hands-on procedures forms the bridge between school and the world of work.
2. The ability to learn math is based as much on our emotions as on our intelligence.
3. Math anxiety can be overcome if we accept our feelings and are willing to find out what we need to learn.
4. Preparation, not panic, is the key to success in your program.
5. The clinical experience is your opportunity to enter the real world of health care.
6. Learning to problem-solve effectively can improve the quality of your life.
7. Creating a personal reference guide can add to the value of your education.

POSITIVE SELF-TALK FOR THIS CHAPTER

1. I am perfecting my skills by the work I do in lab sessions.
2. I can overcome math anxiety and learn what I need to know for health care applications.
3. I am presenting myself competently and professionally in my clinical experience.
4. I use problem-solving techniques to make sound decisions.

REFERENCES

Chester, Gail. *Modern Medical Assisting.* Philadelphia: W.B. Saunders Company, 1998.

O'Toole, Maria, ed. *Miller-Kean Encyclopedia & Dictionary of Medicine, Nursing, & Allied Health,* 6th ed. Philadelphia: W.B. Saunders Company, 1997.

BIBLIOGRAPHY

Kogelman, Stanley and Joseph Warren. *Mind Over Math.* New York: McGraw-Hill Book Company, 1978.

Pauk, Walter. *How to Study in College,* 6th ed. New York: Houghton Mifflin Company, 1997.

7

Developing Your People Skills

OBJECTIVES

THE INFORMATION AND ACTIVITIES IN THIS CHAPTER CAN HELP YOU TO:

- Understand the importance of good people skills.
- Describe ways to better understand people with different backgrounds and beliefs.
- Explain the meaning of empathy and its importance in health care work.
- Become an active listener.
- Improve your effectiveness when speaking.
- Use the various types of questions effectively.
- Become aware of how you and others communicate nonverbally.
- Prepare and present effective oral presentations.
- Practice good teamwork skills.
- Identify the teaching styles of your instructors and describe what you can learn from each.
- Apply effective strategies when dealing with difficult people.
- Explain why criticism is important in the learning process.

KEY TERMS

Debate: Formal discussion in which two people or teams take sides on an issue. Each side tries to persuade the audience to accept its point of view. Debate topics are often controversial.

Diversity: The differences that characterize people in our society. These include native language, religious beliefs, values, and everyday customs.

Empathy: Attempting to understand how another person feels and experiences the world.

Feedback: Techniques used in spoken communication to check your understanding of the speaker's message.

Nonverbal communication: Facial expressions, gestures, nondeliberate movements, and body position. While gestures are usually deliberate, people are mostly unaware of their nonverbal communication.

Organizational culture: The customs and practices of an organization that influence all aspects of how work is accomplished and what is considered appropriate behavior.

Teamwork: Working with other people to accomplish a common goal. Modern patient care depends on teams of professionals working together.

The Importance of People Skills

The last few chapters focused on you as an individual and the personal attitudes, habits, and skills that will influence your academic and career success. In this chapter, we shift our focus to other people and how you relate to them. You can expect to work closely with many kinds of people in performing your health care duties, and your ability to create and maintain mutually beneficial relationships will be an important factor in your job performance.

The quality and consistency of patient care are affected by how well health care professionals communicate among themselves and with patients and their families. Poor communication skills demonstrated by health care professionals are a contributing factor to the growing number of malpractice lawsuits. When patients feel that they are listened to and understood, they are less likely to sue. This is true even if their treatment outcomes are negative.

One of the most frequent complaints from employers today is that their employees lack good people skills. They don't know how to work well with others. More people fail on the job because of poor interpersonal skills than because they lack the necessary technical qualifications.

Good interpersonal skills are also important for academic success. Throughout your studies, you will have opportunities to learn from both your instructors and fellow students. Your ability to communicate effectively will influence both the quantity and the quality of learning. Activities such as working on teams, practicing hands-on skills with other students, and joining study groups are ways you can start now to practice working with others. Most of life's activities take place in relation to other people. Improving the quality of these relationships can improve the overall quality of your life.

RESPECTING OTHERS

Be kind. Remember, everyone you meet is fighting a hard battle.—Thompson

By choosing a career in health care, you have accepted the responsibility to serve others. You must believe in the principle that all human beings deserve to be treated with respect and dignity. Your duties may range from performing an uncomfortable medical procedure to explaining a complicated bill for an office visit. It will be your obligation to serve all patients or clients with an equal level of care and concern, regardless of their appearance, behavior, level of education, or economic status. Not everyone will look, act, behave, or even smell as you would like. They will not all express appreciation for your efforts. The satisfaction you obtain from your work must be based on what you can give to others, not on what you receive from them.

The need to treat all patients equally and fairly has been recognized and endorsed by the American Hospital Association. It is formalized in writing as the Patient's Bill of Rights, briefly summarized in Chapter 1. It includes the right of all patients to be treated with consideration and respect. This principle forms the foundation on which all health care is delivered.

It is also important to demonstrate respect toward your supervisor and coworkers. The quality of work produced in any organization depends on the quality of the relationships among the people who work there, and good relationships are based on mutual respect.

Guidelines for Respectful Communication

Adhering to the following guidelines will allow you to interact respectfully with your patients, supervisor, and coworkers.

- *Be courteous.* Many observers today have noted a trend away from the practice of common courtesy. People often fail to use expressions like "please" and "thank you." These are powerful words that improve the quality of both personal and professional relationships.

- *Maintain professionalism.* As a student and on the job, it is important to project maturity and competence. Examples of inappropriate communication behaviors are chewing gum, arguing, swearing, and yelling.
- *Acknowledge the other person.* No one likes to be ignored. If you are busy working with someone else or talking on the telephone, use eye contact and a quick nod to let the person know that you are aware of his or her presence.
- *Don't interrupt.* Avoid breaking in when another person is speaking. Some people need extra time to compose their thoughts or express themselves. Avoid the habit of finishing sentences for others. This frustrates the speaker, and your assumption about what they planned to say may be incorrect.
- *Guard privacy.* This is always a good practice in your personal life. In health care, patient privacy is protected by law. It is illegal to discuss patient information with anyone who is not working directly with the patient. Make a habit of never sharing anything told to you in confidence by family members, friends, or classmates. (The patient must give written permission before information can be given to insurance companies, other health providers, and so on.)
- *Avoid gossip.* Gossip is a growing and very serious problem in the workplace. It serves no useful purpose and can lead to hurt feelings, broken trust, and strained relationships at school and at work. If it involves confidential patient matters, it can lead to a lawsuit.
- *Show interest.* Look at the other person when you are talking and listening. Show that you are listening by nodding or using confirming sounds or phrases such as "uh, huh," "I understand," "okay," and so on. Don't point yourself toward the door as if to say, "Hurry up. I need to move on to something else."
- *Remain calm.* It is important to behave and speak calmly when you are dealing with situations such as emergencies and angry patients. This provides reassurance to others and allows you to focus on doing what can best help the situation.

PRESCRIPTION FOR SUCCESS 7-1

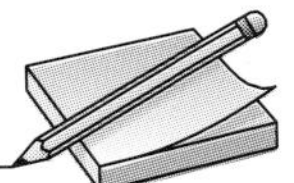

Showing Respect

1. What other ways can you think of to show respect to others when communicating?
2. Describe a situation in which someone made you feel that you were respected. How was respect communicated to you?
3. Why is showing respect to patients an important part of providing health care?

Appreciating Diversity

Commandment Number One of any truly civilized society is this: Let people be different.—David Grayson

The population of the United States is made up of people from all over the world. Immigration has increased dramatically in recent years, and Americans now represent a wider variety than ever of races, religions, lifestyles, languages, and educational and economic levels. These variations are known as **diversity.**

Diversity also refers to differences that are not related to cultural background or race. These include age, sexual orientation, disabilities, and appearance. People who are different are sometimes ignored or cruelly mistreated. Sometimes this is not done intentionally. For example, it is not uncommon for health care professionals to speak to younger relatives who accompany very elderly patients as if the patients were not present.

Our society can benefit from the contribution of people with different customs and ideas. By drawing from a variety of viewpoints, we increase our chances of solving the complex problems encountered in modern society. Differences can be beneficial, as when Americans find pain relief from the ancient Chinese practice of acupuncture. Unfortunately, differences in values and beliefs about life can cause misunderstandings and even violence. Learning to take advantage of the differences and peacefully work out the misunderstandings is one of the major challenges faced by the world today.

Working in health care enables you to work with people from many different backgrounds. There will be opportunities to learn about other cultures and promote mutual understanding. Your personal actions and efforts to understand and serve others can make a difference. These opportunities may occur while you are in school because today's student populations also reflect our diversity. If your own background is different from that of the majority of your classmates, you can serve as a source of information about your culture.

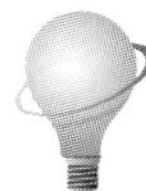

Take a Moment to Think

1. Which cultural groups are represented in your area?
2. How much do you know about their customs and beliefs?
3. How could you learn more?

Promote Understanding

Here are suggestions for ways that students from all backgrounds can benefit from diversity in their classes and on the job:

- *Put fear aside.* Some people are frightened by what they don't understand. Others are afraid that accepting differences among people will somehow result in negative changes in society. In fact, the contributions of people from different backgrounds have resulted in the economic success and political stability of the United States. Different viewpoints provide us with many ways to resolve the problems of living.
- *Listen to other points of view.* Seek opportunities to interact with people whose backgrounds are different from yours. Encourage them to express their ideas and opinions. Listen carefully to what they have to say.
- *Ask questions.* Use questions to learn more, but never challenge the other person. For example, instead of asking, "Why do you believe *that*?" you could say, "That sounds interesting. Could you explain more about that?" Your goal is to learn and understand, not to imply that the other person is wrong.
- *Avoid stereotypes.* Don't make assumptions about people because of their age, race, gender, or other categories. Consider each person as an individual with a unique set of characteristics.
- *Don't judge people by their appearance.* Outward appearances do not always represent who people are. To truly know people, you must talk with them and observe their actions. If you immediately dismiss them based on how they look, you may lose the opportunity to form a friendship or a beneficial working relationship.

- *Explore different cultures.* Many schools and communities sponsor activities that highlight the cultures represented in the local population. Check your local library and the Internet for other sources of information about the backgrounds of your classmates and future patients.
- *Learn about other value systems.* People are defined by their values and beliefs about how they should live. Culture is much more than typical foods and daily customs. Develop a deeper level of knowledge and understanding through conversation and by learning about the religions and important beliefs of the groups in your area.
- *Look for commonalities.* As human beings, we all share many of the same needs, concerns, and goals for our lives. Find out what you have in common with those who seem different.
- *Offer to help others.* Expand your attitude of caring by looking for ways to help others. Extend a hand to those who are different and may suffer from discrimination. Offer to help a classmate who has trouble understanding English.
- *Learn another language.* You may not have time now to study another language formally, but you can learn a few key phrases of any major cultural groups in your area. This can also increase your worth to an employer.

When we learn about others, we also learn about ourselves and what it means to be human. Enrich your life by welcoming diversity and seeking opportunities to learn new ways to see the world.

Cultural Differences in Everyday Life

Everything we do is influenced by our cultural background. Knowing where some of these differences exist can help you to better understand the people you encounter at school and at work. Principles that many of us take for granted, such as "It is important to always be on time," are not important to everyone. Making assumptions can result in misunderstandings. Let's look at an example. A patient has to wait fifteen minutes before you can perform his lab test. In an effort to respect his time and not add to the delay, you keep conversation to a minimum and complete the procedure as quickly as possible. You believe that you have been considerate. The patient, from a culture that does not consider time in the same way, is insulted. His interpretation is that you obviously have more important things to do than work with him, so you are rushing along. The "right thing" in your eyes was the "wrong thing" in his.

Of course, it is impossible to know and accommodate every cultural difference that you encounter. You can, however, be aware of what types of differences exist and strive to be sensitive to them. Ask questions if you are unsure about a person's feelings or understanding of a situation. Table 7-1 contains examples of common areas of differences among cultures.

EXPERIENCING EMPATHY

Empathy means seeing the world through the eyes of others. It means understanding their feelings and experiences. This is not always easy because we are all influenced by our individual set of beliefs, values, and previous experiences. Being empathetic starts with listening carefully to others without judging what you hear. The next step is reflecting on what you heard and, if necessary, asking for clarification or more information. What is the person trying to communicate or trying to hide? What clues can you get from the person's body language? What is important to the speaker?

It is essential for the health care professional to have empathy with patients in order to understand their needs and learn how best to help them. Practicing empathy conveys the message "You are important and worth my time and respect. I will make every effort to know who you are and what you need."

TABLE 7–1 ***Common Cultural Differences***

Time	It is important to always be on time for meetings and appointments Appointment times are just estimations of when they might take place. Time is valuable and should not be wasted. Time is not a resource over which we have control. It just is. Planning and using time productively is important. If something is important, it will eventually get done; there is no reason to rush. The present is more important than the future. The present should be used for planning and preparing for the future.
Personal Space	The distance comfortably maintained when people are talking ranges from a few inches (when you can feel the breath of the other person on your face) to over a foot away.
Age	Youth is valued. People should try to maintain a young appearance and lifestyle as long as possible (exercise, wrinkle creams, and hair dyes). Older people are valued for their wisdom and shown great respect. When elderly people are no longer able to care for themselves, it is appropriate to place them in nursing or retirement homes. Older people should live with and be cared for by family members until they die.
Touching	Shaking hands is okay for everyone. Only members of the same sex can shake hands with each other. Hugging is okay for everyone, even members of the same sex. Kissing is okay between women. When meeting a new person, only a slight bow is permitted, not touching.
Gender	A woman cannot be treated by a male physician. Women and men are equal. Men are dominant. Women act as the head of most families. Women have no economic or political power.
Eye Contact	Direct eye contact is a sign of sincerity, honesty, and interest in the other person. It is a sign of disrespect. Sustained eye contact communicates hostility and aggression or sexual interest.
Personal Control	Each person is in control of his or her own life. Luck, fate, or the will of god determine how things turn out.
Spiritual Practices	There is one god. God helps those who help themselves. God punishes those who sin. God answers all prayers. Unsure about the existence of god. There is no god. Witchcraft and magic exist and can be used to help us.
Definition of Success	Personal and professional achievement. Acquiring material possessions. Living a spiritual life. Achieving inner peace. Raising many children. Being a kind person and helping others.
Health Care Beliefs	Disease is caused by germs, environmental conditions, and personal habits such as smoking. Illness is a punishment sent by god. Illness happens when the body's energy or humors get out of balance. Science has the best answers for preventing and curing disease. The body can heal itself naturally. Herbs are the best remedies. Only god can heal.

PRESCRIPTION FOR SUCCESS 7–2

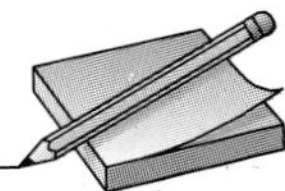

What Would It Be Like . . . ?

Answer the questions that follow for patients in the following conditions:

Paralyzed
In pain
Unable to work
Blind
Poor and without health insurance
Elderly and alone
Unable to speak English
Suffering from a terminal illness

1. What emotions might they be experiencing?
2. What might be their concerns and fears?
3. What are their major needs likely to be, both physical and emotional?
4. How are their conditions likely to affect their quality of life?
5. How could you learn more about each person?

Part of empathy is letting the other person know that you are trying to understand his or her experience. It is best, however, not to say that you know *exactly* how he or she feels. This sounds insincere because, in fact, it is impossible to know precisely how another person feels. In trying to be helpful, we may be tempted to share and compare our own stories—for example, saying, "Oh, I know just what you mean. The same thing happened to me . . ." and then launching into a detailed explanation about what happened to us. This shifts the focus to ourselves and away from the person who needs the attention.

Learning to experience empathy improves all interpersonal relationships, including those with friends, family members, classmates, instructors, coworkers, and supervisors. Our lives are more harmonious when we learn to see the views of others. You can start practicing empathy now at home and in school.

- When you are talking with your classmates, listen carefully. How are their views different from yours? What experiences have they had that explain these differences?
- Are there students who exhibit poor behavior? Why do you think they behave in this way? What are some clues that might explain their actions?
- Why do family members sometimes "act out?"
- What kinds of experiences have shaped the opinions of your friends?

Oral Communication: Creating the People Connection

Many people believe that they are good communicators because they are friendly and like to talk. But the ability to speak is only one part of effective communication. There are three other essential parts to effective communication in addition to what we call "talking." These are listening, requesting feedback, and using and interpreting nonverbal communication (body language and gestures). Successful oral communication takes place when the receiver receives the intended message of the speaker. We all know that this is not always the case! Let's look at how you can increase the effectiveness of your communication.

SPEAKING

Speaking involves creating and sending messages. The first step in creating a clear message is to determine your purpose. Just as when you are writing, it is important to know your communication goal.

- Provide information
  Examples: help a classmate who missed an important lecture, provide patient education, give instructions to a coworker.
- Demonstrate knowledge
  Examples: give a presentation in class, describe your training to a potential employer in a job interview, explain your performance to a supervisor.
- Persuade
  Examples: convince a friend not to cheat on a test, show a potential employer why you are qualified for the job, inspire a patient to follow her exercise program.
- Gather information
  Examples: ask questions in class, ask a professional contact for career information, conduct a patient interview.
- Acknowledge others
  Examples: greeting people, asking how they are, expressing interest in their lives.

Who Is Your Receiver?

Effective messages match the purpose of the speaker with the needs of the receiver. Consider the following factors to create appropriate messages:

- Age
- Level of education
- Cultural background
- Language fluency
- Physical condition
- Emotional state
- Disabilities, such as hearing impairment
- Level of pain and medication

Develop Good Speaking Habits

The following guidelines can help you improve your oral communication skills and ensure that your message gets across.

- Choose a level of language that is appropriate for the receiver. If a person is heavily medicated, for example, use simple words and short sentences.
- Choose appropriate vocabulary. Using medical terminology is an effective way to be precise when speaking with coworkers, but it can be confusing for patients. They may hesitate to tell you that they don't understand because they don't want to look stupid.
- Avoid slang and nonstandard speech. These are often characteristic of certain age and social groups and can cause misunderstandings with people outside those groups. Speech that is appropriate among friends and at social gatherings may not be correct for school and work. For example the current use of "goes" to mean "says" is understood by many young people but may be misunderstood by others.
- Speak clearly and at a moderate speed—not so quickly that you are difficult to understand or so slowly that the receiver's mind wanders. (We listen and comprehend many times faster than we speak.)
- Avoid speaking in a monotone. Speak naturally, but with expression in your voice. Make sure it is appropriate for your message. For example, speak with respect when asking questions in class, friendliness when greeting a new student, reassurance when calming fears, and firmness when giving instructions that affect patient safety.

ACTIVE LISTENING

To listen well is as powerful a means of communication as to talk well.—U.S. Supreme Court Chief Justice John Marshall

Active listening should not be confused with hearing. Listening requires effort, while hearing is more passive. Listening requires that you pay attention, focus on the speaker's words, and think about what you hear. Active listening demonstrates respect for the speaker. It is an essential skill for the health care professional because all patients want to work with someone who will listen to them.

Think about your own listening skills. Do you catch your mind wandering and thinking about other things? Do you think about what you are going to say next? Do you argue mentally when you disagree? These habits can interfere with your attention and prevent you from understanding the speaker's message. Try the following techniques to improve your listening skills:

- Prepare yourself mentally to listen by clearing your mind of other thoughts.
- Control the noise level of your environment as much as possible. Turn off the radio or television, look for a quiet place to talk, or move out of the busiest part of the office.
- Focus on the other person. What are his or her needs? What does the person want to talk about? What are his or her problems? How can you help? What can you learn from this encounter?
- Concentrate on following what the speaker is saying. Sometimes when we think we are listening, looking at the speaker, and perhaps even nodding in agreement, we are actually thinking about something else. Practice being aware of where your attention is directed.
- If you disagree with what you are hearing, try not to engage in mental arguments. Internal self-talk interferes with your ability to listen. It is easy to understand people we agree with. It takes more effort to hear people we disagree with, but only by listening carefully can we begin to understand them.
- Practice making quick mental notes about points you need to clarify. Work on being able to do this without losing track of what the person is saying.
- Focus on what is being said rather than how it is said. Move beyond the speaker's appearance, manners, language level, or even odor. Try not to let unpleasant factors about the person interfere with your ability to concentrate on what he or she has to say.
- Acknowledge the person even if you are taking notes or performing a test or procedure while he or she is talking. Look at the person from time to time and make eye contact.

Listening effectively is one of the most valuable skills you can develop for both personal and professional success. It can increase your learning, your effectiveness in helping others, and even your popularity. At the same time, it is a skill that many people neglect because they assume that they know how to use it. Pay attention to how well you listen. Working on improving your listening skills is one of the most important actions you can take to work well with others.

GIVING FEEDBACK

Feedback is used to check your understanding of what the speaker says. In spite of careful listening, what you hear may not be what the speaker intended. Misunderstandings can occur when we assume that we understand the speaker's message. There are several methods for giving and requesting feedback:

- *Paraphrasing.* This means saying what you heard in your own words so that the speaker can confirm or correct your statement.

  Examples: "Let me make sure that I have it right. We're to do exercises 3 through 7 on page 83 in the workbook and turn them in on Friday?"

  "It sounds like the pain is much worse when you first wake up in the morning but decreases during the day."
- *Reflecting.* This is similar to paraphrasing, but you repeat what the other person says using words as close as possible to his or her own words. This gives the person the opportunity to confirm or add additional information.

  Examples: "You said that you don't have time to join our study group because of your work schedule . . ." (You suspect there may be another reason, and if it is known, arrangements could be made for the person to join the group.)

"You haven't lost any weight because the diet isn't working . . ." (There may be other reasons, such as not following the diet exactly, lack of exercise, and so on.)

- *Clarifying.* Asking the speaker to explain what he or she means.
  Examples: "You said the tests in medical terminology are really hard. Can you give me an example of a question?"
  "Can you explain what you mean when you say your son has been acting 'strangely' since he started taking the medication?"

PRESCRIPTION FOR SUCCESS 7–3

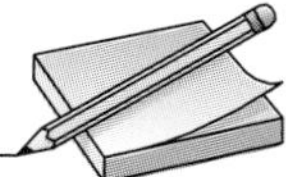

Rate Your Communication Skills

Think about and become aware of your own communication skills.

1. Do any areas need improvement?
2. If so, what can you do to improve them?
3. Who can help you improve your communication skills?

ASKING QUESTIONS

No man really becomes a fool until he stops asking questions.—Charles P. Steinmetz

Scientific discoveries and technological advances are based on people asking questions. What causes . . . ? What would happen if . . . ? How can we . . . ? Asking questions is a powerful tool for learning. In school you can increase your knowledge and understanding by asking questions. Yet many students sit through hours of classes and never ask a single question. Maximize your learning by being prepared to ask good questions in class.

- *Prepare ahead for class.* If you haven't read the assignment or completed the other homework, you won't have the background information on which to base a question.
- *Write questions down.* You did the reading and remember that there were several points you didn't understand. But you didn't write them down, and now you can't remember what they were. During lectures, write down questions as you think of them so that you can ask them at the appropriate time.
- *Don't be embarrassed.* No one wants to ask a stupid question. The fact is, if you already knew everything, you wouldn't be in school, right? Instructors welcome questions in class and are usually pleased when students take an interest in the subject. (Exception: You don't pay attention in class and often ask questions that force the instructor to repeat what he or she just finished saying.)
- *Ask them later.* If all the class time is taken up with the lecture or the instructor never gets around to your lab group, arrange a time to ask your questions later. Be willing to make the extra effort to get the help you need.
- *Be brave.* You find yourself so confused that you can't even phrase a question. This is exactly when you should ask a question. "I'm lost here. Could we go back to . . . ?" Avoid getting so far behind that you don't have a chance of catching up.

On the job, it will be important to know when to ask questions. For example, never proceed with a task if you are unsure about any part of it. It is smarter to ask than to take safety risks, waste supplies, or make it necessary for someone else to redo your work. Questions are also a good way to show interest in your job and gain a better understanding of your duties.

Types of Questions

Gathering information from patients is an important part of most health care occupations. Your ability to ask effective questions, combined with active listening, can increase the amount and quality of information received both at school and on the job. There are four basic types of questions:

1. *Closed-ended.* These can be answered with a "yes" or "no" or in one or two words. They are used for getting specific facts.
   Examples: "What is the date of the math test? Can we use our calculators?" "Have you ever had surgery? In what year?"
2. *Open-ended.* These questions require a longer answer and request explanations, descriptions, examples, and other details.
   Examples: "How would you recommend that we study for the math test?" "What was your understanding of why you needed surgery?"
3. *Probing.* Questions are based on what the other person has already told you. The purpose is to learn additional information.
   Examples: "Could you give us an example of the kind of question that will be on the test?" "After you had the surgery, describe how you found it easier to walk."
4. *Leading.* The question provides a possible answer. These questions should be used with great care because they may encourage the other person to simply agree because he or she doesn't really understand the question or thinks that this is the right answer. Leading questions can be helpful with people who find it difficult to communicate because of injury, language barriers, shyness, or other problems that make communicating difficult.
   Example: "Did you not do the exercises at home because you didn't understand the instructions?"

PRESCRIPTION FOR SUCCESS 7-4

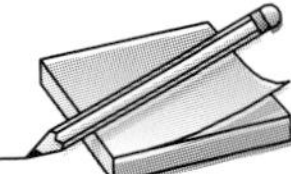

And the Question Is . . .

Create two examples of each of the four types of questions.

1. Closed-ended ______________________
   ____
2. Open-ended ______________________
   ____
3. Probing ______________________
   ____
4. Leading ______________________
   ____

Effective Questions

Using the following techniques can increase the effectiveness of your questions:

- *Plan them in advance.* Be prepared to get the most out of every potential learning situation. Some situations should be approached with questions in mind. Write down questions to ask in class or at your clinical site. Note questions as you think of them about your career area to ask professional contacts. Start a list of questions you might want to ask at job interviews. Sometimes we fail to take full advantage of potential learning opportunities because we don't think of questions until it is too late.
- *Allow silence.* Some people need more time than others to think and prepare a response. Unless it is obvious that they didn't understand the question, don't feel that you must speak in order to fill the silence.

- *Avoid challenging or judgmental questions.* Your choice of words and tone of voice can communicate the negative message "You are wrong, and I demand an explanation." For example, questions like "*Why* did you do that?" or "What *were* you thinking?" may draw a defensive reaction or no response at all. A major purpose of communication is to encourage discussion so that issues can be resolved.
- *Choose the right place.* Some important questions are personal, embarrassing, or potentially challenging. A question for the instructor about a low grade you believe to be unfair is best asked in private, not during class. An interview with a patient with acquired immune deficiency syndrome (AIDS) should be conducted out of the hearing of others.
- *Choose the right time.* Asking your supervisor a question about your performance when he or she is ready to leave the office isn't fair to either of you.
- *Know what not to ask.* There is a difference between showing interest in others and asking questions that are too personal. People can be offended by questions that seem too personal. To show concern without prying, you can say, "You seem really upset. Is there some way I can help?" This allows the person to reveal as much information as is comfortable. If you must ask potentially embarrassing questions, explain why you are asking them and how the information will be used. Assure patients that anything they say will remain confidential, as required by law.
- *Know what's legal.* Some questions, especially when asked in hiring situations, are illegal. These include asking about age, marital status, number of children, and other matters that are not related to job performance.

Nonverbal Communication

More than half of the content of our messages is communicated nonverbally through our movements, posture, gestures, and facial expressions. In fact, **nonverbal communication** is usually more informative than verbal communication because it occurs unconsciously. For example, telling a friend that you are "fine" when you have a worried expression on your face sends a mixed message. The friend is more likely to believe your face than your words. Nonverbal communication can define or distort the content of verbal messages.

Pay attention to your own nonverbal language (Fig. 7–1). The following questions can guide you:

- Do you have nervous habits, such as jiggling your leg or playing with your hair, that distract from or distort your messages? These habits can give the impression that you would rather be elsewhere.
- Is your general posture upright or slouching? Do you face the person you're talking with or partially turn away, as if looking for escape? Leaning forward slightly toward the other person communicates interest.
- Do you assume an accepting body position? Crossing the arms, for example, can be a sign of being closed to what the other person is saying.
- Do you use gestures to emphasize or add meaning to your words? Or are they routine habits that add nothing to your message? Gestures are especially helpful when used for demonstrations and to communicate with people who have limited ability to understand spoken language. Examples include very young children, non-English speakers, and the hearing impaired.
- Does your face express interest or boredom? In class, do you usually face the instructor or look out the window? When an activity is announced, do you roll your eyes and exchange pained looks with other students? Poor attitudes are easy to read and can negatively affect the quality of the class by putting the instructor on the defensive. Learning to control facial expressions is important because, as a health care professional, you will need to maintain expressions that convey caring and reassurance even in difficult situations.
- Do you smile whenever it is appropriate? Does your face send the message "I'm glad to be here talking with you"?

- Do you maintain good eye contact? Looking away while you are speaking communicates a lack of sincerity, interest, or respect. (Exceptions to this include cultures that consider looking down to be a sign of respect.)

In addition to monitoring your own nonverbal communication, practice observing it in others. Learn to "listen between the lines." Do the speaker's words and actions match? Are there nonverbal signs of confusion, fear, or anger that you should take into account? Does your instructor give the nonverbal messages, discussed in Chapter 4, that communicate what is most important for you to learn?

Ask for clarification if verbal and nonverbal messages seem to conflict. Be willing to take the time and make the effort to get the true message. You can improve the interpersonal relationships in all areas of your life by combining an understanding of nonverbal communication with active listening and feedback.

PRESCRIPTION FOR SUCCESS 7–5

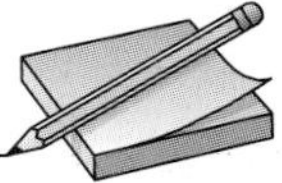

What Does It Mean?

Choose a time and place to observe people as they are communicating.

1. Give at least three examples of nonverbal behaviors.
2. Can you tell what they mean?

   Self-observation
3. How can you become more aware of your own nonverbal communication?
4. Are there habits you often use when speaking?

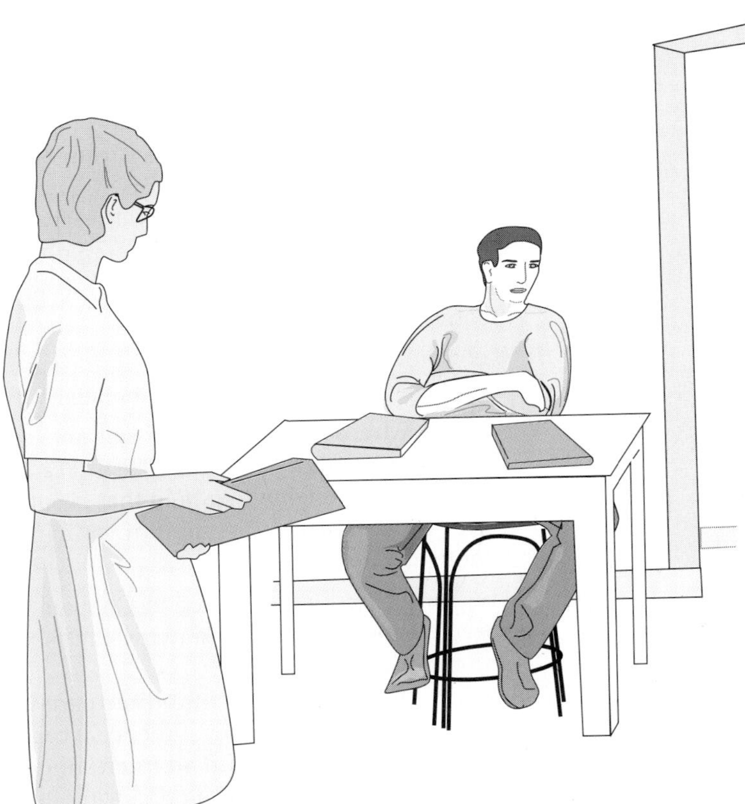

FIGURE 7–1 What message is this student communicating to the instructor?

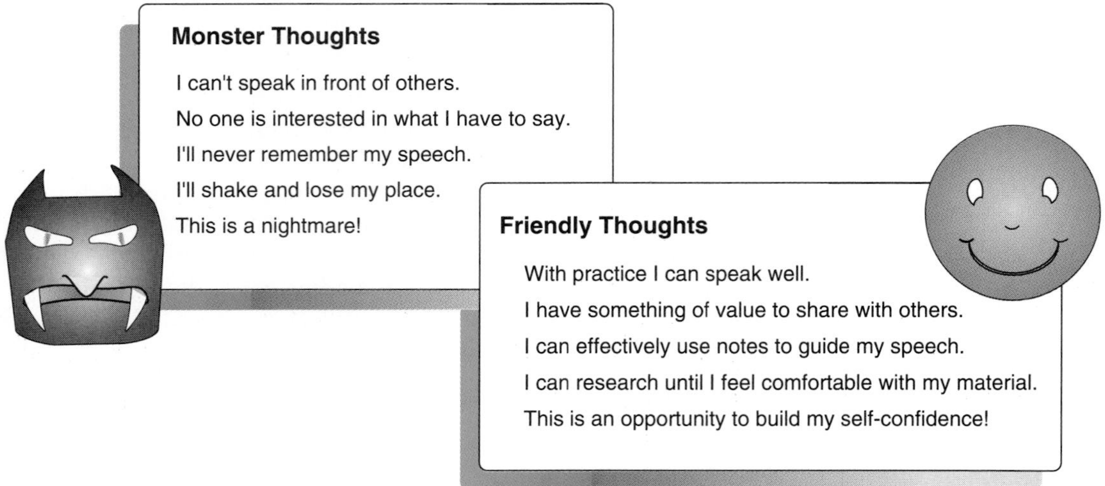

FIGURE 7–2 Turn public speaking monsters into friends.

Giving Presentations with Confidence

Many students find speaking in front of a group a frightening experience. This is a fear worth conquering, because the ability to speak with confidence can increase your opportunities to grow professionally and advance in your career. Proper preparation and a lot of practice can take the terror out of public speaking (Fig. 7–2).

PREPARATION

Preparing an oral presentation requires the same skills needed for writing: research and organization. It is said that an excellent way to learn something is to explain it to someone else. Convert oral presentations into positive experiences by focusing on how you can learn from them.

The steps for preparing a speech are similar to the suggestions given in Chapter 5 for writing a paper.

I. Choose your topic early. It should be something you want to know more about or something you have strong feelings about. (Note: If you must speak on a topic with which you disagree, as sometimes happens with **debates** on controversial subjects, this is a chance to practice seeing other points of view and experiencing empathy.)

II. Be clear about your purpose: inform, persuade, demonstrate, encourage people to take action, entertain.

III. Know your audience. What is their background? How much do they know about the topic? What are their beliefs? What is their interest level?

IV. Identify what you need to find out and do your research. Make sure you have accurate, up-to-date facts. Health care work demands accuracy. This is especially challenging in a field that is constantly advancing and changing. Start now to develop the habit of verifying all information you use or distribute to others.

V. Use the techniques suggested in Chapter 5 to organize the content of your speech. These include mind maps, idea sheets, note cards, the brain dump, and questions.

VI. Divide your presentation into three parts:

   A. Introduction ("Tell the audience what you're going to tell them"). Engage your listeners with an interesting story or fact. Give them a reason to pay attention. Why is this topic important to them? What should they know about it? How does it relate to their lives? Approach your audience with the attitude that you have something to offer them. This helps put both you and them at ease.

B. Body ("Tell them"). This part takes up the most time. In it you explain and develop your ideas; give supporting facts, details, and examples; narrate events; and tell stories. This is the "meat" of your presentation.

C. Conclusion ("Tell them what you've told them"). Briefly review your major points, show how they tie together, and summarize why they are important. Tell the audience what action you want them to take or how they can use what you have told them.

VII. Compose your speech so that it flows smoothly. For example, you might number your major points. Tell your audience how many there will be and then announce each one as you come to it:

"The kidneys have five important functions. The first is the regulation of fluid and electrolytes." (You then explain how they do this.)
"The second function is regulation of blood pressure." (More explanation.)
"The third is . . ." (etc.)

It is especially important that oral presentations be put together in a logical, organized manner. With written material, readers can take their time and go back if they miss a point or don't understand something. Listeners don't have this advantage. You continue talking whether they are following what you're saying or not. You can lose them entirely if you jump from topic to topic, fail to support your ideas, or don't provide clear and complete explanations of the material.

Some students are most comfortable writing out their presentation using complete sentences, as if it were a paper to be turned in. (In fact, some instructors require submission of a written report that corresponds with an oral presentation.) At a minimum, you should write out a fairly detailed outline of your talk. Use this to plan the order of the material and act as a framework for including important facts and examples.

Memory Joggers

It is usually a bad idea to read directly from your paper when giving the presentation. You may be tempted to look only at your paper instead of at the audience. Presentations that are read lack the warmth of human interaction and are less interesting for the audience. You should become familiar enough with your material to use one of the following prompts to help you remember what you plan to say.

- *Note cards* with key points.
  - Advantages: Small and easy to handle. Prevent you from reading directly from your paper. Encourage you to practice the speech beforehand and become familiar with the material.
  - Watch Out For: Having too many cards and getting them confused. Failing to number the cards and getting them out of order. Fiddling with them, which distracts the audience. Not including enough information on them and forgetting what you meant to say about each point.
- *Outline* on full sheets of paper.
  - Advantages: Includes more information than note cards and may increase your confidence in remembering what you plan to say.
  - Watch Out For: Rattling the paper while you speak. Looking at the paper instead of the audience. Holding the paper with both hands and failing to use natural gestures while you speak.
- *Mind map* with major topics and supporting points in graphic form.

- Advantages: Easy to see major points at a glance. Especially helpful if you are a visual or global learner and don't need a lot of notes to remember what you plan to say.
- Watch Out For: May be less room on the page to include detail, so be sure you know your material. Sometimes mind maps have words written at angles and are difficult to read quickly. Make sure that you set it up in an easy-to-read format so that you don't get lost. Nonvisual learners are not likely to find these maps helpful.

- *Key points* written on overhead transparencies, on charts, or listed on the board (Fig. 7–3). They serve both as visual aids for the audience and as a guide for you.
  - Advantages: You and the audience are working together and sharing the experience of looking at the same materials. Listeners become more involved if they are both listening and seeing. This technique also helps visual learners (the majority) follow your presentation.

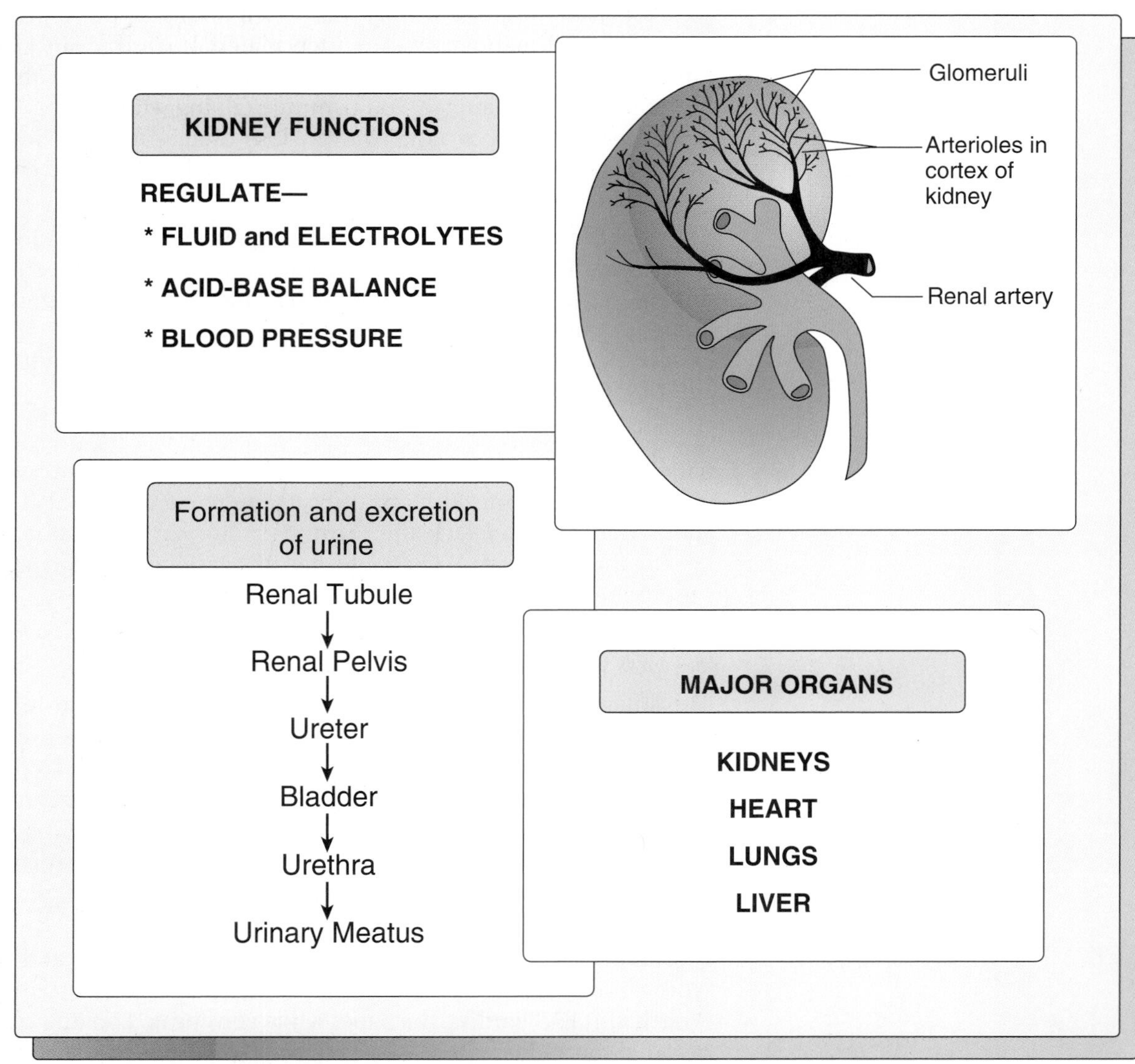

FIGURE 7–3 Effective posters and overheads for presentations. (Chabner, Davi-Ellen. *The Language of Medicine,* 5th ed. Philadelphia: W.B. Saunders Company, 1996, p. 193, with permission.)

- Watch Out For: Poorly prepared visual aids that have too much information or lettering that is difficult for the audience to see. Technology failures such as burned-out light bulbs or no extension cord (or discovering at the last minute that the projector is being used by another class!). Prior planning and consulting with the instructor are critical to prevent being tripped up during your presentation.

Practice

The audience is not the enemy. Lack of preparation and practice is.

Give yourself the best chance possible to give a smooth presentation by practicing it a few times before doing it for real. Friends and family members make a good audience. You will have the reassurance that comes from being familiar with your materials and knowing that you have anticipated any problems *before* you stand in front of an audience.

Should you memorize what you plan to say? Unless you are entering a formal speech contest or it is part of the assignment, this is usually not necessary or even a good idea. First, it is time-consuming. Second, it can make you sound stiff and unnatural. Finally, and perhaps most important, if you forget a line or lose your place, it can be hard to get back on track. Rather than continuing to talk as you would with natural speech, you are in the uncomfortable position of trying to remember exactly where you are. The resulting long pause is very uncomfortable for both you *and* your audience.

The best advice is to practice enough so that you can speak intelligently on your topic while using your prompts as guides. Here are some tips to make the most effective use of your practice time.

I. Practice as if you were presenting the speech in front of an audience: stand up, speak out loud, and use appropriate expressions and gestures.

II. Use the actual materials that will serve as your prompts (note cards, outline, etc.). Are they clear and easy to follow?

III. If the speech has time requirements, use a timer or clock to see if you need to lengthen or shorten your material.

IV. Practice at least once in front of a mirror. Check your expressions and gestures. Do they seem natural? Do you have habits that might distract the audience, such as twisting your hair, shifting your weight back and forth, or staring straight ahead?

V. If you have an opportunity, record yourself and listen for expression and fill-in words ("uh," "you know," "okay," etc.). Are you speaking in a monotone? Too fast or too slow? Too loud or too soft? Do you mumble? Do you know how to pronounce all the words?

VI. Practice in front of a real audience: friends, classmates, or family members. Ask for an honest evaluation.

VII. If you can, practice in the same room in which you will give your speech. If this is not practical, at least check the important details.

   A. Is there a place to set down your cards or outline, or will you have to hold them as you speak? If you are short (like the author), can you see over the podium?

   B. Do you know how to operate the overhead projector? In which direction should the transparencies be placed? How do you adjust the image? Is the machine in working order? Are the transparencies visible from the back row?

   C. Is there chalk or a pen available for the blackboard or white board? Will you have time to write out what you need? Is there an eraser?

   D. Is there a place to hang your charts, graphs, and other illustrations? Will you need tape, tacks, and so on?

E. If you have models, samples, or other objects to show, is there a place to set them? Will the audience be able to see them? Will you pass them around?

PRESENTATION

You've prepared and practiced and feel reasonably ready to give your presentation. There are some techniques that will make it more comfortable:

1. Before you start to speak, take a breath, smile, and look at your audience. Even if you don't *feel* glad to be there, *act* as if you are. Try putting yourself and everyone else at ease.
2. Look at the audience while you are speaking. Make eye contact with them. Look around the audience, not just in one direction. Catch the eyes of people who appear to be listening attentively and are "with you" to increase your feelings of support.
3. Pause briefly if necessary. Some speakers even use pauses for dramatic effect. If you need a moment to gather your thoughts, stay calm. It is better to pause than to nervously ramble on or repeat filler words ("uh") that, if overused, are distracting. Pauses also give the audience time to reflect on what you have said.
4. If you do lose your place or blank out a whole portion of your talk, stop and take a breath. Try not to panic. Acknowledge the audience with a smile or a nod (they may be as nervous as you are), and then concentrate on getting reorganized.
5. Shift your focus from yourself to the audience. Remember that you have prepared well and have something of value to share. The audience needs this information, and you are being of service by sharing it with them.
6. An old trick used by speakers is to imagine the audience in a funny situation: dressed in silly costumes, wearing big fake noses, standing on their heads—anything to change your perception of them as a threat.

Consider organizing a buddy system. If you are already in a study group with classmates, that might do the trick. Practice your speeches for each other and offer constructive suggestions. Ask them to "cheer you on" by making eye contact when you are speaking, signaling when your time is almost up, and letting you know if you need to speak louder. Ask them to help you with handouts or visual aids. You will feel less alone.

Develop Your Teamwork Skills

Modern health care delivery relies on specialized professionals who work together. **Teamwork** refers to the works of individuals who coordinate their efforts to achieve common goals. High-quality patient care depends on how well people communicate and function as team members. People do not always work together easily and naturally. Competition, rather than cooperation, is built into many aspects of our educational system. As students, you compete individually for grades, especially on tests that are scored on a curve. On the job, however, the emphasis shifts to being able to work with others. A health care facility will not survive if it depends on only one excellent worker. All team members must be able and willing to contribute to the overall effort.

One of the most famous sentences spoken by an American president was that of John F. Kennedy: "Ask not what your country can do for you, but what you can do for your country." Kennedy encouraged Americans to work together in activities that ranged from organizing the Peace Corps to putting a man on the moon. Americans achieved both, proving that when people work together, they can accomplish amazing things.

You can begin to practice teamwork in school. Group activities assigned by instructors and lab sessions are excellent occasions to prepare for real work situations. Study groups provide additional opportunities to practice working with others. Apply the techniques presented in this section to develop your teamwork skills.

PRESCRIPTION FOR SUCCESS 7-6

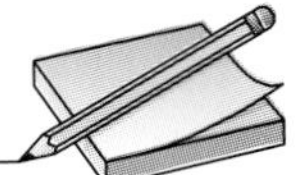

Go Team!

Describe any teams to which you belong at work or school.

What is your role in each?
How is the work assigned?
How are group decisions made?
How could each team be more effective?

MAKING THE TEAM WORK

1. *Understand the ground rules and agreements.* These may not be formally stated or written down, but they are important for keeping communication open and preventing misunderstandings.

2. *Be clear about the purpose and goals of the group.* Everyone should know what is to be accomplished. Have you been assigned a specific project? Or is the goal an ongoing effort related to your role as a student or an employee?

3. *Do your part—and then some.* Follow through and complete any work you have been assigned or have volunteered to do. Let the group know if you run into problems. Ask for help. Someone may be willing to pick up the slack. Letting things go can result in serious consequences: affect the group's grade, endanger patient safety, or cost the facility money.

4. *Listen* to what others have to say. What can you learn from them? What are their ideas about how to accomplish the work? What are their needs? What can they contribute?

5. *Speak up.* Share your ideas and opinions.

6. *Take advantage of differences.* Maximize group efficiency by assigning tasks that are appropriate for each member.

Differences among Team Members

Team members can support each other and make work a pleasant experience. On the other hand, teams in which members don't get along can slow down the work process and make life difficult for their members. People have differences that can interfere with communication, hurt feelings, and disrupt the work flow. Understanding and taking advantage of these differences can help teams flourish rather than fight.

Work Styles

Just as we all have different learning styles, we also have different work styles. Identifying and taking advantage of the styles of each team member can help prevent misunderstandings and allow each one to make useful contributions. There are no right or wrong work styles. Ignoring styles, however, can decrease the effectiveness of the team and reduce the satisfaction of the people on it.

Here are a some common approaches to work. Do any of these characteristics describe your own preferences?

- Work methodically and complete one task or part of a task before moving on to the next.
- Work on several projects simultaneously.
- Work alone and be responsible for your own work.
- Work with others in situations where cooperation determines the success of the project.
- Like working with details. Enjoy striving for accuracy and neatness.

- Think of ideas, but let someone else carry them out.
- Receive assignments with clear deadlines.
- Know exactly what is expected.
- Receive general instructions and a final due date. Figure out yourself how to get it done.
- Generate new ideas, products, and ways to work. Value creativity.
- Receive a lot of guidance: have someone check and approve your work as it progresses.
- Work with little supervision. Ask questions when you need help.
- Prefer quiet and order.
- Find noise and activity stimulating.

Understanding Organizations

Organizations, such as schools and dental offices, have their own personalities, just as individual persons do. These "personalities" are known as **organizational cultures,** and they include the goals, rules, expectations, and customs of the organization as a whole. Schools have cultures. For example, some are formal and emphasize respect for authority. Students are required to address their instructors by title and last name. Uniforms must be worn, and rules are strictly enforced. At other schools, the atmosphere is more casual, with students and instructors on a first-name basis. At some health care facilities, people eat lunch together, celebrate birthdays and holidays, and meet after work. At others, there is a clear distinction between work and social life. Some organizations stress orderliness, engage in detailed planning, and have clear work assignments. Others move at a fast pace, with informal job descriptions and planning done "on the run."

It is important to be aware of the culture you are in—or plan to enter—to see if it matches your preferences or if you can at least adapt to it. Sometimes we can learn from a culture that has values we would like to develop in ourselves. For example, if you have poor study habits and find yourself in a strict school, this can be a great opportunity for getting the encouragement you need to develop new habits.

Understanding Your Instructors

We have discussed how people have different learning and working styles. There is another factor that will impact your academic success: teaching and classroom management styles. Instructors are individuals who have their own ideas about education, preferred teaching methods, and the proper roles of instructors and students. Understanding what is important to your instructors will help you benefit fully from your classes.

Here are some common characteristics of instructors, along with suggestions about what you can learn from each:

1. *Strict.* Rules are emphasized. They are clearly explained, and there are consequences if they are broken.

You learn: Good habits for health care work situations in which rules *must* be followed to ensure patient and worker safety.

2. *Value appearance.* Students must be neat, with clean, pressed uniforms and polished shoes. Points may be deducted from grades for infractions. Students who arrive out of uniform are sent home to change. (In a work environment, improperly dressed employees may also be asked to leave.)

You learn: To practice the habits of excellent hygiene that are critical in health care work. (Remember: Your professional career began when you started school.)

3. *Believe students should be responsible.* Instructors with this philosophy may allow you to go all term without ever mentioning that you haven't handed in all your homework assignments. You interpret this as meaning that it's not important and are shocked to receive a final grade of F. Never assume that no nagging means "not important." The same can happen at work. An employee may not be told about unsatisfactory work performance until the day of an official evaluation—or dismissal!

You learn: To take responsibility for yourself and what you must do. On the job, supervisors won't have time to remind you constantly about your tasks. It will be up to you to get them done.

4. *Believe they must monitor students closely.* Some instructors believe it is their responsibility to prompt students to complete their work. They give constant reminders, check their progress frequently, call students who are absent, and generally provide "super-support." They are like supervisors who are very organized and nurturing and are willing to tell employees what's to be done. They give a lot of feedback.

You learn: To work with frequent deadlines and a hands-on manager. How to meet deadlines and avoid falling behind in your work. Be careful, however, that you don't become dependent on continual help, because you can't always count on it being there for you.

5. *Value order.* The classroom is neat and tidy, lectures follow a clear pattern, and class activities are well planned.

You learn: To practice orderly habits when necessary. While your home may be comfortably chaotic, order is necessary in many areas of the health care environment. Forms must be filled out in a very specific way, tests performed in a prescribed order of steps, and disinfecting procedures carried out precisely.

6. *Value creativity over order.* Classes may seem disorganized. Lectures are mixed with interesting stories and don't follow an orderly plan. Group activities and creativity are emphasized over doing things the instructor's way.

You learn: To be creative and think for yourself. To work with classmates and practice the teamwork activities discussed in this chapter.

The teaching styles chosen by instructors are usually a reflection of their own learning styles or the way they remember being taught themselves. Instructors may rely on lectures to teach because they are auditory learners or because they believe that their role is to tell students what they know. You can take advantage of teaching styles to help you improve your weak areas. For example, if an instructor uses a lot of group activities and you prefer to work alone, you now have an opportunity to increase your ability to work with others, something you might not choose to do if it weren't required.

If you have difficulty with an instructor, the first step in resolving the problem should be to speak privately with him or her. If you go straight to a school administrator, neither you nor the instructor has a chance to explore the problem and try to work out a solution. Furthermore, the administrator doesn't have personal knowledge of the situation. The problem has been moved away from its source. If speaking with the instructor fails to resolve the situation, inquire about the proper procedure to follow at your school.

Most instructors decide to teach because they want to share what they have learned about their profession. They are motivated by concern for their students. This does not necessarily mean that they are liked by their students, because this is not the purpose of their job. Their job is to train students to be excellent health care professionals. You may not like all of your instructors, but given a chance, they all have something of value to share with you.

Take a Moment to Think

1. How would you describe your instructors?
2. Do they represent types other than those listed in the previous discussion?
3. What can you learn from each?
4. Which do you find easiest to learn from?

Dealing with Difficult People

People problems cannot be avoided entirely. There will be classmates who annoy you, don't do their share of the work on a group project, or take up a lot of class time with questions because they never read the assignments. Family members may criticize you because they are upset about the amount of time you spend studying. Friends may be jealous of your future career possibilities. Some of your future patients, clients, coworkers, and supervisors will be challenging, too. Learning to get along with difficult people helps make life more pleasant and productive. Here are a few hints:

1. *Separate your role from yourself as a person.* It is often your position with which the other person has a problem. For example, your family may be annoyed with your role as a student because of the time it takes away from them. Or a patient may take his anger out on you as a representative of the clinic with which he has a problem.

2. *Listen carefully to the other person.* Try to see the world from his or her point of view. What might explain the person's behavior? Are there personal problems that you don't know about? Is there a chance that you have done something unintentionally that hurt his or her feelings?

3. *Remain calm and courteous.* This is an opportunity to practice professionalism. Reacting negatively will only make the situation worse. (This does not mean that you have to take verbal or physical abuse. If necessary, seek the assistance of your instructor, other school personnel, or your supervisor.)

4. *Be honest.* Tell the other person what the problem is and how it is affecting you. For example, with a lab partner who is never prepared to practice the assigned procedures, say, "I feel really frustrated when you continually come unprepared. I'm worried that I'm losing valuable learning opportunities, and I can't afford to do that."

5. *Seek solutions.* Simply venting or arguing—or even stating the problem as suggested in suggestion 4—won't solve the problem. Try to reach an acceptable agreement. With the lab partner you might ask: "Can you agree to come to class prepared?"

6. *Set limits.* In situations that have serious consequences for you (your grade or work performance), let the other person know what you plan to do if the situation is not resolved. Tell the lab partner, "If I can't depend on you to come prepared to work with me, I'll have to ask the instructor to let me change lab partners."

7. *Keep a positive attitude.* Remember from our discussion of attitude that it doesn't make sense to give an unpleasant person the right to ruin your day completely. Do what you can to seek a positive solution and then move on.

We learn and develop professionally when we engage in all types of relationships, both positive and negative. Expressing kindness toward a troublesome classmate or giving an instructor the benefit of the doubt is a sign of maturity. It is easy to be professional when things are going well. True professionals can also deal effectively with challenging situations.

Dealing with Criticism

Criticism and constructive suggestions about your work present you with opportunities to learn. In school, you are paying for instruction that includes correction of your work. Your instructors would not be acting responsibly if they awarded inflated grades or withheld criticism to avoid hurting students' feelings. It is unfair to allow students to perform work incorrectly, because this only sets them up for failure on the job.

If you receive criticism that seems harsh, try to focus on the content and not on the way it is delivered. Not all instructors and supervisors are skilled at giving suggestions. If you don't understand what you did incorrectly, ask for clarification. It is your responsibility to learn as much as possible. Feelings must be put aside, if necessary, to ensure your development as a competent health care professional.

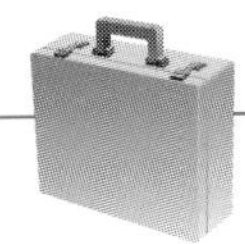

PEOPLE SKILLS ON THE JOB

A medical office manager in California tells the following story: The receptionist, Grace, was a very efficient woman who treated all patients courteously. One of the patients, William, was a gay man with AIDS. Grace was courteous but stiffened visibly whenever he came for appointments. She had trouble accepting his lifestyle. One day William learned that Grace's son had been a missionary in Africa. On his next visit, William brought in a scrapbook that showed **his** experience working with missionaries in Africa. After that, Grace was warm and friendly to William. When asked why seeing the scrapbook had changed her behavior, she said that now she was able to see William as a **person** and not simply as a gay man with AIDS.

SUMMARY OF KEY IDEAS

1. The ability to get along with others is critical to career success.
2. All human beings deserve to be treated with respect.
3. We are all *people,* in spite of our differences.
4. Empathy is an essential trait of the caring health care professional.
5. The ability to listen well is as important as the ability to speak well.
6. The keys to effective oral presentations are preparation and practice.
7. Understanding the work, learning, and teaching styles of others will increase your ability to work with them effectively.
8. You can learn from difficult situations.

POSITIVE SELF-TALK FOR THIS CHAPTER

1. I respect other people and try to learn something from everyone I meet.
2. I value differences and strive to promote understanding among people.
3. I practice empathy with others.
4. I have good communication skills.
5. I prepare well and speak confidently in front of groups.
6. I work well with others and make valuable contributions to teams.

BIBLIOGRAPHY

Purtilo, Ruth and Haddad, Amy. *Health Professional and Patient Interaction,* 5th ed. Philadelphia: W.B. Saunders Company, 1997.

8

Beginning the Job Search

OBJECTIVES

THE INFORMATION AND ACTIVITIES IN THIS CHAPTER CAN HELP YOU TO:

- ➢ Understand how a positive attitude contributes to a successful job search.
- ➢ Use a variety of organizational techniques to conduct an effective job search.
- ➢ Know what skills you have to offer an employer.
- ➢ Identify your employment goals and income needs.
- ➢ Use a variety of resources effectively to locate health care job leads.

KEY TERMS

Cover letter: Letter of introduction sent along with your resume to a potential employer.

Fax machine: Device that allows you to send documents over telephone lines. Many computers are equipped with fax capability.

Job lead log: An organized list of the information you gather about job leads from various sources.

Job line: Recorded list of jobs available at a facility that is accessible by telephone.

Mailing lists: Subscription services that send messages on specific topics via e-mail. For example, people interested in pediatric nursing can form a newsgroup and share information among the subscribers.

Newsgroups: Collections of articles on specific topics accessible in a special section of the Internet called the Usenet.

Reference sheet: A written list of your references that includes their titles and telephone numbers. It is given to potential employers after the interview if they request it.

The Search Is On

Employment is nature's physician, and is essential to human happiness.—Galen

Congratulations! All the studying, assignments, labs, and clinical experience are about to pay off. You are ready to focus on the job search and on reaching your goal of working in the health care field. Completing your education and graduating represent important personal achievements. Your attitude played a large part in your success. In the same way, attitude will play an important role in helping you obtain the right job.

THE BIG A—ATTITUDE!

Remember that your own resolution to succeed is more important than any one thing.—Abraham Lincoln

Attitude is the single most important factor in determining whether a student finds a job. In Chapter 3 we discussed how we control our own attitudes and noted that any situation can be approached either positively or negatively. For example, some people are nervous and fearful about looking for a job. They worry about lacking the qualifications needed by employers and see each interview as a chance to be rejected. A more positive approach is to look at the process from the employers' point of view. Think about it: health care facilities cannot function without good employees. Employers must fill positions with well-trained individuals who can help them serve their patients. You are a recently trained person ready to fill one of these positions.

Knowing your skills and competencies is the first step in presenting yourself successfully as the person who will fit an employer's needs. Students sometimes don't realize just how much they have learned. They tend to underestimate their abilities and the amount of practice they have had in applying their skills. Being aware of your accomplishments builds self-confidence and enables you to present yourself positively at interviews. Take some time now to review your knowledge and give yourself credit for what you have learned and what you have to offer.

PRESCRIPTION FOR SUCCESS 8-1

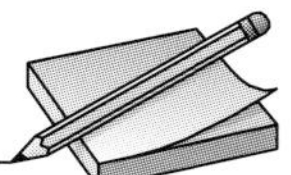

Inventory of Technical Skills

1. Refer back to Prescription for Success 2-6, in which you began to collect lists of the skills learned in school.
2. If necessary, gather additional sources of information needed to complete your inventory: lab checklists, course objectives, clinical performance evaluations, textbooks, and class handouts.
3. Create categories, such as the following, that are appropriate for your occupational area. List your specific skills under each heading:

   Equipment I Can Use

   Lab Procedures I Can Perform

   Tests I Can Perform

   Patient Procedures

   - Care
   - Diagnostic
   - Treatment
   - Therapy

   Administrative Procedures

   - Computer Skills and Applications
   - Medical Records

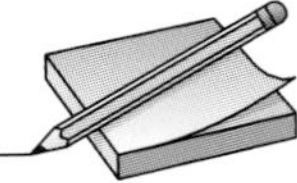

Documentation and Charting

Medical Insurance

Billing

Communication

Oral

Written

4. Think of examples that demonstrate your mastery of each skill. These may include practice in class or in the lab, completing special projects, or applying the skills during your clinical experience. Think about how well you can perform each one. You will use these examples to present your qualifications to potential employers.

PRESCRIPTION FOR SUCCESS 8-2

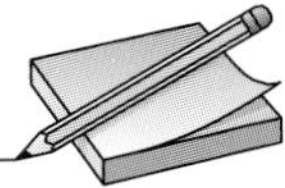

Updating Your Self-Assessment

You rated yourself on the SCANS Competencies in Prescription for Success 1-4. As you recall, these are the general skills and qualities that employers have identified as important when hiring employees. Reviewing this exercise will help you prepare to sell yourself to potential employers.

1. Review your self-ratings in Prescription for Success 1-4 for each of the SCANS Competencies listed.
2. Think of at least two examples to illustrate how you have demonstrated each competency. Draw from previous employment, school, or your personal life.
3. Identify any areas that still need improvement.
4. What are some things you can do to improve in these areas?

Competency	*Examples*
1. Creative thinking:	________________
2. Decision making:	________________
3. Problem solving:	________________
4. Continuous learning:	________________
5. Reasoning:	________________
6. Responsibility:	________________
7. Self-worth:	________________
8. Empathy:	________________
9. Self-management:	________________
10. Integrity:	________________
11. Honesty:	________________

FOCUS YOUR SEARCH

To find out what one is fitted to do, and to secure an opportunity to do, is the key to happiness.—John Dewey

Knowing what type of job and facility you prefer is the next step in carrying out a successful job search. In Prescription for Success 2-2 you began to identify your job preferences. While completing your educational program, you may have changed your mind about what you want in a job.

PRESCRIPTION FOR SUCCESS 8–3

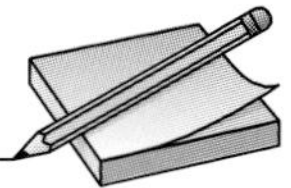

What Do I Want? An Update

Review Prescription for Success 2-2 and note any changes you have made.

1. Type of facility: large, small, urban, suburban, rural, in-patient, out-patient

   ____

2. Type of population served: economic status, age range, gender, ethnic groups

   ____

3. Work schedule: steady employment, per diem, flexible hours, fixed hours, overtime, days only, evenings and weekends

   ____

4. Specialty area

   ____

5. Type of supervision

   ____

6. Work pace: fast, moderate

   ____

7. Interaction with others (*All* health care professionals are part of a team, although some work more independently than others.)

   ____

8. Range of duties: wide variety, concentrate on a few

   ____

As we discussed in Chapter 2, it is sometimes necessary to set short-term goals in order to achieve long-term career success. Remember that when seeking an entry-level position, it is important to be open to a variety of possibilities. School career services personnel report that students can lose good opportunities by setting limits that are too restrictive. For example, some students don't want to face long commutes. But passing up a good position at an excellent facility by refusing to consider jobs outside your immediate area may not be a good career move. Driving an extra ten minutes may be worth the inconvenience in the long run.

CALCULATE YOUR NEEDS

An important part of preparing for the job search is to determine the salary you will need to support yourself and your family. While many occupations have salaries set within a certain range, knowing how much you need to live will help you identify appropriate positions.

This may seem like a lot of work, but it is smart to know your financial situation. If you have a computer, there are several software programs, such as Quicken, that can help with budgeting.

Making a Commitment to the Job Search

You can't try to do things; you simply must do them.—Ray Bradbury

Obtaining a job has been compared to working at a job. It takes a lot of time and effort. You must dedicate a portion of each day to your search and be on call to

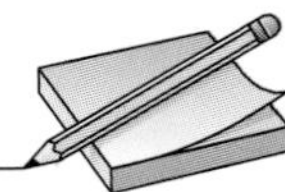

How Much Do I Need?

Write down all of your regular expenses for a three-month period. Include items that you are not paying now but can expect in the future, such as student loan payments.

Item	*Amount* Month 1	Month 2	Month 3
Mortgage or Rent	______	______	______
Utilities			
Gas & Electricity	______	______	______
Television	______	______	______
Telephone	______	______	______
Online Access	______	______	______
Water	______	______	______
Food	______	______	______
Student Loan (Future)	______	______	______
Payments			
Car	______	______	______
Credit Card	______	______	______
Other	______	______	______
Transportation			
Gas	______	______	______
Fares	______	______	______
Nonfood Grocery Items			
Cleaning Supplies	______	______	______
Paper Goods	______	______	______
Personal			
Grooming	______	______	______
Clothing	______	______	______
Entertainment	______	______	______
Totals	______	______	______

Add the three monthly totals and divide by 3 to calculate your average regular monthly expenses. Now list expenses that occur less frequently.

Item	*Annual Amount*
Insurance	
Homeowners or Renters	______
Car	______
Health	______
Life	
Other	

(Note: Health and disability insurance may be offered as employment benefits. This is discussed in Chapter 11.)

Car	
Registration	______
Other Fees	______
Repairs	______

continued

PRESCRIPTION FOR SUCCESS 8–4 *(continued)*

Item	*Amount*		
	Month 1	*Month 2*	*Month 3*
Property Taxes	______		
Total	______		
Divide by 12	______		
Average Monthly	______	+ Average monthly total = Total amount needed each month ______	

follow up quickly on leads. Employment professionals recommend that job seekers spend between twenty and forty hours per week on job search efforts. In this and the following chapters, you will learn about the many activities necessary to conduct a successful search:

- Preparing skills' inventories and examples
- Networking
- Finding leads
- Conducting searches on the Internet
- Writing and revising your resume
- Assembling your portfolio
- Writing letters
- Contacting references
- Creating a **reference sheet**
- Preparing for and attending interviews
- Writing thank-you notes

Failure to spend adequate time on these activities is one of the major reasons that people fail to get hired (Fig. 8–1). Many of the time-management techniques suggested in Chapter 3 can be applied to the job search:

- *Prioritize.* Becoming employed must be your main focus. Dedicate sufficient time and attention to achieving this goal. Looking for a job *is* your job. Determine which activities are most productive and spend the majority of your time on them.
- *Keep a calendar.* Missing—or even being late for—an interview is a sure way to lose a job even before you are hired. Nor do you want to arrive much too early. Take care to note all appointments and follow-up activities accurately, and check your calendar daily. If you haven't developed a calendar system yet, *now is the time to start.*
- *Plan a weekly schedule.* Decide what needs to be done each week, and create a to-do list to serve as a guide to keep you on track. It's easy to reach the end of the week and discover that you accomplished only half of what needed to be done.
- *Plan ahead.* This is critical. Suppose that one morning you are notified that a hospital where you want to work is scheduling interviews for later that day. You don't want to miss out because you haven't completed your resume or don't have a clean shirt to wear. Being prepared leads to being hired.
- *Plan for the unplanned.* The unexpected tends to strike at the worst possible moment. Keep an extra printer cartridge on hand. Have extra copies of your resume printed. Leave early for interviews in case you get lost. (Better yet, take a dry run a day or two in advance to learn the route.)

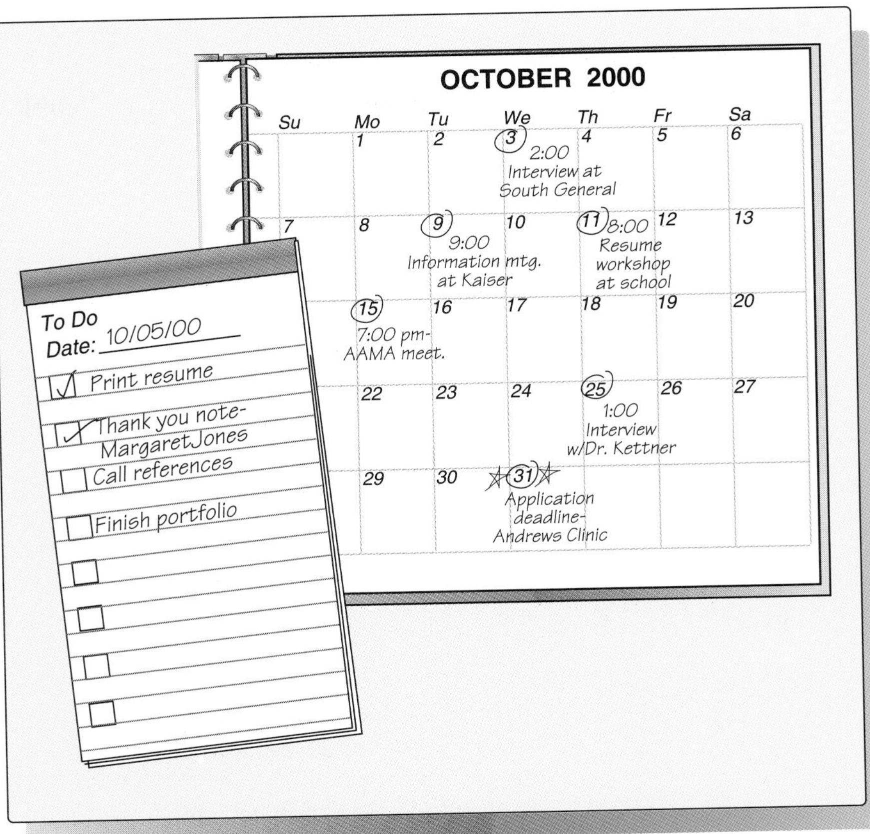

FIGURE 8–1 Apply your time management skills to conduct a successful job search.

Setting up Job Search Central

Create a personalized employment headquarters by designating a space for job search activities. Save time and prevent the loss of important information by gathering your resources and supplies in one location. The following items will be helpful:

- Telephone
- Telephone directories, including Yellow Pages
- Computer, printer, and supplies
- Dictionary
- Good-quality paper for resume and **cover letters**
- Matching envelopes
- Extra copies of resume
- Notepaper or thank-you cards
- Calendar
- Job search notebook

JOB SEARCH NOTEBOOK

Each person's job search is different and requires different information. Creating a personalized job search notebook will help you focus your efforts and keep track of phone numbers, web page addresses, and the name of the office manager at the office where you last interviewed. A three-ring binder gives you the flexibility to add pages and keep everything organized. Choose content that will best support your efforts. The purpose of this notebook is to save you time and effort, not to create another assignment to complete. Here are suggestions for information you might find useful:

- List of professional contacts (from your Personal Reference Guide, discussed in Chapter 6)
- List of professional organizations (also from your Personal Reference Guide)
- Prescriptions for Success 8-1, 8-2, and 8-3

- Resume content lists discussed in Chapter 2 ("To Do Now" suggestions)
- **Job lead log**

  Pages for recording all job leads and contacts. They should include the following information:
  Lead Source (personal contact, ad, referral, Internet, etc.)

  ____
  Facility Name ______________________________
  Contact Person ______________________________
  Telephone Number ______________________________
  Address ______________________________
  Fax number ______________________________
  Web site address ______________________________
  Follow-Up Action (call, send resume, thank-you note, etc.) ____________
  ____
  ____
  ____
  ____

DIALING FOR JOBS

The telephone provides a vital link with potential employers and job lead sources. The telephone can be one of the job seeker's best friends. It can also be a barrier if not used properly. Employers form an impression of you based on your telephone manners, so it is essential to ensure that they hear you at your best. The following suggestions for making calls will apply to your telephone habits *on* the job as well as during the search to get a job:

- Be courteous, never pushy. If the receptionist cannot connect you to the person you wish to speak with, leave a clear message and ask for a good time to call back.
- Speak clearly and distinctly. Don't mumble or use slang or nonstandard speech that the listener may not understand.
- Prepare what you plan to say ahead of time, and be as brief as possible without rushing and speaking too quickly.
- When making appointments or gathering important information, listen carefully and repeat to make sure that you have the correct date and time, address, suite or office number, and so on.
- Always thank the other party and end the call graciously.

It is important that your school, potential employers, and other contacts be able to reach you in a timely way. Be sure that the telephone number you distribute is accurate and includes your area code. If you have an answering machine, call your number to make sure it is working properly. The outgoing message should be simple and professional. Avoid the use of music, jokes, and clever remarks ("You know what this is and you know what to do"). Instruct everyone who might answer the telephone about proper telephone manners and how to write down a message. Every contact represents *you,* and employers don't have time to deal with rude adults or untrained children. If you are away from the telephone during office hours and don't have an answering machine, give out an alternate number where someone reliable can take messages for you. Don't lose out on jobs because you can't be contacted.

COMMUNICATING BY FAX

An increasing number of employment ads read "Fax resume to . . ." If you don't own a **fax machine** or a computer that has fax capability, find a print, postal, or business supply store that provides this service. Some schools will fax student resumes to potential employers. When sending documents by fax, the print on the original should be clear and dark for maximum quality transmission. Be sure that there is at least a one-inch margin on all sides so that nothing gets cut off.

When faxed resumes are requested, it is best to follow the employer's instructions. Mailed resumes may arrive too late to be considered. Demonstrate that you are resourceful and can follow instructions. If you don't hear from the employer in a couple of days, call to ensure that your resume was received.

Setting up a Support System

Your job search will be easier and more pleasant if you have people available who care about your success and are willing to help you. They can provide technical support or offer friendly encouragement. Your supporters can help you with the following tasks:

- Proofread your resume and other written materials (more than one person should proofread).
- Role play for practice interviews.
- Discuss postinterview evaluations.
- Act as a cheerleader.
- Help you keep things in perspective.

You may want to work with just one other person who is qualified to help you in many areas. Or you can enlist the help of several "specialists." Be sure that the people you choose are qualified to spot spelling and grammatical errors and are comfortable giving you constructive feedback. They should know when you need a push and when you need a hug. Consider drawing from friends, family members, classmates, school personnel, and health care professionals. If you have a mentor, this person might be an excellent choice.

Most people are happy to support your efforts to secure employment. Take care to keep your support system intact. Be considerate of everyone's time, be prepared for meetings with them, and show appreciation for their help.

Some schools and communities have job clubs or support groups for people seeking employment. Consider using these to supplement your support system. They can offer additional viewpoints, encouragement, and helpful suggestions.

PRESCRIPTION FOR SUCCESS 8-5

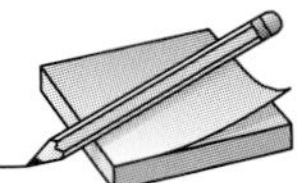

Your Support System

Think about the people in your life who are qualified to help your job search efforts. Who can you ask to help you with each of the following?

1. Proofreading __________
2. Interview practice __________
3. Postinterview evaluations __________
4. Encouragement __________

Understanding the Job Market

Economic and employment conditions change frequently. The following factors should be considered when planning your job search strategies:

- Local employment customs
- Current economic conditions
- Current employment rate
- Trends in health care delivery
- Medical advances
- Changing government regulations

Local customs vary in what is considered acceptable dress for the workplace. In some parts of the country, physicians may dress casually, sport long hair, and even wear an earring. In other areas, anyone who showed up for work looking like this would be sent home to change—or worse, sent home for good!

Local and national economic conditions affect the job seeker. When the economy is strong and unemployment is low, job seekers have the advantage. When the economy slows down, competition heats up and it becomes more difficult to find a position.

Health care occupations are also affected by state and federal laws. The demand for certain occupations is influenced by the reimbursement policies of both government and private insurance carriers. Knowing what's happening in your local area as well as being aware of national trends is important when planning both your initial job search and your long-term career strategy.

Your local newspaper is a good source of information. Look in the business section for articles about the economy and local employment trends. Health care trends and major facilities are often featured. For example, an article in a southern California newspaper in October 1999 described a new state law that increased the required nurse-to-patient ratios in hospitals. The predicted result was a shortage of registered nurses to meet employer needs. This information is valuable for the recent nurse graduate or a student who is considering nursing as a career. Articles about major health care employers can give you an edge when choosing where you want to work. Knowing about the facility where you are applying enables you to present yourself at interviews as a candidate who has taken the time to learn about a prospective employer.

Many newspapers also publish a special weekly or monthly section dedicated to employment issues. These are good sources of information. They contain articles about resume writing, lists of local agencies that assist job seekers, and announcements of job fairs. News magazines such as *Newsweek, Time,* and *US News and World Report* also contain many articles about health care topics. And the Internet provides access to a wide variety of topics from many sources. The research techniques discussed in Chapter 4 can be applied to your job search.

PRESCRIPTION FOR SUCCESS 8–6

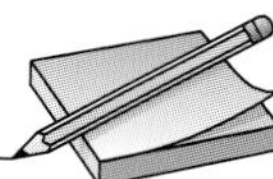

What's Going On?

Use your research skills to find answers to the following questions:

1. What is the unemployment rate in your area?
2. Who are the major health care employers?
3. What are the general hiring trends in health care?
4. How will these conditions affect your occupation?
5. How will they affect your job search strategies?

Locating Job Leads

There are many ways to find job leads, ranging from personal contacts to the Internet. Increase your chances of finding the job you really want by using a variety of lead sources. Do not limit yourself to the one or two methods you find easiest or most comfortable to use. We discussed self-marketing in Chapter 2. People who work in sales know that it usually takes many calls to make a sale. Likewise, the more sources you use in your job search, the greater your chances of finding the right job for you. Employment experts recommend that no more than 25% of your time be spent on any one job search method. See Figure 8–2.

When unemployment is high and there are few job openings, networking and developing personal contacts can be the most effective methods for finding a job. You may not find the perfect job under these conditions. Looking for an opportunity to gain experience will be the best strategy. When unemployment is low or there is a shortage of workers in your field, you will have a larger selection of opportuni-

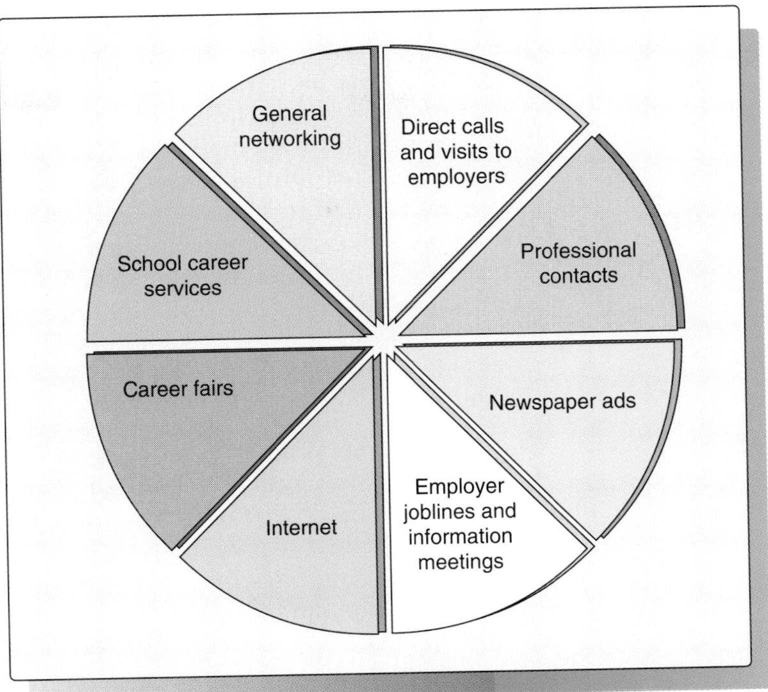

FIGURE 8–2 Use a variety of job lead sources.

ties. Under these conditions, you may find that responding to newspaper ads and directly contacting potential employers are very effective methods. It is a sure thing that you will experience all types of job markets during your career. The economy runs in cycles, and you must be prepared to deal with changing conditions.

NETWORKING

More people become employed through personal contacts than any other method. In Chapter 2 it was recommended that you start early to meet people in the health care field. In addition to providing you with useful information about your occupational area, they can be a source of job leads and referrals. If you have already met people through professional networking, let them know that you are launching your job search. Don't be shy about asking for their advice about where you might apply, as well as about the job search in general. People who are successful in their careers are generally happy to help newcomers. Show consideration for their time, and send a thank-you note when they put forth extra effort on your behalf. It is critical that you follow up on any leads given to you by professional contacts. Failure to do so is not only rude, it is likely to result in the withdrawal of their support.

In addition to professional contacts, general networking can be an effective way to get the word out about your search efforts. Let the people in your life know that you are seeking employment in health care. By telling 10 people who each know 10 other people, you create a network of 100 people who know you are looking for a job. Of those 100, it is likely that a few work in health care. And most people use health care services. The chances are good that someone will know something that can help you.

Keep in touch with your classmates. Being in the field themselves, they can be valuable sources of information. Those who are hired may be willing to pass on your name to their employers.

When speaking with others about your career goals, present yourself positively and express enthusiasm about your field. People want to feel confident about passing your name along.

CAREER SERVICES AT YOUR SCHOOL

The staff at your school wants you to succeed. The goal of health care educators is to train future workers, and a sign of *their* professional achievement is that every graduate becomes satisfactorily employed. Schools have special personnel who are trained to help students find jobs. These people work to develop relationships with local employers. Your school may be contacted about job openings before they are even advertised. This is because it is expensive for employers to place help-wanted ads in the newspapers. It is also time-consuming to review resumes, set up appointments, and interview large numbers of applicants. The success of a health care facility depends on the quality of its employees, so it is important that they find and hire the right people. Considerable time, expense, and doubt can be avoided if employers know they can count on local schools to provide qualified candidates. How can you be among those who are recommended by your school?

- Get to know the career services staff. Introduce yourself early in your program. Don't wait until you are beginning the job search. Seek their advice about how you can best prepare ahead for successful employment.
- Treat school staff with the same courtesy and respect you would an employer. They cannot risk the school's reputation with employers by recommending students who are rude or uncooperative.
- Maintain an excellent attendance record. Schools report that this is the question asked by nearly every employer about students. It ranks far above inquiries about grades.
- Participate fully in any career development classes or workshops that are offered. Attend every session and complete all assignments. Conduct yourself in practice interviews as if they were the real thing.
- Follow up on any leads you are given, even if you don't think the job is for you. Attend all interviews scheduled for you. Failure to do so embarrasses the school and may result in a denial of help in the future. Take advantage of all opportunities to meet potential employers. You will get valuable confidence-building interview practice. Even if the job isn't the one for you, the employer may know about one that is.
- Keep the school informed about how to contact you. If you move and career services can't find you, they can't help you.
- Let the school know when you are hired. Many agencies that regulate and accredit schools require annual reports to monitor graduation and job placement rates. These act as school report cards and are important for schools to stay in good standing. If the staff has taken the time to help you, return the favor by giving them the information they need to complete their reports.

CAREER FAIRS

Schools, community agencies, and large health care facilities organize activities to connect job recruiters and job seekers. In a single day, you can meet dozens of potential employers. You can gather information, ask questions, and submit your resume. Here are suggestions for taking full advantage of job fairs:

- Dress as you would for an interview. If the event takes place at school and you will go directly from class in uniform, be sure that it is clean and pressed.
- Prepare a list of questions in advance. It is easier to think of them beforehand than to try to remember them all in a noisy room. Good questions to ask include:
  - What types of jobs does your facility offer?
  - How can I find out more?
  - What are the most important qualifications that you look for when hiring employees?

  - Is it possible to get a job description?
  - Who do I contact to set up an interview?
- Take copies of your resume. Carry these in a large envelope or folder so that they will stay clean and neat.
- Smile, make eye contact, and introduce yourself to recruiters. Thank them for any information they give you. Leave graciously by telling them that it was nice meeting them, you appreciate their help, and you look forward to speaking with them again.
- Take something in which you can collect brochures, job announcements, and business cards. A small notebook is helpful for taking notes.
- As soon as possible after the fair, organize what you collected and make additional notes about the people you met and what you learned. Prepare a list of follow-up activities, such as people to call and resumes to send.

EMPLOYER INFORMATION MEETINGS AND JOB LINES

Some large facilities that do a lot of hiring have public meetings at which they explain their application process. Contact personnel departments, watch the local newspaper, and visit employer Internet sites to find announcements. You may not have a chance to meet personally with the hiring staff, but it is important that you make a professional impression. Be prepared to take notes and ask questions.

The telephone can provide you with a link to job leads through employer **job lines,** taped announcements of current openings. Many large facilities maintain job lines that include information about how to apply for the jobs described. Check the help-wanted ads for telephone numbers or call the personnel department at the facility in which you are interested.

EMPLOYMENT ADS

Many people think that looking for a job only means reading the help-wanted section of the newspaper. This is, after all, one of the most traditional methods of locating openings. While it can result in success, it suffers from overexposure. So many people see the same ad that employers may receive dozens—or even hundreds—of responses. This makes it difficult for a single resume to get attention. This doesn't mean that you shouldn't respond to ads. After all, someone will be hired and it might be you! Writing a cover letter and mailing or faxing a resume is worth the time and expense that it takes. Every action taken increases your chance of being hired.

The Sunday edition of the newspaper usually has the largest number of employment ads. When reviewing them, look under every category that might contain jobs for which you are prepared. For example, while "nursing assistants" will most likely appear in the "nursing" section, they may also be listed under "medical" or "health care." If your training has prepared you for multiple outcomes, be sure to check all possible job titles For example, graduates of health information programs may be qualified for many positions: coding specialist, health information technician, managed-care specialist, medical records coordinator or supervisor, and patient records technician. New job titles are constantly being created to describe the many activities performed in the modern health care facility. The skill inventories you created earlier in this chapter will help you identify all the jobs for which you might apply.

Don't be discouraged if you find only a few ads—or none—for your occupation. This may actually mean that there is such a shortage of applicants that employers have given up placing expensive ads.

When you respond to an ad, point out how you meet the employer's needs. You can do this in the cover letter, which will be discussed more fully in Chapter 9. For now, let's look at a couple of sample ads and see how to encourage the employer to read your resume. Even very short ads contain information you can use.

The following ad for a medical assistant gives three requirements that can be addressed in the cover letter you send with your resume.

AD: MEDICAL ASST—75% CLERICAL, 25% CLINICAL. COMPUTER LITERATE.

Your Response

YOUR REQUIREMENTS	HOW I MEET THEM
75% clerical	I enjoy and am proficient in front office duties. I received top grades in my administrative classes. I understand the importance of efficiency, accuracy, and confidentiality when performing clerical functions in the medical office. My written and oral communication skills are excellent.
25% clinical	I have up-to-date skills in all medical assisting back-office procedures.
Computer literate	I have basic computer literacy skills, can work in a Windows environment, and am proficient in Medical Manager, WordPerfect, and Excel.

AD: DENTAL ASST—RDA

We are looking for the best! If you understand quality, modern dentistry, appreciate excellent patient care and are dedicated to true teamwork, please fax your resume to . . .

Your Response

I am a registered dental assistant who recently completed a program of study at Dental Technical College in Health Town. My training program was patient-focused. In all courses, we learned the importance of considering the needs of each patient and delivering the best care possible. I also understand the importance of teamwork, having worked closely with other students throughout both the theory and lab portions of the program. During my clinical experience with Dr. Frank Samuels, I enjoyed sharing responsibilities with his five-member office staff.

There is no set formula for creating an effective response to an ad. Highlight your qualifications with a format that best suits the content of the ad. It isn't necessary—or even desirable—to repeat what's in your resume. A few quick highlights about how you meet the requirements mentioned in the ad are sufficient.

PRESCRIPTION FOR SUCCESS 8–7

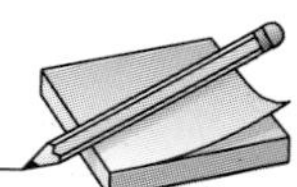

Create a Targeted Response

Find an ad in the employment section of your local newspaper. Identify the employer's requirements and write a response that demonstrates how you meet these qualifications.

(Attach ad) ____

____

____

Response: ____

____

____

____

____

Reviewing employment ads can also help you track employment trends and see which facilities are hiring and for what types of positions. They may also be a source of job line telephone numbers and employer web site addresses.

PRESCRIPTION FOR SUCCESS 8-8

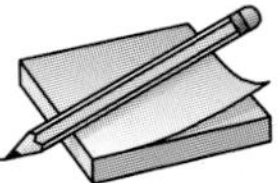

Learning from the Ads

Read the health care employment ads in a recent Sunday newspaper. They may be listed under dental, medical, nursing, rehabilitation, occupational and physical therapy, and so on. Answer as many of the following questions as possible based on what you learn from the ads.

1. In which occupation do employment opportunities seem to be growing the fastest in your area?
2. Which of the following employment settings have the most job openings?

   Home care

   Long-term care

   Acute care

   Private offices

   Other ______
3. How much experience is generally required for the position you have targeted as your long-term career goal? ______
4. Where might you acquire this experience? ______
5. How many positions are seeking bilingual applicants? ______

   Which language(s)? ______
6. Do any of the ads contain job line numbers? ______
7. If you answered "yes" to question 5, call the job line. What information is given on the tape? ______

   ______

   ______
8. Do any of the ads contain web site addresses? ______
9. If you answered "yes" to question 6, and you have access to an online service, look at the sites. What information is available? Can you submit an application online?
10. Are there announcements of job fairs, open houses, or informational meetings?

    ______

DIRECT EMPLOYER CONTACTS

Calling or visiting employers to inquire about job openings can be a successful strategy. These actions demonstrate motivation and self-confidence. These very qualities can help win you a job. When making telephone calls, find out the name or title of the person who does the hiring. Use your best telephone manners, and be considerate of the person's time. He or she may be busy with patients or paperwork and not have time to answer more than a quick inquiry. Your goal is to find out if there are job openings, how to apply, and whether you can schedule an interview.

Telephone calls are especially helpful if you are relocating to a new area. They provide an efficient way to contact a large number of employers. Explain that you will be moving and are unfamiliar with the area. If the facility contacted has no openings, ask if they can refer you to anyone else in the area.

Dropping in on employers gets the word out that you are looking for a job. Visiting all the offices in a large medical facility can be a productive way to spend a day. It gives you a chance to introduce yourself to at least one staff member and personally distribute your resume. If the person who greets you has time, ask for information about the facility. If this is not possible, ask who does the hiring, leave your resume, and express your appreciation. While you should be dressed as if you were attending an interview, *do not* ask for one at this time if you don't have an appointment.

Large medical facilities, such as hospitals, often coordinate all hiring through the personnel office. All resumes and applications must be submitted to this office. It can be very effective, however, to also visit the department where you wish to work. Ask for the supervisor and, if available, let him or her know that you have applied for work through personnel and are very interested in working in that department. Explain why you want to work there and ask that your application be given consideration. If the supervisor is not available, ask to make an appointment.

CLINICAL EXPERIENCE

Students who perform well during their clinical experience are sometimes offered jobs at the site. Some employers even create new positions for graduates who impress them with their attitude and skills. While it is not appropriate to ask your clinical site for employment before completing your training, you should work as if this were your goal. Even if the site is unable to offer you a position, your clinical supervisor can serve as a valuable reference and may recommend you to another employer.

Using the Internet

The Internet is the newest job search tool. It expands your possibilities by being available twenty-four hours a day. It offers a wide range of how-to information, job postings, and facts about specific occupations and employers. So much information is available that it is easy to become overwhelmed or find that you have spent three hours moving from one interesting site to another without actually adding much to your job-search efforts.

GETTING STARTED

An excellent place to start learning about using the Internet for the job search is *The Riley Guide* (http://www.dbm.com/jobguide/). This is a highly rated and reliable site whose purpose is to teach the job seeker to use the Internet effectively. It contains links to many other informative sites. It does not post jobs or resumes, although it contains tips for using these services effectively at other sites.

GENERAL JOB SEARCH INFORMATION

A number of web sites cover the economy, employment trends, and specific occupations. Others offer useful advice on topics such as resume writing, interviewing, and negotiating a salary offer. The following sites are a good start for the job seeker:

- America's Career InfoNet
  http://www.acinet.org
  Includes employment trends and information about specific careers. The site is well organized and easy to use.
- JobSmart
  http://www.jobsmart.org
  Contains job posting information for California cities. In addition, it contains loads of useful information for job seekers everywhere.
- Quintessential Career and Job-Hunting Resources Guide
  http://www.quintcareers.com/
  Many links to helpful advice and how-tos, online job fairs, and other valuable information.

HEALTH CARE FACILITIES

Many large health care facilities have web sites that include photos, maps, information about the services they offer patients, job postings, and forms to fill out to apply for jobs online. There are several ways to find these sites. If you know the names of facilities you want to learn about, conduct a web search using the facility name as the key word. For a listing of health care facilities, use a directory such as ComFind (http://www.comfind.com). Using this directory, you can conduct a worldwide search or limit it to your home town.

JOB POSTINGS

Job openings are available at both general and specialty health care sites. At the time of this writing, listings in allied health care are rather limited. Some sites, for example, list openings at only a few facilities. As use of the Internet grows, it is expected that an increasing number of facilities will advertise. The following are only a few examples of the many sites that offer job lists for all types of occupations:

- CareerPath.com
  http://www.careerpath.com
  Provides lists of help-wanted ads from the country's largest newspapers. Especially helpful if you are moving to a new area.
- The Monster Board
  http://www.monster.com/
  Jobs are grouped by occupational field, geographic location, and salary range. In addition to job lists, this site offers extensive job-search advice on topics ranging from writing effective resumes to answering tough interview questions.
- America's Job Bank
  http://www.ajb.dni.us/
  This site is a partnership between the U.S. Department of Labor and state employment offices. Job listings are available, as well as opportunities for registered users to submit their resumes.

The following sites are specific to health care:

- Allied Heath Opportunities
  http://www.gvpub.com
  In addition to job listings, this site includes guidelines for job seekers and links to professional organizations.
- Call24 Online
  http://www.call24online.com
  Jobs are posted for employer subscribers in the eastern part of the United States. Additional geographic areas are likely to be covered in the future. This site contains helpful information about seminars for health care professionals, professional organizations, and licensing boards, and allows job seekers to post resumes at no cost.
- Health Careers Online
  http://www.healthcareers-online.com
  Jobs are listed for specific employers who subscribe to the service and submit openings. The listings are organized by geographic region for easy searching.

Most professional organizations maintain web sites, and some offer placement assistance for members. For example, the American Health Information Management Association (AHIMA) maintains job postings online for members (http://www.ahima.org). See the Appendix.

There are dozens of sites for specific cities and states. Many of these include job lists and opportunities to post your resume. The number of jobs posted varies, but these sites are worth checking. Many contain valuable information, such as job fair announcements and facts about local employers.

A good way to find potentially useful sites is to use a directory such as *The Guide to Internet Job Searching,* listed in the bibliography at the end of this chapter. It is well organized and contains hundreds of suggestions.

Keep in mind that new web sites are being developed all the time and old ones are merging, being deleted, or being moved to a different "address." Some of the addresses given above and in other books may have changed by the time you try them. It is certain that many others will have been created. Those that remain will contain more information than ever.

NETWORKING

The Internet provides opportunities for sharing information and ideas with others through mailing lists and newsgroups. **Mailing lists** operate through e-mail. Each list is devoted to a specific topic: occupations, hobbies, health conditions, and so on. Once you have subscribed, you receive information via e-mail related to the topic. Some mailing lists allow subscribers to interact electronically, exchanging information and ideas. Mailing lists offer a way to learn what other job seekers are doing and what's happening in your field around the country. A comprehensive directory of mailing lists (there are over 65,000!) is available from Liszt (www.liszt.com). This site also includes detailed information about how to access and use mailing lists, including proper Internet etiquette.

Newsgroups also provide information about specific topics. However, the articles are not sent to you by e-mail. Rather, you must access them through the Usenet, a special section of the Internet. This is done using special software which is now included in both Netscape Navigator and Microsoft Internet Explorer. Books such as the *Student Resource Guide to the Internet,* listed in the bibliography, contain step-by-step instructions for using mailing lists and newsgroups.

PRESCRIPTION FOR SUCCESS 8–9

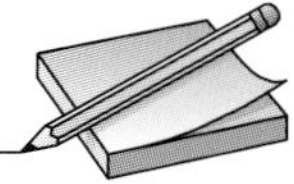

Traveling the Information Highway

Conduct Internet searches to locate the following:

1. Articles about using networking to learn about job openings
2. Major health care employers in your town or city
3. A list of jobs for which you qualify
4. The web site of a professional organization related to your occupation

USING THE INTERNET EFFECTIVELY

The following tips can increase your effectiveness when using the Internet:

- *Learn more.* If you are not already proficient at using the Internet, take a class or consult one of the books in the bibliography at the end of this chapter. If your school does not offer instruction, look for adult education classes in your community. Many are offered free of charge.
- *Be patient.* The Internet is a developing technology and still has a few bugs. You may get bumped offline just as you find what you are looking for. A promising site may have disappeared. But the wealth of information available is worth the time it takes to search.
- *Monitor where you are.* It's easy to get lost in a maze of links that takes you far from the original site. When you access a major site, write down its name and address so that you can find it again.
- *Mark favorite sites.* Most Internet-access software allows you to create personalized lists of useful sites so that you can find them easily later.
- *Be polite.* If you subscribe to a mailing list or newsgroup, be sure to follow proper Internet behavior. Experts suggest that you read the group's messages for at least two weeks before submitting anything. That way, you'll know the type and quality of material that is expected. It is also recommended that you check the "Frequently Asked Questions" section to avoid asking something that has already been covered. This is because all subscribers, not just you, will receive the answer. Keep your messages short and to the point. *Never* send advertising or use these groups to ask for a job.
- *Watch the time.* Using the Internet can be addictive. You can wander for hours linking and looking and actually accomplishing very little. If you find sites that look interesting but are unrelated to the task at hand, note their addresses and return to them later.

- *Don't exceed* 25%. Remember that the Internet is only one tool for your job search. Use it wisely as a supplement to other methods.

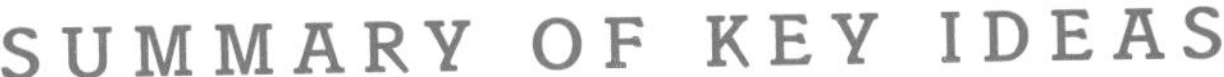

SUMMARY OF KEY IDEAS

1. Know yourself: what you want and need and what you have to offer an employer.
2. Get to know the employment climate.
3. Increase your chance of finding the right job by using a variety of lead sources.

POSITIVE SELF-TALK FOR THIS CHAPTER

1. I am confident and competent.
2. I have valuable skills to offer an employer.
3. I am organized and have a good search plan.
4. I will find the job that's right for me.

BIBLIOGRAPHY

Dickel, Margaret Riley, Frances Roehm, and Steve Oserman. *The Guide to Internet Job Searching.* Chicago: VGM Career Horizons, 1998.

Drake, John. *The Perfect Interview: How to Get the Job You Really Want,* 2nd ed. New York: American Management Association, 1997.

Leshin, Cynthia B. *Student Resource Guide to the Internet: Student Success Online.* Upper Saddle River, NJ: Prentice Hall, 1998.

Levitt, Julie Griffin. *Your Career: How to Make It Happen.* Cincinnati: South-Western Educational Publishing, 1996.

Locke, Robert D. *Job Search: Career Planning Guide, Book II,* 3rd ed. Pacific Grove, CA: Brooks/Cole Publishing Company, 1996.

Yena, Donna J. *Career Directions,* 3rd ed. Chicago: Irwin/Times Mirror, 1997.

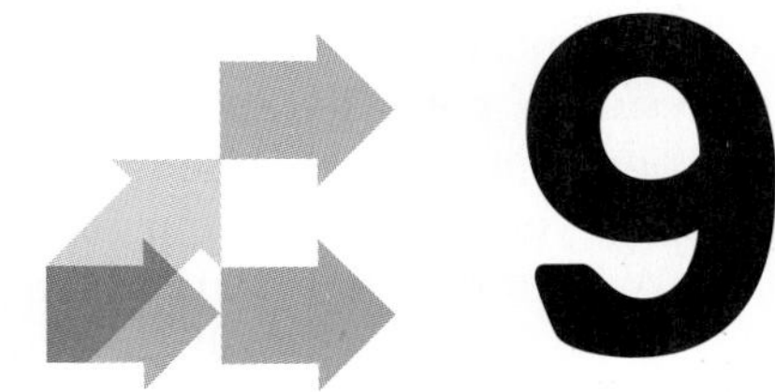

9

Finalizing Your Employment Presentation Materials

OBJECTIVES

THE INFORMATION AND ACTIVITIES IN THIS CHAPTER CAN HELP YOU TO:

- Write an effective resume.
- Write appropriate cover letters.
- Fill out employment applications correctly and accurately.
- Secure good references who will support your job search efforts.
- Prepare a reference sheet correctly.
- Create a professional portfolio that supports your qualifications.

KEY TERMS

Application: A form containing questions and spaces for information that employers need in order to make a decision regarding an applicant's qualifications for a job.

Objective: The job seeker's job or career goal. It may be general or specific and can include the job title and type of facility desired.

Portfolio: A collection of items that provide evidence of your job-related skills and capabilities. Examples include work samples, certificates of achievement, and employment evaluations.

Resume: A written document that summarizes your professional skills and capabilities. Its main purpose is to persuade potential employers to interview you.

Targeted objective: An objective that matches the requirements of a specific employer.

Presentation: Putting Your Best Pen Forward

The door of opportunity won't open unless you do some pushing.—Anonymous

Preparing high-quality written materials is an essential part of a successful job search. The purpose of some materials is to outline your qualifications clearly. These include **resumes, cover letters,** and **applications.** Other materials are designed to support your claims and include **reference sheets** and **portfolios.**

Anything you submit in your bid for employment is a form of personal advertising. Written materials serve as a reflection of who you are and what you can do. They speak on your behalf, and for this reason, it is critical that you apply your best writing, organizing, and spelling skills to their creation. Keep in mind that written materials are, in a sense, permanent. What is on paper stays there. You cannot change, correct, or explain that "what I really meant to say was . . .". Once they are sent, they are all prospective employers have to go by. Prepare all written materials thoughtfully and carefully so that they represent you at your best.

PRESCRIPTION FOR SUCCESS 9–1

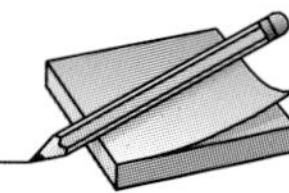

First Impressions

1. Imagine yourself behind the employer's desk. You have placed an ad for a medical receptionist. You receive a large number of resumes, and among them you find:

   Misspelled words

   Pages lightly printed so that they are difficult to read

   Lack of information about relevant training or experience

   No telephone number for the applicant

   No mention of what type of work the applicant is interested in

2. Answer the following questions:

   What is your impression of these applicants?

   What do each of these errors say about the person who submitted the resume?

   Would you call any of them for an interview? Why or why not?

   Is it significant that this is a job in health care? Explain why or why not.

Your Resume: A Vital Sales Tool

The resume gets you the interview. The interview gets you the job.

Selling yourself as a qualified job candidate begins with a well-prepared resume. The purpose of the resume is to convince prospective employers to interview you. To accomplish this, you must show them that you have the qualifications they need. Health care employers are looking for employees who will contribute to the success of their facility. They depend on finding good employees. Your well-constructed resume is a way to show them that you are the kind of person they are looking for.

The building blocks of the resume were presented in Chapter 2. They are listed here in the same order for easy reference. Apply the results of the "To Do Now" sections from Chapter 2 to construct the resume you will now use in your job search.

COMPLETING THE BUILDING BLOCKS OF YOUR RESUME

Objectives may be quite general—"Seeking a position as a licensed practical nurse"—or more specific—"Seeking a position as a front-office medical assistant in an urgent care facility." The more restrictive the objective, the fewer the number of

Career Objective

positions likely to be available. Consider the following questions when deciding how to write your objective:

- Are you *only* willing to accept jobs that meet your specific requirements?
- Are you more interested in a specific facility or a specific type of work?
- What are the current economic conditions? If the competition for jobs is great, being willing to consider a variety of positions will increase your chance of being hired.
- What are the current conditions for your occupational area? Are there many applicants or is there a shortage?
- What is your skill base and amount of experience? What advantages do you have over other applicants?
- Are you responding to an advertised position? Does your objective match the requirements of the position?

Consider writing a **targeted objective** when applying for a specific job. This type of objective mirrors the employer's language. It draws attention to how you fit that particular job. The following example demonstrates how to write a targeted objective:

AD: X-RAY TECH. WITH STRONG PATIENT RELATIONS SKILLS FOR ORTHOPEDIC PRACTICE. GREAT OPPORTUNITY TO JOIN AN ESTABLISHED TEAM ENVIRONMENT.

Key Words: patient relations skills, orthopedic, team
Objective: Position as an x-ray tech in an orthopedic office where I can apply my excellent human relations skills working with patients and fellow workers.

PRESCRIPTION FOR SUCCESS 9-2

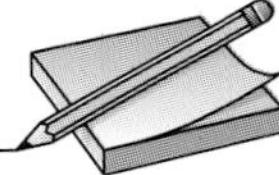

Writing Your Objectives

Consider the preceding factors and then write at least one objective that will be appropriate for your resume.

____

____

PRESCRIPTION FOR SUCCESS 9-3

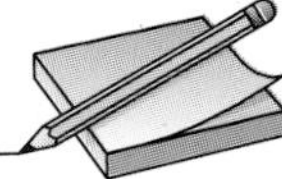

Writing a Targeted Objective

1. Find an advertised position in your occupational area.
2. Underline the portions of the ad that describe what the employer is looking for.
3. Write a targeted objective that responds specifically to the ad.

____

____

Education

Up-to-date training is likely to be the strongest employment qualification of recent graduates. It is important that this section of your resume be well prepared and contain more than a simple list of schools attended. For example, the following items are appropriate to list in the education section:

- Name of the program of study
- Degree, diploma, or certificate earned
- Grade point average, if at least 3.0 (on a 4.0 scale)

- Licenses, certifications, and other documentation of preparation
- Additional courses, workshops, seminars, and special training
- Educational honors, awards, and achievements
- Special projects that demonstrate job qualifications

Some program titles do not clearly communicate the types of skills acquired by the student. For example, the program entitled "Patient Care Assistant" varies in content from school to school throughout the country. In cases like this, it is a good idea to list the courses completed. This gives the employer a better idea of what the applicant is qualified to do.

List all schools you have attended, starting with the most recent one. Include high school only if high school graduation or its equivalent is a job requirement.

Sample Education Section

EDUCATION

Mental Health Technician Certificate, 2000
Wellness College, Salem, OR

- Graduated with Top Honors
- GPA 3.9 on a 4.0 scale
- Received Perfect Attendance Award

Nursing Assistant Certificate, 1997
Saddler Health College

- GPA 3.6 on a 4.0 scale
- Maintained perfect attendance
- Completed CPR training
- Organized musical program presented by students at Christmas to local nursing home patients

Workshops completed at Sunnyville Psychiatric Institute, 2001

- Updated Review of Research on Depression (25 hours)
- Suicide Prevention Measures (20 hours)
- Managing Assaultive Patients (25 hours)

PRESCRIPTION FOR SUCCESS 9–4

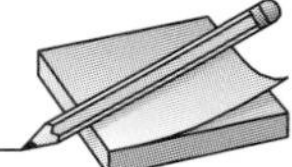

Complete the education section for your resume.

EDUCATION

____

____

____

Professional Skills and Knowledge

Occupational skills acquired from training or experience are listed in this section. Recall from Chapter 2 that these may be listed individually or in clusters of related skills. See the following examples:

Example 1: Creating Skill Clusters

MEDICAL ASSISTANT SKILLS

- Front Office
  Schedule appointments, handle phone calls, greet patients, maintain medical records, code and fill out insurance forms, perform billing and bookkeeping functions.

- Back Office
  Assist physician, prepare and administer medications, perform venipuncture and ECG, take vital signs, practice aseptic technique
- Laboratory
  Perform urinalyses, hematological tests, various specialty tests
- Computer
  Medical Manager, Word, Quattro

Example 2: Listing Individual Skills

MEDICAL INSURANCE TECHNICIAN*

- Abstract medical information from patient records
- Code diagnoses and procedures accurately
- Complete insurance forms correctly and accurately
- Submit and monitor insurance claims
- Process payments
- Maintain patient accounts
- Keep abreast of changes in coding, fee schedules, and other third-party requirements

PRESCRIPTION FOR SUCCESS 9–5

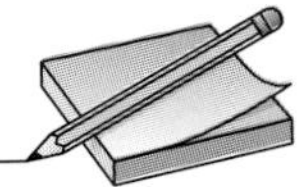

Review your occupational skills. Decide whether they are best listed separately or organized into clusters. Create headings for the clusters.

PROFESSIONAL SKILLS

____

____

____

____

____

Work History

A record of your previous employment, this section is more than a simple listing of jobs and the duties you performed. As discussed in Chapter 2, this section can be strengthened by including accomplishments and emphasizing transferrable skills that support your job target.

Use active verbs when describing job duties and achievements. For example, "Taught students to swim" is a stronger and more effective statement than "Responsible for teaching students to swim." Even better is "Successfully taught students to swim so that 97% passed the Red Cross swim test for their level." See Box 9–1 for suggestions of active verbs.

Military service and your clinical experience can be included in this section. It is not necessary to include very short-term or temporary jobs. Consider including these only if they are directly related to your job target. Do not include your reasons for leaving each job. This may be asked for on employment applications, but it should not be part of the resume.

---

*Adapted from Fordney, Marilyn. *Insurance Handbook for the Medical Office*, 5th ed. Philadelphia: W.B. Saunders Company, 1997.

BOX 9–1. ACTIVE VERBS FOR USE ON RESUMES

Achieved
Administered
Assisted
Billed
Budgeted
Calculated
Cared for
Coded
Communicated
Composed
Constructed
Controlled
Coordinated
Created
Demonstrated
Designed
Developed
Directed
Documented
Educated
Encouraged
Established
Expanded
Generated
Greeted
Handled
Helped
Hired
Implemented
Improved
Increased
Influenced
Informed
Initiated
Inspired
Instructed
Introduced
Justified
Launched
Led
Maintained
Managed
Monitored
Motivated
Negotiated
Obtained
Operated
Ordered
Organized
Participated
Performed
Planned
Prepared
Presented
Produced
Provided
Purchased
Recorded
Regulated
Repaired
Reported
Represented
Revised
Scheduled
Secured
Set up
Showed
Sold
Supervised
Taught
Tested
Trained
Verified
Word processed
Wrote

Example of Work History Entry

CASHIER, PETAMERICA BIGDOG, GA 1998–2000

- Assisted customers and informed them about products
- Performed cashier duties
- Closed out registers at end of day
- Named "Most Helpful Employee" for 1999
- Maintained perfect attendance for two years
- After one year, was promoted to head cashier
- Trained newly hired cashiers

PRESCRIPTION FOR SUCCESS 9–6

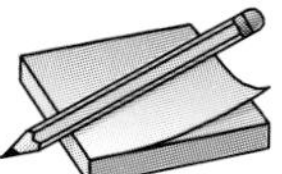

List your employment history, beginning with the most recent job held. List duties and accomplishments for each job.

WORK HISTORY

___

___

___

Licenses and Certifications

This section is necessary only if this information is not listed in the Education section or elsewhere. Be sure that dates and numbers are accurate.

Examples

Certified Occupational Therapist Assistant, 2001
American Occupational Therapy Association

Registered Nurse
California State Nursing License, #123456

PRESCRIPTION FOR SUCCESS 9-7

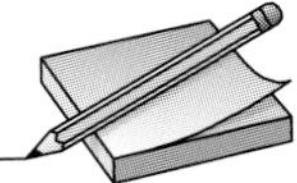

If this section applies to you, write out here with an appropriate heading:

CERTIFICATION/LICENSE/REGISTRATION

____

____

Honors and Awards

When listing these items, include information about why they were awarded if this is not clear from their names.

Example

Parent Volunteer of 2000 for James Madison Middle School
Recognition for organizing activities that raised over $200,000 to purchase school equipment and library books.

PRESCRIPTION FOR SUCCESS 9-8

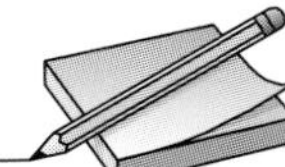

If this section applies to you, list any awards and honors that you did not already include in the Education section or elsewhere.

AWARDS AND HONORS

____

____

Special Skills

Recall that these should relate to your value as an employee.

PRESCRIPTION FOR SUCCESS 9-9

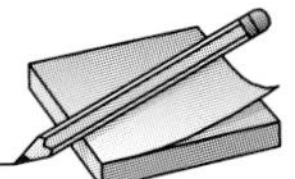

List any skills you did not include in the Professional Skills section.

SPECIAL SKILLS

____

____

____

Community Service and Volunteer Work

This can be work other than that related to health care. Any volunteer work that demonstrates responsibility, the willingness to contribute to society, or the development of teamwork skills is appropriate. It may have been performed at school, at a religious organization, or with any organization devoted to promoting the good of the community. Write brief phrases to describe what you did, if necessary. Use active verbs, as in the Work History section.

Examples

March of Dimes, 1995–present
Participated in annual fund drives

Boy Scout Troop Leader, 1992–2000

PRESCRIPTION FOR SUCCESS 9-10

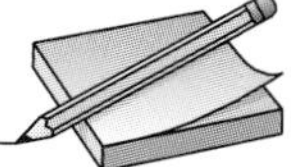

Include any activities that you did not list in the Education section. Choose an appropriate heading.

COMMUNITY SERVICE/VOLUNTEER WORK

____

____

____

Membership in Professional and Civic Organizations

Briefly describe any organizations that might not be familiar to prospective employers. If you took an active part, such as serving on a committee or as an officer, briefly describe what you did. On the resume, this heading can be shortened to "Memberships" or "Affiliations."

Example

California Association of Medical Assistants, Riverside Chapter
Chair of membership drive for 2000
Served on continuing education planning committee

PRESCRIPTION FOR SUCCESS 9-11

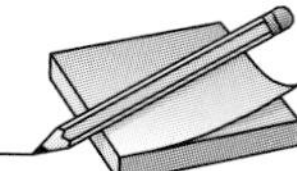

List any that apply.

MEMBERSHIPS/AFFILIATIONS

____

____

Languages Spoken

Examples

Spanish: speaking and reading—good. Writing—fair.

Vietnamese: Very basic conversational ability. Some knowledge of health care terms for conducting patient interviews.

PRESCRIPTION FOR SUCCESS 9–12

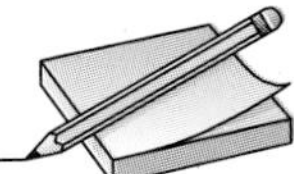

List, if this applies to you.

LANGUAGES

____

CONSTRUCTING YOUR RESUME

You are now ready to gather up your resume building blocks and construct a finished product. Just like actual blocks, the content created in Prescriptions for Success 9–1 through 9–10 can be put together in a variety of ways. The steps described in this section will help you create a document that best highlights your qualifications.

You will see as you progress through this chapter that there is no one best way to put together a resume. Each of us has a different set of characteristics and experiences. Even students who graduate from the same health care program at the same time will bring a variety of backgrounds that can be presented in different ways. For example, a young person who completed high school shortly before beginning a dental assisting program will benefit from emphasizing different areas than those featured by someone who worked in sales for thirty years before entering the same program.

There are also local customs and employer preferences regarding resumes. Seek the advice of your instructors, school career service personnel, and professional contacts. They keep in touch with employers and can offer sound guidance.

At this busy time in the job-search process, it may be tempting to use a standard resume format. Filling in the blanks on a "one-type-fits-all" resume may appear to be a fast and easy way to complete this task and get the interviews going. However, the time spent customizing your resume will pay off in several ways. It will:

- Help you recognize and review your own qualifications
- Demonstrate your initiative and creativity
- Respond to employers' specific needs
- Showcase your relevant skills and strongest qualifications
- Support your claims with examples
- Present your organizational skills

An effective way to increase your efficiency when creating your resume is to use word processing software, such as Microsoft Word or WordPerfect. Word processing offers several advantages because it enables you to:

- Try different layouts and formats
- Change and reorganize content quickly and easily
- Check for spelling errors
- Change the wording to match specific jobs
- Enable the use of special features such as boldfacing and changing the size and style of the font (letter)

If you don't know how to word process, now is a good time to learn. Windows-based programs are easy to learn. Even nontypists can produce great-looking documents by knowing a few basic computer commands. For example, spacing, boldfacing, underlining, moving text, and printing can be accomplished with the click of a button. Taking a few hours now to learn the basics of a word processing program is a good investment of your time. Not only will it support your job-search efforts, it will provide you with a valuable workplace skill, regardless of your occupational area. Even health care professionals who dedicate most of their time to hands-on patient-care activities can benefit from knowing how to word process.

THE 10-STEP GUIDE

Step 1 *Write the heading.* It is not necessary to write the word "Resume." Instead, clearly label the top of the page with your name, address, and telephone number. Centering your name is good for both appearance and practicality. Placing it on the far left side makes it more difficult to find if it is placed in a stack of other resumes. Capitalizing your name and using a slightly larger font size than the rest of the document helps it to stand out.

Capitalize and boldface name
Consider using a larger font size for your name
Include zip code and area code

JAIME RAMIREZ

3650 Loma Alta Lane
San Diego, CA 92137
(619) 123-4567

Be sure all numbers are accurate

The following format is an option if your resume is long and you are trying to conserve space:

JAIME RAMIREZ

3650 Loma Alta Lane   San Diego, CA 91237   (619) 123-4567

Step 2 *Add the objective.* The objective should be near the top so that prospective employers can quickly see if there is a potential match between your goals and their needs. This part of the resume may change if you are attempting to match your objective with the stated needs of each employer. It will stay the same if you have specific requirements which you are not willing to change or if you have written a very general objective that fits many job targets.

Step 3 *Select the best type of resume for you.* The three basic types are chronological, functional, and combination. They provide different ways to present your work history and professional qualifications. Your particular background determines which type you should choose.

Chronological Resume

The chronological resume emphasizes work experience and highlights the progression of jobs to demonstrate an accumulation of knowledge and experience and/or increasing responsibility that is relevant to the targeted job. This type of resume is recommended if you have:

- Held previous jobs in health care.
- Held jobs in other areas in which you had increases in responsibility or a strong record of achievements.
- Acquired many obvious transferrable skills.

In the chronological resume, each previous job is listed, followed by the duties performed and accomplishments achieved. The Work History section is well developed and likely to be longer than most of the other parts of the resume. This is the format you used to complete Prescription for Success 9–6. See Figure 9–1 for an example.

Functional Resume

The functional resume emphasizes skills and traits that have been acquired through non-health-care jobs and experiences. Qualifications can be pulled from a variety of sources. Related personal experiences, such as caring for a sick relative for an extended period of time, are appropriate. Once identified, qualifications are organized into three or four clusters with descriptive headings. This type of resume is advantageous if you:

- Are entering the job market for the first time
- Have held jobs that are unrelated to health care

- Have experiences that relate to the targeted job but were not gained through paid employment

The Work History section in a functional resume consists of a list of job titles with each employer's name, city and state, and dates of employment. The clusters of qualifications are fully developed and contain the strongest bid for employment. See Figure 9–2.

WORK HISTORY

Registered Nurse III, Surgical Unit 1998-Present
Gladstone Hospital, Happy Valley, OR

- Serve as charge nurse, providing high quality nursing care without supervision
- Develop and implement patient care plans based on individual needs
- Evaluate and revise plans as needed
- Conduct patient care conferences with care team members
- Serve as a patient advocate to ensure provision of appropriate and high quality care
- Provide teaching and counseling to patients and their families for home care procedures and maximation of wellness
- Serve as preceptor for ADN and LPN nursing students

Registered Nurse II, Surgical Unit 1992-1998
Gladstone Hospital, Happy Valley, OR

- Identify patient care problems
- Implement nursing interventions and evaluate the results
- Administer medications without error
- Teach patients pre- and post-operation procedures
- Carry out procedures as ordered by physician
- Communicate clearly to patients, their families, co-workers, and physicians
- Orient new employees

Staff Nurse 1988-1992
Sunnyville Community Hospital, Sunnyville, OR

- Provide direct patient care
- Carry out nursing care plans
- Complete prescribed treatments
- Give medications
- Document all care given on patient charts
- Call physicians as needed in response to patient's conditions

FIGURE 9–1 Work history section of a chronological resume of an experienced applicant for the position of registered nurse. Note the increasing complexity of tasks and levels of responsibility.

COMPUTER SKILLS

- Created electronic spreadsheet to track fund raising for Lewison Elementary School PTA
- Taught self to effectively use leading brand software programs in the following areas: word processing, database, spreadsheets, and accounting
- Set up and managed electronic accounting system for family construction business
- Teach computer classes at Girl Scout summer day camp

ORGANIZATIONAL SKILLS

- Created system to monitor all church collections and fund raising projects
- Initiated and developed computer career awareness program for Girl Scouts
- Secretary for college HIT student organization
- Completed HIT associate degree program with record of perfect attendance while working part-time and managing family life

CLERICAL/ADMINISTRATIVE SKILLS

- 7 years bookkeeping experience
- Keyboarding speed of 78 wpm
- Excellent written communication

WORK HISTORY

Bookkeeper 1998-Present
Buildwell Construction Company, Yuma, AZ

Bookkeeper 1994-1998
Perfect-Fit Cabinetry, Yuma, AZ

Secretary 1990-1994
Caldwell Insurance Company, Yuma, AZ

FIGURE 9–2 Work history section of a functional resume for a recent graduate seeking a health information technology position. Note the clustering of skills that support this position.

A functional resume may take more time to develop than a chronological one, but the extra effort can really pay off for the creative person who learns to relate a variety of experiences to health care job goals.

Combination Resume

The combination resume, as its name implies, combines features of both the chronological and functional types. The details of the job(s) related to health care may be listed, along with clusters of qualifications or a list of supporting skills. This resume is appropriate if you:

- Have held a limited number of jobs in health care *and*
- Have important qualifications that you gained through other, non-health-care jobs and experiences *or*

- Have held a number of relevant jobs in health care for which you performed the same or similar duties

Let's look at the example of a recent nursing graduate who worked for a year as a nurse's aide and for seven years as a kindergarten teacher. She could:

- Include the duties performed in the nurse's aide position.
- Create clusters to highlight her teaching, human relations, and communication responsibilities.
- Pull skills from teaching and other experiences to fill in the clusters.

See Figure 9–3 for an example.

NURSING ASSISTANT 1998-2000
GoodCare Nursing Home, Denver, CO

- Encourage patients to achieve their maximum level of wellness, activity and independence
- Demonstrate interest in the lives and well-being of patients
- Assist patients with prescribed exercises
- Organize and participate in activities with patients
- Help patients carry out basic hygiene and dressing

TEACHING

- Teach swim classes to all ages at YMCA
- Conduct CPR instruction for the American Heart Association
- Organize holiday programs and outings for nursing home residents (volunteer)
- Planned and supervised craft and play activities for pre-school children
- Tutored ESL students at Salud College while in OTA program

INTERPERSONAL SKILLS

- Provided daily care for parent with Alzheimer's disease for 18 months
- Answered telephone, directed calls and took messages for busy sporting goods manufacturer
- Received Connor Memorial Award for graduating class for making positive contributions and assisting classmates at Salud College

WORK HISTORY

Preschool Aide 1997-2000
Bright Light Preschool, Denver, CO

Swim Instructor 1997-Present
YMCA, Denver, CO

Receptionist 1994-1997
Sportrite Manufacturing Co., Denver, CO

FIGURE 9–3 Work history section of a combination resume for a recent graduate seeking an occupational therapy assistant position. The one health care–related job is detailed, and clusters have been developed for skills that support the new career.

Choosing the Best Resume for You

Review your skills and experiences and use the information in this section to choose the type of resume that is best for you. If you select a chronological presentation, copy what you prepared for your Work History.

If a functional resume would serve you better, use the following guidelines to create the occupational clusters:

1. Consider the current needs of employers. Sources to use include help wanted ads, the National Health Care Skill Standards (see Chapter 1), and the SCANS competencies (see Chapter 1).
2. Think about the skills and traits that contribute to success in your occupational area.
3. Assess your work history, clinical experience, personal experience, volunteer activities, and participation in professional organizations.
4. Refer to your completed Prescriptions for Success 8-1 and 8-2 for skills and traits that can be used in clusters.
5. Use the information gathered in steps 1-4 to create three or four headings for clusters that support your job target and give you an opportunity to list your most significant qualifications. The following list contains examples of appropriate health care cluster headings:

   Communication Skills
   Organizational Skills
   Teamwork Experience
   Interpersonal Relations
   Computer Skills
   Clerical Skills

Step 4 *Consider creating a qualifications section.* This is an optional section. Its purpose is to list any skills that support your bid for employment but do not fit in other sections. For example, you may have chosen to use a chronological format but have additional experiences that don't belong in the Work History section. Or you have experiences in addition to those listed in the clusters on a functional resume. Here are some examples:

Excellent time-management skills
Work calmly under pressure
Proven problem-solving ability
Cost conscious
Enthusiastic team player
Work well without supervision
Enjoy learning new skills

Another version of this section is a summary of highlights that draws attention to your most significant features. Such a summary might look like this:

- Eight years' experience working in health care
- Up-to-date front and back office medical assisting skills
- Current CPR certification
- Fluent in spoken Spanish
- Excellent communication skills

Popular titles of the section for listing qualifications include "Summary of Qualifications," "Professional Qualifications," and "Professional Profile." Review the same information sources recommended in step 4 for preparing the functional clusters. The difference in preparing the qualifications section is that it can consist of a mixed list of items. These items need not fall into categories, but only demonstrate capabilities, traits, and special skills that relate to the targeted job and support your objective.

Step 5 *Decide which resume sections you will use.* Your resume needs to be comprehensive and, at the same time, avoid duplication. For example, if you are using a functional format and have listed a special skill in one of your clusters, do not repeat it under another heading. Try to group items in each section rather than having many headings with only one item listed. Think about what items can logically be gathered into each section. The following areas are those most appropriate to combine:

- Licenses and Certifications can be included in the Education section or listed as a Professional Qualification.
- Honors and Awards earned in school can be listed under Education. If you have a variety, it might be better to list them all together under their own heading.
- Memberships can go under Education if they are limited to school groups or your health care professional organization. If you have been active in the organization in significant ways or are involved in several organizations, highlight them by creating a separate section.
- Clinical experience can be listed under Education or Work History. In either place, it should include some detailed information about your duties. For career changers and new graduates, this may be a significant employment qualification. Be sure to indicate clearly that the work was unpaid and part of an educational program.
- Languages spoken other than English can be listed under Qualifications, Special Skills, or Languages.

Deciding on headings and the location of content depends on the amount of content, how directly it is related to the targeted job, and your own organizational preferences. Suppose that you speak two languages other than English. If they are spoken by people in your geographic area, they are likely to be valuable job qualifications and can be listed there. If they are not commonly spoken in your area, they might best be listed under Languages—skills that you want known but that are not directly related to the job. Think about the relative importance of items as you decide how best to group and label them.

Step 6 *Plan the order of your sections.* Place the sections that contain your strongest qualifications first. For example, if you are changing careers and recent education is your primary qualification, list that section before Work History.

Step 7 *Consider adding a personal touch.* In their book *Career Planning,* Dave Ellis and coauthors suggest adding a positive personal statement at the bottom of the resume. This provides an opportunity to make a final impression and add an original touch. It is a way to say "Here is something personal and interesting about me that might help you, the employer." If you decide to create a personal statement, be sure that it is a sincere reflection of you and not simply something that sounds good. And, as with the entire resume, be sure that it is related to your job target. Here are some examples:

> "I enjoy helping in difficult situations where I can make a positive contribution by using my ability to remain calm and work efficiently under stressful conditions."
>
> "I get great satisfaction working with people from a variety of backgrounds who need assistance in resolving their health care problems."

Review your reasons for choosing a career in health care to help you develop an effective personal statement.

Step 8 *Know what to leave out.* Don't include personal information such as age, marital status, number of children, and statements about health status. And *never* make false claims about your education or experience. If these are discovered later, they can be grounds for dismissal.

While it is essential to have a Reference Sheet to give to potential employers who request it, there is disagreement among employment experts about whether "References Available Upon Request" should be stated on the resume. The author recommends that you include the phrase only if you have extra room. Otherwise, the space is best used for presenting information of interest to employers. (Preparing a Reference Sheet is discussed later in this chapter.)

Step 9 *Plan the layout.* Each section of your resume, except the heading and personal statement, should be labeled: Objective, Education, and so on. Headings can be flush (aligned) with the left margin, with the content set to the right.

OBJECTIVE: XXXXXXXXXXXXXXX Note: placing colons after each heading is a personal preference

EDUCATION: XXXXXXXXXXXXXXX

Alternatively, headings can be centered, with the information listed beneath and flush left. The second method uses up more space and may be most appropriate if your resume is short.

OBJECTIVE

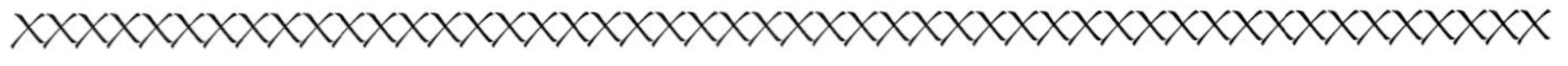

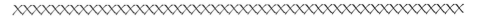

EDUCATION

XXXXXXXXXXXXXXXXXXX Note: in this type of layout, do not use colons

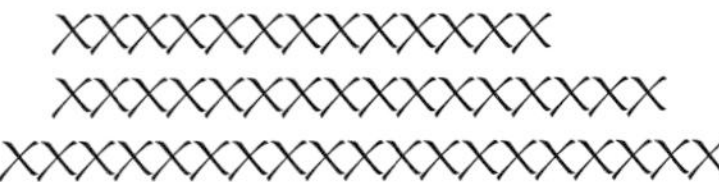

Information listed under headings can be arranged in various ways. The design should be based primarily on whether you need to use or save space on the page. The second consideration is personal preference. Whichever method you choose, strive for a balanced, attractive look. Note the varied use of capitalization and boldface to draw attention to the job title.

WORK HISTORY	Medical Transcriptionist 1997–Present Hopeful Medical Center, Better Health, NJ	
OR	MEDICAL TRANSCRIPTIONIST Hopeful Medical Center, Better Health, NJ	1997–Present
OR	**Medical Transcriptionist** Hopeful Medical Center, Better Health, NJ 1997–Present	

Step 10 *Create an attractive document.* Selecting and organizing content is the most time-consuming part of writing your resume. Don't waste your efforts by failing to attend to the details of appearance. The following tips will help achieve a professional look:

- Leave plenty of white space so that the page doesn't look crowded. Double-space between sections and single-space within them.
- It is highly recommended that you limit your resume to one page. It is better to use two pages, however, than to crowd too much information on one page. If two pages are used, write "More" or "Continued" at the bottom of the first page and your name and "Page 2" or "Page Two" at the top of the second.
- Capitalize headings.
- Use bullets to set off items in lists.
- Try using boldface for emphasis.
- Make sure that spelling and grammar are *perfect.*

- Leave at least a one-inch margin on all sides.
- Use good-quality paper in white, ivory, or very light tan or gray.
- Whether printing from the computer or using a copy machine, make sure that the print is dark and clear. If you don't have access to either a computer or a copy machine, consider paying to have the resume printed. While this limits your flexibility in customizing the resume for various employers, it will provide professional-quality copies.

Once completed, your basic resume can serve you throughout your health care career. Think of it as a living document on which you record your experiences and acquisition of skills. With additions and changes, it can continue to represent you to a variety of employers. See Box 9–2.

NEW DEVELOPMENTS IN RESUME WRITING

Preparing a Scannable Resume

Some employers enter all resumes received into a computerized database. Each resume is scanned electronically and categorized by key words that match words in job descriptions. When there is a job opening, the database searches for resumes that contain appropriate key words. If there is a possibility that your resume will be scanned, make the following revisions to ensure that it has the best chance of being selected from the database for the jobs you want:

- Prepare a list of key words that relate to your job target. Fifteen to thirty words are recommended. Place this list at the top of the resume in place of the objective. Think about which key words most nearly describe the jobs for which you want to be considered. If possible, secure job descriptions from potential employers. Read ads or job announcements and visit facility web sites. The *Dictionary of Occupational Titles,* a government publication which contains descriptions of thousands of jobs, as well as the *Occupational Outlook Handbook,* are also good sources.
- Don't use special features such as boldface, italics, or special styles of type. These do not always scan well.
- Do not fold or staple the pages.
- Make sure that the print is clear and sharp so that the scanner can read it accurately.

Posting Your Resume on the Internet

A number of web sites allow you to post your resume on the Internet. If you decide to do this, it is extremely important that your resume be error-free. Once posted, it is on display for literally millions of viewers. Follow the web site's instructions carefully for posting. There may be a required standard format.

BOX 9–2. RESUME CHECKLIST

____ Dates and numbers are complete and accurate.
____ Your phone number is included.
____ The objective is clear.
____ Content supports the objective.
____ Content is organized in order of importance.
____ All important qualifications are included.
____ Information is not repeated.
____ Spelling is perfect.
____ Grammar is correct.
____ Layout is consistent.
____ The page is attractively laid out.

DISTRIBUTING YOUR RESUME

Make the best use of your resume by distributing it to the following:

- Employers who place help-wanted ads
- Employers who have unadvertised openings
- Your networking contacts
- Friends and relatives
- Anyone who indicates that he or she knows someone who might be hiring
- Your school's career services department

Keep enough copies of your resume on hand to respond to unexpected opportunities. Take copies to interviews (even if you have sent a copy in advance), career fairs, and personnel departments. Be sure to have plenty on hand if you decide to drop in on employers, as described in Chapter 8. A well-prepared resume in many hands is an effective way to get the word out that you are a serious job candidate.

It is usually not recommended, however, that dozens of resumes be sent to lists of employers in the hope of locating one who has a job opening. One exception to this recommendation is when there are more job openings than applicants. When there is a shortage of applicants, you are more likely to receive responses when sending unsolicited resumes. A second exception is if you are moving to a new area. Sending a large number of resumes may be more economical and direct than calling potential employers.

Introducing Your Resume: Cover Letters

Cover letters are sent out with the resume. Their purpose is to provide a brief personal introduction and tell the recipient why you are submitting your resume. They should be short, informative, persuasive, and polite. The fact that you write the letter can be persuasive in itself. It shows that you took the time and effort to consider why and how you meet this particular employer's requirements. You did more than simply put a resume in an envelope.

Cover letters are customized for different circumstances. Before discussing the different types, let's look at a few to-dos that are common to all cover letters:

- Use a proper business letter format. See Figure 9–4.
- Be sure to use correct spelling and grammar.
- Print the letter on the same paper as your resume.
- Direct it to a specific person, whenever possible. Look for a name in the ad, ask your contact for the appropriate person, or call the facility and ask. If you are writing in response to an unadvertised position or sending a letter of inquiry, this is especially important. Letters without names can get misdirected or discarded. Busy facilities don't have time to determine to whom to direct your inquiry.
- Write an introduction: explain who you are, why you are writing, who referred you or what ad you are responding to, and what position you are applying for. Employers may have more than one position open, so don't assume that they will know which job you are applying for.
- Develop the body of the letter: explain why the employer should interview you. Summarize your qualifications for the job. Do your best to match these with what you believe the employer is seeking. Avoid repeating the same information that is on your resume.
- Include a closing paragraph in which you ask the employer to call you for an interview or state that you will call for an appointment.

LETTER FOR AN ADVERTISED POSITION

In Chapter 8 we discussed responding to employment ads and demonstrating how you meet the employer's needs. Use language that mirrors that used in the ad or job announcement. Review the examples in Chapter 8; then see Figure 9–5, which shows a complete cover letter.

You may learn about openings through your school or networking contacts. Mention your source of information in the letter's introduction. Be sure that you obtain

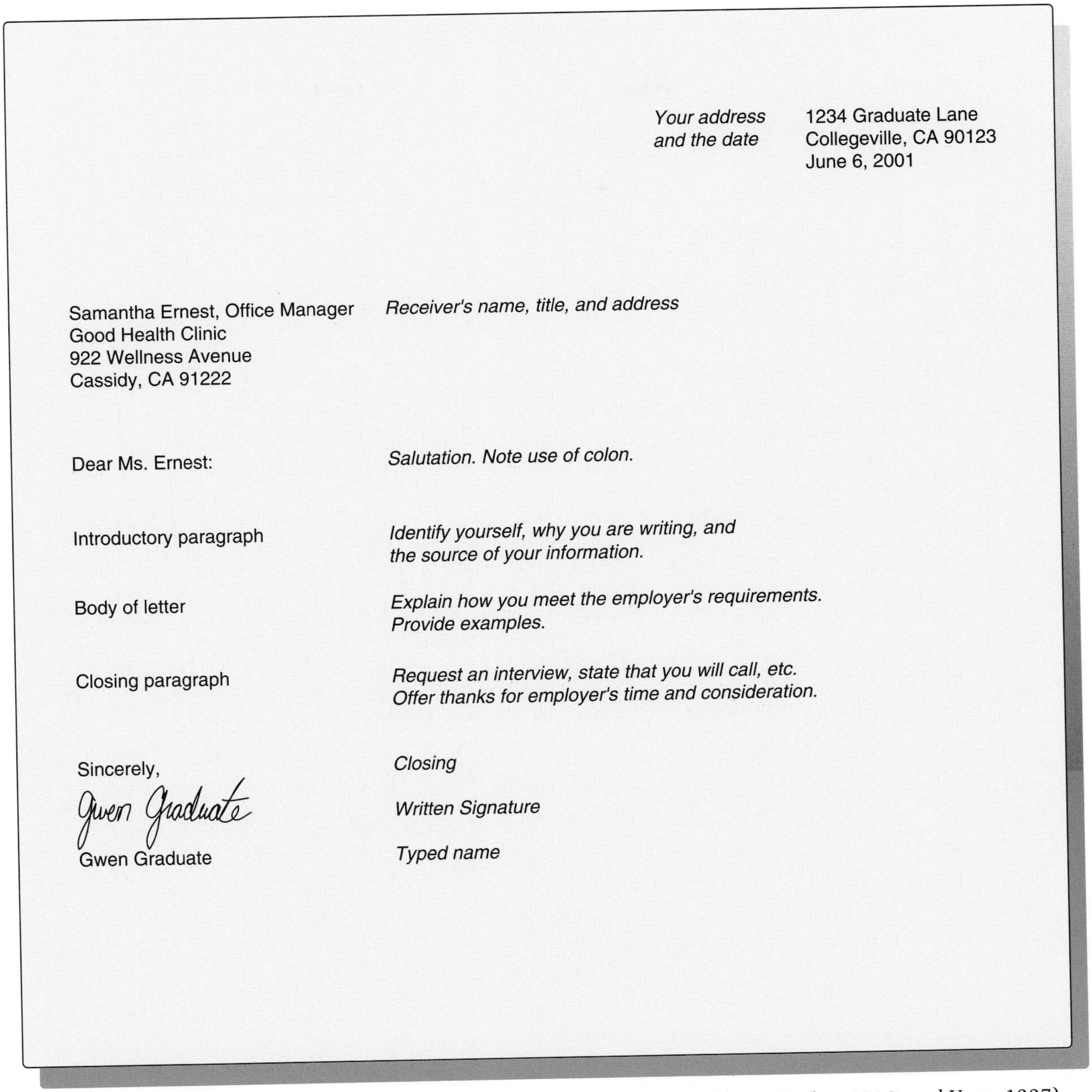

	Your address and the date	1234 Graduate Lane Collegeville, CA 90123 June 6, 2001
Samantha Ernest, Office Manager Good Health Clinic 922 Wellness Avenue Cassidy, CA 91222	*Receiver's name, title, and address*	
Dear Ms. Ernest:	*Salutation. Note use of colon.*	
Introductory paragraph	*Identify yourself, why you are writing, and the source of your information.*	
Body of letter	*Explain how you meet the employer's requirements. Provide examples.*	
Closing paragraph	*Request an interview, state that you will call, etc. Offer thanks for employer's time and consideration.*	
Sincerely,	*Closing*	
Gwen Graduate	*Written Signature*	
Gwen Graduate	*Typed name*	

FIGURE 9–4 Format of a business letter. (Adapted from Hacker, 1999, and Yena, 1997).

PRESCRIPTION FOR SUCCESS 9–13

Respond to an Ad

1. Find an ad for a job in your occupational area.
2. Write a complete cover letter, in mailable form (contains all features mentioned above and has no errors), that responds to the requirements stated in the ad. (Attach the ad to your letter.)

LETTER FOR AN UNADVERTISED OPENING

permission from the contact person before using his or her name. Before writing the letter, learn as much as possible about the job. Sources include the person who told you about it, the employer's web site, or an inquiry call to the facility. See Figure 9–6 for an example of this type of letter.

1234 Graduate Lane
Collegeville, CA 90123
June 6, 2001

Samantha Ernest, Office Manager
Good Health Clinic
922 Wellness Avenue
Cassidy, CA 91222

Dear Ms. Ernest:

I was excited to see your ad in the Cassidy Times on June 5 for a medical assistant. As a recent graduate of Medical Career College, I believe I can make a positive contribution to your health care team. In addition to submitting my resume for your review, I would like to point out how I meet your needs for this position.

Your requirements:	How I Meet Them:
75% clerical duties	I enjoy and am proficient in front office duties. I received top grades in all my administrative classes. I understand the importance of efficiency, accuracy, and confidentiality when performing clerical functions in the medical office. My written and oral communication skills are excellent.
25% clinical duties	I have up-to-date skills in all medical assisting back-office procedures.
Computer literate	I have basic computer literacy skills, can work in a Windows environment, and am proficient in Medical Manager, WordPerfect, and Excel.

I am an energetic, detail-oriented person with good interpersonal skills. I appreciate the need to maintain high-quality patient relations in today's health care environment and know that I am capable of providing efficient, caring service.

Good Health Clinic has an excellent reputation in Cassidy and it would be a privilege to have the opportunity to discuss my qualifications with you in person. I will call next week to schedule an appointment or you can contact me at (760)123-4567. Thank you for your time and consideration.

Respectfully,

Gwen Graduate

Gwen Graduate

FIGURE 9–5 Format of a targeted cover letter.

LETTER OF INQUIRY

There may be a facility where you would like to work, but you are unaware of any job openings. Perhaps you have a friend who is happily employed there and has recommended it as a great place to work. Or it may have a reputation for excellent working conditions and educational and promotional opportunities. When you cannot respond to a specific job opening, state your general qualifications that meet the current needs in health care work. Explain why you are interested in working at that specific facility. Be sure to include contributions you can make, not just what

5687 Success Avenue
Schoolville, MI 48755
September 10, 2001

Joseph Featherstone, Laboratory Supervisor
North Valley Medical Laboratory
4657 Flanders Road
Schoolville, MI 48757

Dear Mr. Featherstone:

Kim Lee, the academic director of the Laboratory Technician Program at High Tech Institute, told me that your facility has an opening for a laboratory technician. North Valley has an excellent reputation for performing high-quality work and providing learning opportunities for employees. As a recent graduate of High Tech, I am enthusiastic about starting my career in an environment in which I can make a positive contribution and at the same time, continue to acquire new skills.

I am dedicated to performing my work accurately and efficiently. High standards are important to me and I earned top grades in all my classes at High Tech. At the same time, I maintained near-perfect attendance and served as president of the student council.

My resume is enclosed for your review. As it can only partly communicate my qualifications, I would appreciate the opportunity to meet with you personally. I will call you on Friday to arrange a time that is convenient for you. I can be contacted at (906) 123-4567.

Sincerely,

Sandy McDougal

FIGURE 9–6 Format of a cover letter for an unadvertised position.

you hope to gain. Learn as much as possible about the facility so that when stating your reasons, you can make specific statements rather than vague, self-centered comments such as "I heard that Caring Clinic is a really good place to work." See Figure 9–7 for an example of a letter of inquiry.

Applications are commonly required of job applicants, even when they have submitted a resume. They provide the employer with complete, standardized sources of information for comparing candidates. Once you are hired, the application is placed

10752 Learning Lane
Silver Stream, NY 10559
July 22, 2001

Ms. Sandra Walters, Manager
Caring Clinic
7992 Oates Road
Greenville, NY 10772

Dear Mrs. Walters:

I am writing to inquire about job openings at Caring Clinic. My husband and I are relocating to Greenville in September and I am looking for a position in which I can apply my up-to-date skills as a phlebotomy technician. Caring Clinic has a reputation for excellent service to the health needs of the Greenville community and I would be proud to be a contributing member of your team.

As a recent graduate of Top Skill Institute, I had the opportunity to perform my internship at Goodwell Laboratory Services, an affiliate of Caring Clinic. I understand the importance of combining technical excellence with attention to customer service. While at Goodwell, my technical skills were highly praised by my supervisor, Mr. Jaime Gutierrez. In addition, I consistently received top ratings on patient satisfaction surveys.

My resume is enclosed for your review. I will call you in early September to see if I can set an appointment to meet with you. Thank you for your consideration.

Respectfully,

Carla Martinez

Carla Martinez

FIGURE 9–7 Format of a letter of inquiry.

PRESCRIPTION FOR SUCCESS 9–14

Inquire about Possibilities

1. Select a facility in your area where you might like to work.
2. Learn as much about it as possible. Sources of information include networking contacts, the Internet, acquaintances who work there, school personnel, and published information such as brochures and newspaper articles.
3. Write a complete cover letter in mailable form.

Applications

in your personnel file and serves as a legal document and record of important information about you and your previous employment.

Some applications contain important statements that you are required to read and sign. For example, employers of home care personnel may restrict their liability (obligation for damages or loss) for employees when they are driving to and from job assignments. Read all statements carefully before signing. Applications may contain legal language and unfamiliar words. Ask for an explanation of anything you don't understand.

After the work of constructing a resume, filling out an application may seem easy. But don't take it for granted. Take time to read the instructions, and fill it out as accurately and neatly as possible. This is particularly important when applying for health care positions, in which neatness and accuracy are important job requirements. Use this opportunity to demonstrate that you meet these requirements.

The following actions will ensure that your applications present you at your best:

- Read the entire application before you begin to fill it in.
- Fill all sections out completely. *Do not* say "See resume" in the Work History section.
- Use black or blue pen, never pencil.
- Print neatly.
- Go to interviews prepared to fill out an application. Take complete information about the following:
  - Social security number
  - Education
  - Work history, including names of employers and dates of employment
  - Military service
  - References
- Proofread what you have written before submitting it.
- Be honest when answering questions. Giving false information can be grounds for dismissal if you are hired.
- For questions that do not apply to you, write "N/A" instead of leaving them blank. This way it is clear that you saw the question and didn't accidentally skip over it.
- Unless the salary is set, it is best to write "negotiable" in the section marked "salary."
- Be sure to sign and date the application.

ELECTRONIC APPLICATIONS

Some employers now have application forms on their web sites. When applying online, be sure to follow the directions carefully and proofread your entries before hitting the "send" button. Once the application is sent, it is difficult to change incorrect information. As with traditional written materials, what you submit is a reflection of you as a professional.

Reference Sheet

As we discussed in Chapter 2, references are people who will vouch for your qualifications as an employee. Good references can be a key factor in tipping the hiring scales in your favor. Give careful consideration to who you ask to serve as references. They must be considered believable. Friends and relatives are not generally accepted as good work references because they may be biased in your favor and not really knowledgeable about your professional competence. In addition to being credible, references must:

- Have the time and be willing to speak on your behalf to potential employers

- Be able speak positively about you
- Have personal knowledge of your work, skills, and/or character

As discussed in Chapter 2, the following people are good candidates:

- Instructors
- Other school personnel
- Clinical supervisor(s)
- Previous employers
- Supervisors at places where you performed volunteer work
- Professionals with whom you worked on committees or projects

Call or speak personally to each person you wish to serve as a reference. Do this *before* you begin the job-search process. Never give out a name and then ask. This puts the person on the spot and makes it difficult if he or she prefers not to be a reference. Inform them about the types of jobs you are applying for and what qualifications are important. This gives them the advantage of being prepared to respond to the potential employer's questions. Have several people in mind. Some may be willing, but unavailable when the potential employer calls them.

Create a written list of at least three references. At a minimum, include their names, titles, and telephone numbers. You may also want to include their addresses. Ask them if they mind being contacted at work. If not, provide a telephone number and recommended times to call. It is essential that these be current and accurate. If you list a work number and the person is no longer employed there, your credibility can be questioned. Potential employers don't have time to call you back or make numerous calls trying to locate your references. Make it easy for them. This makes it easier for them to hire *you.*

Organize the list in an easy-to-read format and print it on the same paper as your resume. Write "References for ______ (your name)" at the top of the page. The reference sheet should not be mailed out with your resume unless it is specifically requested in an employment ad or job bulletin. Take copies with you to interviews to give to potential employers who request it. If you are visiting a personnel department, have a copy available, because many employment applications have a section for listing references.

Be sure to let your references know when you are hired. Thank them for their willingness to assist you. Keep them posted of your career progress. In the future, you may be in a position to assist them, and that is what true networking is all about—mutual career support.

Letters of Recommendation

Another type of reference is provided through letters of recommendation. These letters are generally written by supervisors or people in authority, such as instructors, who provide statements about your work record, skills, and personal qualities. It is a good idea to request reference letters from employers throughout your career.

Reference letters can serve as a record of endorsements and achievements over the years. As you leave each job (on good terms, it is hoped!), request a letter of recommendation from your supervisor.

Make copies of these letters to place in your portfolio or give to potential employers who request them. It is appropriate at interviews to mention that you have them available.

As with other references, show consideration. Ask only those people who you believe can write a positive letter. Also, give people enough time to compose a letter. Avoid giving one day's notice. Finally, if you are requesting letters to support your effort to secure a specific type of job, advise them of the qualities they should emphasize.

Your success depends mainly upon what you think of yourself and whether you believe in yourself.—William J.H. Boetcker

The Portfolio: Supporting What You Say

Review the items you have been collecting for your portfolio. (See the suggestions in Chapter 2.) Choose the ones that represent your best work, and support the qualifications needed in your target jobs. Use your imagination to think of others. For example, consider adding a list of the courses you took if your educational program included courses not commonly part of your occupational area or if your training has prepared you for a variety of positions.

Organize the materials in a logical order, grouping related items together in sections. Place them in a binder or presentation folder using plastic protection sheets. It is not necessary to go to a lot of expense, but the holder should be well made and in a plain, conservative color. Prepare a title page labeled "Professional Portfolio" and include your name, address, and telephone number. If you have a large number of items, number the pages and prepare a table of contents.

Prepare only one portfolio. It is not intended to be sent with your resume. Take it with you on interviews and mention that you have it available for the interviewer to review. Never simply hand it to the employer and expect him or her to read it (unless you are asked for it, of course). It is to be used during the interview to demonstrate your capabilities. For example, if you are asked about your knowledge of coding, you could show assignments in which you accurately coded many diagnoses and procedures.

Portfolios for health care are more widely used in some parts of the country than others. Some employers don't know what they are, so you may need to explain their purpose.

SUMMARY OF KEY IDEAS

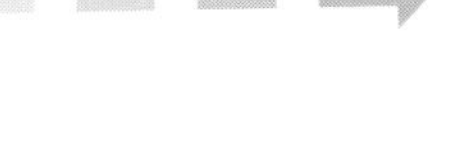

1. Preparing high-quality written materials is a key part of the successful job search.
2. Your resume is an important advertisement of your qualifications.
3. The main purpose of a resume is to secure an interview.
4. Cover letters can increase the effectiveness of the resume.
5. Written materials for health care jobs should reflect the job requirements of accuracy, neatness, and orderliness.
6. References are vital links to future employment.
7. A portfolio gives you a chance to support your capabilities.

POSITIVE SELF-TALK FOR THIS CHAPTER

1. My resume is a good presentation of my skills and qualifications.
2. I write effective cover letters.
3. I fill out applications accurately and neatly.
4. My portfolio supports my claims.

BIBLIOGRAPHY

Dictionary of Occupational Titles, 4th ed. Indianapolis: U.S. Department of Labor, Employment and Training Administration. JIST Works, Inc., 1991.

Ellis, Dave, Stan Lankowitz, Ed Stupka, and Doug Toft. *Career Planning,* 2nd ed. New York: Houghton Mifflin Company, 1997.

Hacker, Diana. *A Writer's Reference,* 4th ed. New York: Bedford/St. Martin's Press, 1999.

Marino, Kim. *Resumes for the Health Care Professional.* New York: John Wiley & Sons, 1993.

Occupational Outlook Handbook. Indianapolis: JIST Works, Inc., 1998.

Yena, Donna J. *Career Directions,* 3rd ed. Chicago: Irwin/Times Mirror, 1997.

10

The Interview

OBJECTIVES

THE INFORMATION AND ACTIVITIES IN THIS CHAPTER CAN HELP YOU TO:

- Explain why the interview should be considered a "sales opportunity."
- Determine the employer's needs.
- Anticipate and prepare to answer common interview questions.
- Know what type of appearance and behavior create a positive first impression.
- Communicate courteously and effectively.
- Demonstrate how to use your portfolio to support your qualifications.
- Deal with difficult situations, including illegal questions.
- Know what types of questions you should ask and avoid.
- Make a gracious exit when the interview is over.

KEY TERMS

Illegal questions: Requests for information that cannot be used to make a hiring decision about a candidate. This information includes age, race, marital and financial status, and religion.

Interview: A meeting, usually in person, in which a job applicant and an employer or representative exchange information. The goal of employers is to determine if the applicants meet their needs. The goal of applicants is to demonstrate that they *do*.

Mirroring: A communication technique in which you match your communication style to that of the other person in order to improve mutual understanding.

The Interview—Your Sales Opportunity

Finally! The words you have been hoping to hear: "When can you come in for an **interview**?" Your job search efforts are paying off. But wait a minute! You begin to worry: "What if I can't think of anything to say?" "What if I don't have the skills they are looking for?" "What if they ask me about . . . ?"

The purpose of this chapter is to help you put the "what if's" to rest and see the interviewing process as an opportunity to present yourself at your best. In Chapter 3 we discussed the power of attitude and how you can choose your reaction to any

At The Interview:
How To Show You've Got What It Takes

Employers want to hire someone who is:	How to show that you are that someone:
Qualified to perform the job	1. Be familiar with and able to document all your skills 2. Create a portfolio that contains evidence of your qualifications
Reliable	1. Arrive on time to the interview 2. Send any requested follow-up materials
Trustworthy	1. Have a good handshake 2. Maintain appropriate eye contact 3. Include only accurate information on your resume and job application 4. Do not lie during your interview 5. Avoid saying anything negative about a previous employer 6. Do not engage in any type of gossip
Professional	1. Dress appropriately 2. Be clean and well-groomed 3. Bring needed materials to interview
Motivated and willing to learn	1. Know something about the facility and why you want to work there 2. Ask questions about the job 3. Inquire about learning opportunities on the job 4. Have a plan for professional development
A good communicator and able to work well with others	1. Show consideration for everyone at the interview site 2. Introduce yourself 3. Behave courteously 4. Listen actively throughout the interview 5. Use feedback appropriately to check your understanding of the speaker's message 6. Answer all questions completely but concisely 7. Speak clearly and with proper expression
Likeable	1. Smile 2. Be enthusiastic 3. Have a sense of humor 4. Show interest in job 5. Express interest in employer's needs 6. Be comfortable with yourself 7. Show respect for interviewer 8. Avoid showing impatience, annoyance
A problem-solver	1. Describe examples of problems solved in the past 2. Be prepared and willing to participate in any problem-solving exercises given 3. Suggest specific ways you can help the employer

FIGURE 10-1 The interview—your sales opportunity.

situation. Interviews can be viewed as opportunities to be rejected. Many applicants approach them with this expectation. But you have another choice. You can view an interview as an *opportunity to determine an employer's needs and show how you fill them* (Fig. 10–1).

Think about it. Employers are busy people who don't have time to conduct interviews with people who are unlikely job candidates. You obviously meet the minimum qualifications. The interviewer wants to see if you are a likable person who can back up your qualifications, communicate, and fit in at the facility.

By learning what will be expected of you at an interview and practicing your presentation skills, you can attend each interview with confidence. The most common reason for not being hired is lack of preparation for the interview. And this is a factor over which you, not the interviewer, has control.

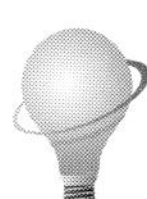

Take a Moment to Think

1. Am I comfortable about attending interviews?
2. If not, what are my biggest concerns?
3. Are they reasonable?
4. What can I do to resolve them?

The Customer's Needs

Good sales presentations are based on showing customers—employers—how they can benefit by buying a product—in this case, hiring *you*. Recall from Chapter 2 that identifying the customer's needs is an important step for students who are beginning a program of career preparation. As was pointed out, it doesn't make sense to create a product that no one needs.

In the same way, attending an interview without knowing what the employer is looking for puts the applicant at a disadvantage. This is because in order to be at your best *during* the interview, the following preparations must be completed *in advance:*

- Anticipate what types of questions might be asked.
- Practice answering them.
- Create examples to demonstrate your mastery of desirable skills.
- Prepare appropriate questions to ask.

All employers have general qualities they look for in applicants. These were identified in the SCANS report. And health care employers have expressed their needs through the National Health Care Skill Standards. (See Chapter 1 to review highlights of the SCANS and NHCSS Skills.)

In addition, each employer has requirements that are based on factors such as patient population, services offered, size of facility, budgets, and so on. It is important for the applicant to learn as much as possible before attending the interview. Depending on the size of the facility, the following sources may be helpful:

- Direct contact by phone or in person: ask questions, request a job description, observe the facility
- Brochures
- People who work there, such as friends, classmates, or networking contacts
- Research in the local newspaper: large facilities are sometimes the subject of news articles
- The facility's Internet site
- School's career services department
- Chamber of Commerce and other organizations that have information about large employers

- The local chapter of your professional organization
- Information gathered at career fairs and employer orientation meetings
- Employment ad if position was advertised

If the facility is small, such as a one-physician office, you should know, at a minimum, the type of specialty practiced and the patient population served. When you are unable to learn very much before the interview, it is especially important that you *listen carefully* to the employer and ask good questions. These topics are discussed later in this chapter.

Research into interviewing shows that the person conducting the interview is often more stressed than the candidate.—Allan-James Associates

PRESCRIPTION FOR SUCCESS 10-1

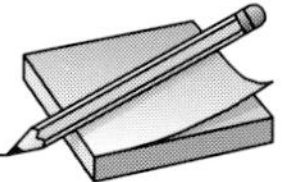

Be Prepared

1. Select a facility where you might want to work.
2. Use the resources described to learn as much about it as possible. Suggested questions:

   What type of work do they do?

   What is their patient population or client base?

   How many employees are there?

   What are the duties of the job for which you might apply?

The Interviewer Is Human, Too

In addition to knowing the employment needs of the employer, consider the personal situation of the interviewer. Many applicants view the interviewer as a person of great confidence who has all the power in the hiring process. Applicants mistakenly see themselves as the underdogs in a game they have little chance of winning. In reality, interviewers may face a number of pressures:

- Concern about finding the right candidate who can perform the job as needed
- An extremely busy schedule
- Lack of interviewing skills
- A demanding supervisor who will hold them responsible for the performance of the person who is hired
- Concern about finding time and resources to orient and train a new employee

Understanding the interviewer's point of view requires empathy—attempting to see the world through the eyes of others (see Chapter 3). This may not seem easy in a job interview when you are nervous and concentrating on presenting yourself well. But it is this very shift of focus—from yourself to the interviewer—that leads to a more successful interviewing experience. For it is through this very attempt to understand and then show how you can help resolve the employer's problems that you best present yourself as *the* candidate for the job.

Heads Up! Knowing What to Expect

Help yourself; 25% of new graduates forget the basics.—Brenda Bracken, Healthcare Staffing Solutions, Inc., San Diego

Some interviews are highly structured; each candidate is asked the same set of prepared questions. Or they may take place as a conversation, with topics and questions generated freely. Most interviews fall somewhere between these patterns, with interviewers preparing at least a few questions in advance. Some questions have become the "golden oldies" of the employment world, and knowing them gives you an opportunity to plan possible responses. It is essential, however, that you focus your answers on the needs of the health care industry in general *and* the specific needs of the employer. This means that even if you are asked the same question, the same answer will not necessarily be appropriate at every interview.

GENERAL INTERVIEW QUESTIONS

QUESTION	RESPONSE GUIDELINES
1. Why are you applying for this job?	Explain your interest in health care and the specific type of work performed at this facility.
2. What do you consider your greatest strengths?	Choose from among technical or personal traits. Show how they relate to the job and will benefit the employer.
3. What are your weaknesses?	It is not a good idea to say "none," as this is unrealistic and gives the impression that you don't know yourself very well. Prepare an honest answer that displays a weakness that has a positive side or for which you have an improvement plan in place that you can describe.
4. What do you know about this organization/facility/specialty?	Do your research! And be clear about what it is that interests you *and* how you believe you can make a contribution.
5. Why should we hire you?	Explain how you can make a positive contribution to the organization: skills, attitude, interest, personal characteristics, and so on.
6. What did you enjoy most in school?	Relate your favorite class/subject/activity to the job you are applying for.
7. Where do you want to be in five years?	This is a good opportunity to think about your long-term goals (*before* the interview, of course). Examples: seek increasing responsibility in the same profession, move into supervisory work, or pursue additional education to move up the career ladder. You don't want to give the impression, however, that you plan to stay at this job for only a short time.
8. How do you work under pressure? Manage your time well? Work well with others? And so on.	Be prepared to give examples showing *how* you have worked well under pressure, used your time well, and so on. Use examples from work, school, or personal life.

These are only a few of many commonly asked questions. You can see that a thorough knowledge of your skills and personal characteristics, along with an awareness of employer needs, are the sources of good answers.

PRESCRIPTION FOR SUCCESS 10-2

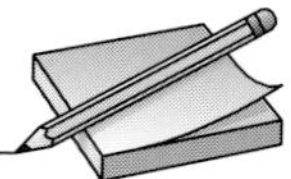

Answering General Questions

1. Create ten questions.
2. Choose a specific job and facility (real or imaginary) and prepare an appropriate response for each question.
3. Say your answers out loud.
4. Continue to repeat the exercise out loud until you can answer the questions smoothly, but without sounding "canned" or phony.

WORK PREFERENCE QUESTIONS

You may asked be about your job preferences. Review your answers to Prescription for Success 8-3, "What Do I Want?" In addition, be prepared to answer applicable questions about:

- Whether you want full- or part-time work
- The hours you are willing to work
- The length of shift you prefer
- The days and time of day you can work

Remember to be realistic when applying for jobs. Don't waste employers' time interviewing for jobs with conditions that you already know are absolutely impossible for you to meet.

PRESCRIPTION FOR SUCCESS 10-3

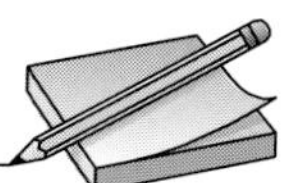

Answering Questions about Your Work Preference

1. Create five questions an employer in your occupational area might ask.
2. Choose a specific job and facility (real or imaginary) and prepare an appropriate response for each question.
3. Say your answers out loud.
4. Continue to repeat the exercise out loud until you can answer the questions smoothly, but without sounding "canned" or phony.

OCCUPATION-SPECIFIC QUESTIONS

Questions in this category explore your specific knowledge, skill mastery, willingness to learn new procedures, and content of your training. The type of question will vary:

- Describe how to perform a specific procedure.
- Explain how to operate certain equipment.
- Describe appropriate action to take in a given situation.
- Suggest how to solve a health care problem.
- Explain how you plan to keep your skills updated.
- Discuss how you would resolve a conflict with a coworker or supervisor.
- What do you know about . . . ? (a theory, new procedure, etc.)
- Why do you want to work in pediatrics/dermatology/children's dentistry, and so on?

Some employers give practical skill tests or ask you to physically demonstrate your knowledge. These might include a keyboarding speed test, filing or record-keeping exercise, spelling test, or demonstration of a procedure. If you are asked to perform a practical test that is appropriate for your level of training, do so willingly. Don't apologize that you "might not do well" or give signs of annoyance. Use the request to show that you have confidence in your abilities and can handle stress.

PRESCRIPTION FOR SUCCESS 10–4

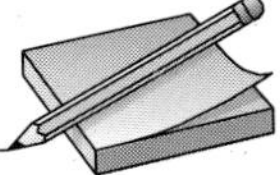

Answering Occupation-Specific Questions

1. Create five questions that apply to your field.
2. Choose a specific job and facility (real or imaginary) and prepare an appropriate response for each question.
3. Say your answers out loud.
4. Continue to repeat the exercise out loud until you can answer the questions smoothly, but without sounding "canned" or phony.

Practice—Your Key to Success

Successful interviews usually depend on good preparation.—John D. Drake

Of course, you cannot anticipate the exact questions that interviewers are going to ask. What you *can* do is prepare yourself to answer a variety of questions. You should practice the following skills to increase your answering abilities:

- Listen carefully to the question.
- Ask for clarification when necessary.
- Think through your "inventory" of capabilities and characteristics that apply (created in Prescriptions for Success 8–1 and 8–2).
- Use examples to back up your answer.
- Feel confident of your ability to deal with questions, and present yourself at your best.

Preparation means practice—actually answering questions, out loud, under conditions as close to those of an actual interview as possible. The best way is to role-play with someone who acts as the interviewer. This can be an instructor, mentor, networking contact, friend, or family member. Many schools require mock (pretend) interviews as part of professional development classes. Take advantage of these opportunities, and do your best to conduct yourself as if you were at a real interview. Videotaping or having an observer take notes can be helpful, even if it's a little nerve-wracking. It's better to make a few mistakes now and avoid them at interviews.

If you believe that you might be asked to demonstrate skills, include them in your practice sessions. The career services personnel at your school may be familiar with the interviewing practices of facilities in your area and can give you additional information about what to expect and how to best prepare.

The goal of "interview rehearsals" is *not* to memorize answers that you can repeat. It is to develop a level of comfort about the process and have facts fresh in your mind that you can call on as needed to respond intelligently and confidently.

PRESCRIPTION FOR SUCCESS 10-5

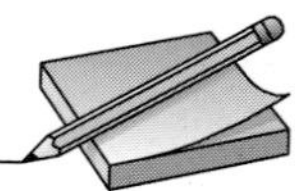

Dress Rehearsal

1. Choose someone who will help you role-play. Give him or her a list of questions to ask you in random order. (Better yet, find someone with interviewing experience and have this person surprise you.)
2. If possible, record the session or have a third person observe.
3. Discuss how you did with your partner and the observer.
4. Make a list of what you need to work on.

Be Prepared—What to Take Along

Having everything you might need at the interview will help you feel pulled together. It will also demonstrate to the employer that you are organized and think ahead, valuable qualities for health care professionals. While your own list may be different, here are some suggestions for what to take along:

- Extra copies of your resume
- Your portfolio
- Copies of licenses, certifications, and so on
- Proof of immunizations and results of health tests
- Reference sheet
- Any documentation of skills and experience not included in your portfolio (or if you have chosen not to create a portfolio)
- Pens
- Small notepad
- Your list of questions (discussed later in this chapter)
- All information needed for an application (see Chapter 9)
- Appointment calendar
- Anything you have been requested to bring
- For your eyes only: extra pantyhose, breath mints, other "emergency supplies"

A small case or large handbag is a convenient way to carry your papers and supplies. It can be inexpensive, but it should be a conservative color, in good repair, and neatly organized.

PRESCRIPTION FOR SUCCESS 10-6

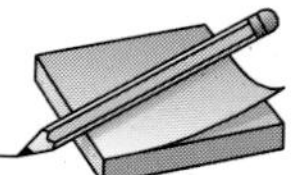

Packing List

1. Check the items on the preceding list that you will take to interviews.
2. Are there others? ______

____

____

First Impressions—Make Them Count!

The way in which we think of ourselves has everything to do with how our world sees us.—Arlene Raven

Just thirty seconds! That's how long you have to make a lasting impression. The average person forms a strong opinion of another in less than one minute. This is why so much emphasis is placed on professional appearance both during the job search and later, on the job. While it is possible to reverse a negative first impression eventually, it's a lot easier to make a good one in the first place.

In Chapter 2 we discussed the messages that dress and grooming communicate. When applying for a job in health care, appropriate appearance can let the interviewer know that you:

- Appreciate the impact of appearance on others (patients, other professionals).
- Know what is appropriate for the job.
- Understand the principles of good hygiene.
- Respect both yourself and the interviewer.
- Take the interview seriously.

There is no universal agreement about the proper clothing to wear when applying for certain health care jobs. In some areas, students are encouraged to wear a clean, pressed uniform. In others, they are advised to wear business attire, which means:

- For women: a suit consisting of a skirt and matching jacket, worn with a blouse, *or* a skirt and blouse, *or* a simple dress.
- For men: a suit consisting of matching pants and jacket, *or* pants and a sport coat, *or* pants and a plain white or light-colored shirt.

The best choices are conservative colors and simple styles. Never wear jeans or clothing that is revealing or extremely casual. Don't wear a hat or sunglasses during the interview. If you're not sure about what to wear, ask your instructor or career services for help. If extra money for interview clothes presents a problem, ask if your school has a clothes-lending program. Many cities have excellent thrift shops that sell nice clothes at reasonable prices. Some specialize in helping people dress for job interviews.

You may arrive at the interview to find that most people at the facility are dressed very casually. Don't worry. It is far better to be overdressed in this situation than underdressed. You can adjust your style later, *after* you get the job.

Here are some additional guidelines that apply to all health care job applicants:

- Be squeaky clean. Take a bath or shower, wash your hair, scrub your fingernails, and use a deodorant or antiperspirant.
- Save the fashion trends for later. Hair and nails should be natural colors, tattoos covered up, and visible rings and studs from piercings removed. Limit earrings to one set. Women should apply makeup lightly for a natural, not painted, look.
- Show that you know what is acceptable for the health care professional. Avoid long fingernails, free-flowing hair, and dangling accessories that can be grabbed by patients or caught in machinery. Wear closed-toe shoes. Strive to be odor-free. Don't smoke on the way to the interview. Even the fragrances in perfumes and other personal products, intended to be pleasant, should not be worn because many patients find them disagreeable or have allergic reactions.
- Men who wear facial hair should groom it neatly.

PRESCRIPTION FOR SUCCESS 10–7

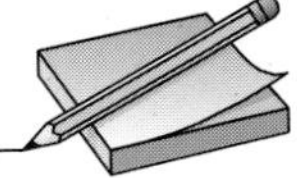

Planning the Look

1. Select an appropriate outfit for interviewing, including shoes. Make sure everything is clean, pressed, and ready to go on short notice.
2. If in doubt, ask your instructor, mentor, or career services staff for input.

Your appearance may be perfect, but if you arrive late for an interview, it may not matter. Being late is a sure way to make a poor impression. Time management is an essential health care job skill, and you will have failed your first opportunity to demonstrate that you have mastered it. In addition, arriving late is a sign of rudeness and inconsideration for the interviewer's time. Make a few advance preparations to ensure that this doesn't happen to you:

- Write down the date and exact time of the appointment.
- Verify the address and ask for directions, if necessary.
- If the office is in a large building or complex, get additional instructions about how to find it.
- Inquire about parking, bus stops, or subway stops.
- Allow extra time to arrive, and plan to be there about ten minutes before the appointed time.

If there is an emergency that can't be avoided (a flat tire or unexpected snow storm), call as soon as possible to offer an explanation and reschedule the interview.

Many job applicants don't realize that the interview actually starts *before* they sit down with the person asking the questions. That's right. From the first contact you made to inquire about a job opening or set the appointment, you have been making an impression. If you arrive for the interview and are rude to the receptionist, you may have already failed in your bid for the job. You cannot know what information is shared with the hiring authority. (Keep in mind, too, that these may be your future coworkers!)

Learn the name of the person who will be conducting the interview. Be sure you have the correct spelling (for the thank-you note, discussed in Chapter 11) and pronunciation. When introduced, the following actions express both courtesy and self-confidence:

1. Make and maintain eye contact.
2. Give a healthy (not limp or hesitant) handshake.
3. Express how glad you are to meet him or her and that you appreciate the opportunity to be interviewed.
4. *Do not* sit down until you are offered a chair or the other person is seated.

PRESCRIPTION FOR SUCCESS 10–8

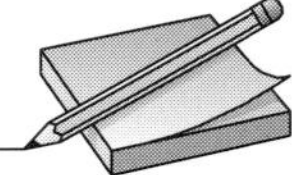

Practice Until It Comes Naturally

1. In front of a mirror, practice your smile and posture.
2. With a partner, practice your handshake.
3. Rehearse the meeting: approach, smile, handshake, sitting down, feeling at ease in the chair.

COURTESY DURING THE INTERVIEW

Maintaining eye contact (without staring, of course) when the other person is speaking indicates that you are interested in what he or she is saying. When *you* are speaking, it is natural to look away occasionally. Most of the time, however, you should look at the listener. This is a sign of openness and sincerity. Review the guidelines for respectful communication in Chapter 7. Following is a summary of behaviors to definitely *avoid* (even if the interviewer engages in them):

- Interrupting
- Cursing
- Gossiping, such as commenting on the weaknesses of other facilities, professionals, or your previous employer

- Telling off-color jokes
- Putting yourself down
- Chewing gum
- Appearing to snoop by looking at papers or other materials on the interviewer's desk, shelves, and so on
- Discussing personal problems

You don't want to come across as stiff or stuffy, but interviewers may be testing your ability to remain professional. Or they may consider behavior that is appropriate for them to be unacceptable in others—especially job applicants! Try to be at ease and act natural, but at the same time, play it safe and maintain your best "company manners."

Apply Your Communication Skills

A successful job interview depends on the effective use of communication. It is essentially a conversation between two people who are trying to determine if they fit each other's employment needs. As a job applicant, you must take responsibility for making sure that you understand the interviewer's needs, questions, and comments, as well as expressing yourself clearly so that he or she understands *you*.

ACTIVE LISTENING

Understanding begins by *listening actively.* The importance of carefully listening to the interviewer cannot be overemphasized. Most of us are so occupied thinking about what we are going to say next that we fail to fully hear—let alone actively listen—to the other person. This is especially true in an interview when we are nervous and worried about whether we are saying the right thing. But this is the very situation where we can most benefit from listening carefully and basing what we say on *what we hear*.

Recall from Chapter 3 that active listening consists of *paying attention, focusing on the speaker's words,* and *thinking about the meaning of what is said.* This takes practice. When you participate in the mock interviews suggested earlier, do not look at the questions the person role-playing the interviewer is going to ask. This will force you to listen carefully. Remember that pausing to think and compose an appropriate response will be appreciated by interviewers. You will be evaluated on the quality of your answer, not on how quickly you gave it.

MIRRORING

An effective communication technique for interviews is known as **mirroring.** This means that you observe the communication style of the interviewer and then match it as closely as possible. This does *not* mean mimicking or appearing to make fun of the other person. It *does* mean adapting a style that will be most comfortable for the interviewer. The following examples illustrate the concept of mirroring.

IF THE INTERVIEWER IS	IT IS BEST TO
Very businesslike. Direct and to the point.	Answer questions concisely, quickly getting to the point. Avoid long introductions, wordiness, and unnecessary detail.
Warm and friendly. Conversational tone.	Reflect the interviewer's warmth without becoming too casual. Include human interest and details, when appropriate, in your answers.
Seemingly unhurried. Spends time describing the job in detail and explains what is meant by the questions.	Include details to support your answers and fully explain yourself (without giving unnecessary or unrelated information).

FEEDBACK Whatever the style of the interviewer, use feedback when necessary to ensure that you understand the message. Feedback, as you recall from Chapter 7, is a communication technique used to check your understanding of the speaker's intended message. It is not necessary—or even desirable—to repeat everything the speaker says. It is annoying to speakers to have everything they say repeated (you don't want to sound like a parrot). And requesting feedback unnecessarily will use up time that should be spent learning about the job and presenting your qualifications. Used when needed, it will enable you to understand the speaker and respond appropriately and intelligently.

ORGANIZATION When speaking, do your best to present your ideas in an organized manner so that they are easy for the listener to follow. This can be difficult when you are nervous, so take your time to think before you speak. Sometimes we feel uncomfortable with silence and feel compelled to talk in order to avoid it. But taking a few moments to consider your content will result in better answers. Saying something *meaningful* after a pause is more important than quickly saying *something*.

PRESCRIPTION FOR SUCCESS 10-9

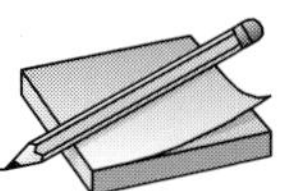

Develop Your Communication Skills

Apply your communication skills at every opportunity: active listening, mirroring, and feedback. These are not just interview skills. Making an effort to use them consistently will benefit every aspect of your relationships with others.

Nonverbal Communication: It Can Make You or Break You

If you want a quality, act as if you already had it.—William James

You can speak smoothly and answer questions correctly and yet completely fail in your communication efforts. What has gone wrong? Your *actions* have betrayed you. That's right: what you *do* communicates as much as—or even more than—what you *say*. As we discussed in Chapter 7, our movements, posture, gestures, and facial expressions reveal our true feelings. You can enthusiastically claim that you would *love* the challenge of working in a fast-paced, think-on-your-feet clinical environment. But if your face and body language reflect fear, anxiety, or subtle expressions of "yuck!," your verbal message will not ring true. Remember that more than half of the content of our messages is communicated nonverbally. This is why videos are very helpful when practicing your interview skills. You can observe your nonverbal language, and catch inappropriate facial expressions and other behaviors that you will want to work on.

The author is not suggesting that you try to mask your true feelings and put on an act to impress the interviewer. On the contrary. The purpose of this discussion is to encourage you to be aware of how important your actions are and what they say about you. Developing a positive attitude about the interviewing process and confidence in your own abilities will help ensure that your body language communicates positive messages. And conversely, developing the body language of a positive, confident person will help you *become* such a person.

There are ways to communicate both self-confidence and respect for the other person:

- Stand up straight, with your head held up and shoulders back.
  Message: "I am a candidate worthy of your consideration."

- Maintain eye contact.
  Message: "I am sincere in what I am saying."
- Avoid nervous actions such as jiggling a leg or fidgeting with your hands.
  Message: "I want to be here."
- Lean forward slightly in your chair.
  Message: "I am interested in what you are saying."

PRESCRIPTION FOR SUCCESS 10-10

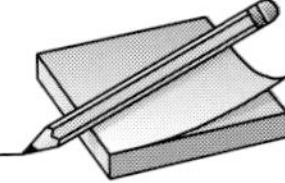

Become Aware of Nonverbal Messages

1. Observe the behavior of others throughout the day. Can you find examples that communicate cooperativeness? Self-confidence? Respect for others?
2. Describe the specific behaviors that communicate positive messages.

PRESCRIPTION FOR SUCCESS 10-11

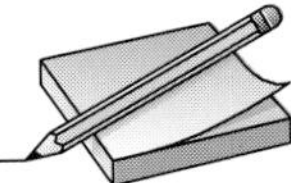

Would You Hire This Person?

1. Check you posture and smile in a full-length mirror. Do you look confident? Approachable? Like a person *you* would choose to work with?
2. Explain why or why not.
3. Is there anything you would like to change?
4. If yes, what is your plan?

Using Your Portfolio Effectively

Portfolios are gaining popularity among jobs seekers, including those in the health care field. They can be a very effective way to back up your claims of competence by providing evidence of your accomplishments and qualifications.

Not all employers are familiar with portfolios. Announcing at the beginning of interviews that you have brought one and asking interviewers if they would like to see it may not be the most effective way of using it to your advantage. Remember that one of your main goals at the interview is to show how you meet the employer's needs. You won't know enough about these needs until you spend a little time listening. Then you can use your portfolio constructively, as in the following situations when the interviewer:

1. Asks a question about your skills and abilities
   "Can you . . . ?"
   "Have you had experience . . . ?"
2. States what skills are needed or provides a job description
   "This job requires . . ."
   "We need someone who can chart accurately, use medical terminology correctly, and so on."
3. States a problem or concern
   "One of our problems has been with ensuring accurate documentation . . ."
   "We have difficulties with . . ."
4. Isn't familiar with the contents of your training program
   "Did your program include . . . ?"
   "What skills did you learn . . . ?"

5. Asks for verification of licenses, certifications, and so on.
   "Have you passed the _____ exam?"
   "Are you a certified medical assistant?"
   "Are you licensed in this state?"

It isn't necessary—or even a good idea—to try to back up *everything* you say with your portfolio. In fact, if overused, a portfolio loses its effectiveness. And many questions are better answered with an oral explanation and/or an example.

Become very familiar with your portfolio's contents so that you can find items quickly. Create an easy-to-read table of contents. Frantically flipping through pages to find something will make you look (and feel) unprepared and disorganized. You will also waste valuable time, a very limited resource in most interviews.

You can use your portfolio to give a brief summary presentation if you are given an appropriate opportunity at the end of the interview. Use this presentation to quickly review your qualifications or to point out those that haven't been mentioned. For example, the interviewer might say "Tell me why I should choose you" or ask "What else should I know about you?"

You may attend interviews where you are unable to use your portfolio at all. This is okay. It is always better—both during the job search and on the job—to be *over*prepared. This prevents you from missing opportunities when they occur.

PRESCRIPTION FOR SUCCESS 10–12

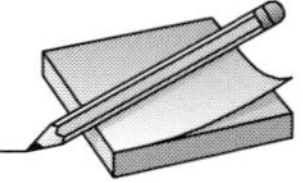

Portfolio Role-Play

1. Write a list of five questions that a potential employer might ask in which you could use your portfolio to support your answer.
2. Role-play with a partner. Have him or her choose the questions at random. Answer each question, and use your portfolio to document your answer.

Handling Sticky Interview Situations

In spite of your best efforts, some interviews can be a little rocky. As mentioned earlier, not everyone is skilled at interviewing. Consider this: you may have prepared and practiced far more than the person conducting the interview! Table 10–1 contains difficult situations and suggestions for handling them gracefully.

DEALING WITH ILLEGAL QUESTIONS

It is illegal for employers to discriminate (use as a reason for not hiring) against an applicant on the basis of any of the following:

- Age (as long as the applicant is old enough to work legally)
- Arrests (without a conviction—being proven guilty)
- Ethnic background
- Financial status
- Marital status, children
- Physical condition (as long as the applicant can perform the job tasks)
- Race
- Religion
- Sexual preference

Questions that require the applicant to reveal information about these factors are illegal. They are sometimes asked anyway. Some employers are ignorant of the laws. Or the interview becomes friendly and conversational, and personal information is shared. ("Oh, I went to Grady High School, too. What year did you graduate?") Employers may take the chance that applicants won't know the questions are illegal. And a few will ask because they know that most applicants will not take the

TABLE 10–1 ***Handling Difficult Interview Situations***

If the Interviewer	What You Can Do
Keeps you waiting a long time.	If you are interested in the job, *do not* show annoyance or anger. It is best not to schedule interviews when you have a very limited amount of time. Remember, this person may be overworked, and that's exactly why there is a potential position for you! Keep in mind that health care work does not always proceed at our convenience. A patient with an emergency, for example, will certainly have priority over an interviewee.
Allows constant interruptions with phone calls and/or people coming in.	Again, do not show that you are irritated. This person may be very busy, disorganized, or simply having a difficult day. (This may be another good sign that this employer really needs your help.)
Does most of the talking and doesn't give you an opportunity to say much about yourself.	Listen carefully and try to determine how you can relate what you have to offer to what has been said. In this case, being a good listener in itself may be the most important quality you can demonstrate.
Seems to simply make conversation. Doesn't discuss the job or ask you questions.	Try to move the discussion to the job by asking questions: "Can you tell me about what you are looking for in a candidate?" "What are the principal duties that this person would perform?" It is possible that this is a test to see your reaction, so take care to be courteous.
Tries to engage you in gossip about other professionals, facilities, your school, etc.	Say you don't really know about the person or situation and cannot comment. Ask a question about the job to redirect the conversation.
Allows long periods of silence.	This may be a test to see how you react under pressure. Don't feel that you have to speak, and do your best to remain comfortable. (Say to yourself: "This is just a test, and I'm doing fine.") If it goes on too long, you can ask: "Is there something you'd like me to tell you more about? Discuss further?"
Doesn't seem to understand your training or qualifications.	Explain as clearly as possible. Use your portfolio, as appropriate, to illustrate your skills.
Makes inappropriate comments about your appearance, gender, ethnicity, etc.	Depending on the nature of the comment and your interpretation of the situation, it may be best to excuse yourself from the interview. For example, comments of a sexual nature or racial slurs should not be tolerated. You should discuss this situation with your instructor or career services for advice on how to proceed.
Is very friendly, chatty, and complimentary about you.	Why in the world, you ask, is this a problem? It may not be. But be careful not to get so comfortable that you share personal problems and other information that may disqualify you for the job.

time to report them for discrimination. It may not be obvious from the questions that answering them will, in fact, reveal information that cannot be considered when hiring.

QUESTION	WHAT IT CAN REVEAL
What part of town do you live in?	Financial status
Do you own your home?	Financial status
Where are your parents from?	Ethnic background
Which holidays do you celebrate?	Religion

Illegal questions put you in a difficult situation, and there are no easy formulas for handling them. In deciding what to do, you need to ask *yourself* several questions:

1. Is the subject of the question of concern to me?
2. Do I find the question offensive?
3. Does the interviewer appear to be unaware that the question is illegal?
4. What is my overall impression of the interviewer and the facility?
5. How badly do I want this particular job?
6. If this person is to be my immediate supervisor, is the question an indication that this is a person I don't really want to work with closely?
7. What do I think the interviewer's real concern is? Is it valid?

Based on your answers, there are several ways that you can respond:

1. Answer honestly.
2. Ask the interviewer to explain how the question relates to the job requirements.
3. Respond to the interviewer's *concern* rather than to the question.
4. Ignore the question and talk about something else.
5. Refuse to answer.
6. Inform the interviewer that the question is illegal.
7. State that you plan to report the incident to the Civil Rights Commission or Equal Employment Opportunity Commission.

Employers do have the right—as well as the responsibility—to ensure that applicants can perform the job requirements both legally and physically. There is sometimes only a small difference in wording between a legal and an illegal question:*

ILLEGAL	LEGAL
How old are you?	Are you over eighteen?
Where were you born?	Do you have the legal right to work in the United States?
What is your maiden name?	Would your work records be listed under another name?
Have you ever been arrested?	Have you ever been convicted of a crime?

Are you beginning to understand how employers can get confused and ask illegal questions? It is possible to be an excellent dentist or physical therapist but not an expert in the details of employment law. However you choose to respond to questions you believe are illegal, it is best to remain calm and courteous. You may decide you don't want to work here, but conduct yourself professionally at all times.

Many employment experts recommend that you respond to the employer's con-

*Adapted from Lock, 1996.

cerns rather than the questions. This requires that you determine what the concerns are. Here are some examples:

QUESTION	POSSIBLE CONCERN	SUGGESTED RESPONSES
Do you have young children?	Your attendance and dependability	Explain your childcare arrangements, good attendance in school and on other jobs, and dedication to employers.
Where do you live?	Reliable transportation, punctuality	Describe your transportation/good attendance record in school.
Which religious holidays are you unable to work?	Scheduling problems	Explain that you are a team player and committed to ensuring that all work days are covered. You will trade with others when they have a holiday.

One recommended strategy for handling common employer concerns is to bring them up before the interviewer does. This gives you the opportunity to present them in a positive light. Employers may be uncomfortable addressing certain issues and will simply drop you from the "possible hire" list.* By taking the initiative, you gain the opportunity to defend your position and stay on the list. Here are some suggestions for finding the positive aspects of various employment "problems":

THE PROBLEM	THE BRIGHT SIDE
You're very young, with little work experience.	Energetic, eager to learn, "trainable," looking for long-term employment ("One of the advantages of being young is . . . ").
You have a criminal record.*	Have learned from mistakes, eager to have an opportunity to serve others
You're over age forty.	Experienced, good work habits, patient
You've had many jobs, none for very long.	Variety of experiences, flexible, can adjust to the working environment, have now found a career to which you want to dedicate your efforts

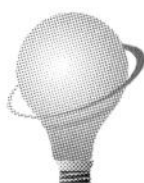

Take a Moment to Think

1. Is there anything you think employers might see as an obstacle to hiring you?
2. How can you turn the obstacle into a positive characteristic?

* Note: Some states do not allow individuals who have been convicted of specific crimes to work in certain health care occupations.

Stay Focused on the Positive

Employers are hiring based on attitude: "Give me a 'C' student with an 'A' attitude."—Melva Duran, Maric College, San Diego

Interviews are a time to do your best to stay positive. They are *not* the place to bring up problems, or what you can't do or don't want to do. Be positive and future-oriented and stress:

- What you can do
- How you can help
- Ways you can apply what you've learned

As mentioned before, you should never criticize a previous employer, instructor, or anyone else. Potential employers realize that they may someday be your previous employer and don't want to be the subject of your comments to others in the profession. Alternatively, these people may be friends and get together regularly at dinner parties.

Remember that the interview is a sales presentation. A sales presentation is not the time to point out the product's faults. You want to emphasize the positive aspects of your skills and character, not your weaknesses. However, if you sincerely feel that you are not qualified for a job (and this is an important consideration in health care), you should never pretend that you are. Lacking needed skills is not a negative reflection on you as a person. It simply means that this job is not appropriate for you. Others jobs will be. In fact, there may be many reasons why jobs and applicants do not match. After all, that's the whole purpose of job interviews—for you and the employer to make that determination.

Personal problems should always be avoided. You are there to help solve the *employer's* problems, not find solutions to your own. Employers are looking for independent problem solvers. Bringing your own problems to the interview will not give them a good impression of your capabilities in this area.

Focusing on your own needs is negatively received by employers. Giving the impression that you are more concerned with what you can get from the job than what you can give is a sure way to get *nothing at all*. The following questions send the message "What's in it for me?" and should be avoided until you know you are actually being considered for the job:

- What are the benefits?
- How many paid holidays will I get?
- Is Friday casual day?
- Can I leave early if I finish my work?
- When will I get a raise?

It is acceptable to inquire about the work schedule, duties, and other expectations. You can attempt to negotiate specific conditions after you have been offered the job (discussed in Chapter 11). It is worth repeating—again—that the purpose of the interview is not to state your needs but to determine those of the employer. The ability to focus on the needs of others is a valuable career skill. Effective health care professionals are able to attend fully to the needs of patients, whether they work in direct patient care or support services.

It's Your Interview, Too

Interviews are not only for the benefit of employers. You have the right—and the responsibility—to evaluate the opportunities presented by the jobs you are applying for. This may seem to contradict what we discussed in the previous section, but it doesn't. In fact, well-stated questions about the job communicate motivation and interest.

When you are in class, it is true that "there are no stupid questions." However, at a job interview, the quality of your questions *does* count. There is a difference between the ones that should be avoided and ones that demonstrate that you:

- Have a sincere interest in the job
- Want to understand the employer's needs

- Understand the nature of health care work
- Have thought about your career goals
- Want information that will enable you to do your best

What you ask will depend on the job, the interviewer, and how much you already know about the job and the facility. It is a good idea to prepare, in advance, a list of general questions, along with a few that are specific to the job and the facility. This will assist you in remembering what you want to ask. As we noted earlier, it is easy to forget when we feel under pressure, as may happen in the interview situation. Not everyone is skilled at "thinking in the seat," especially when it feels like the hot seat!

Here are some suggestions to get you started:

1. How could I best contribute to the success of this facility?
2. What are the most important qualities needed to succeed in this position?
3. What is the mission of this organization/facility?
4. What are the major problems faced by this organization/facility?
5. How is the organization structured? Who would I be reporting to?
6. What values are most important?
7. I want to continue learning and updating my skills. What opportunities would I have to do this?
8. How will I be evaluated and learn where I need to improve?
9. Are there opportunities for advancement for employees who work hard and perform well?

It is perfectly acceptable to ask questions throughout the interview where they fit in. This will be more natural and lead to a smoother interview than asking a long list at the end. You don't have to wait until you are invited to ask them.

PRESCRIPTION FOR SUCCESS 10–13

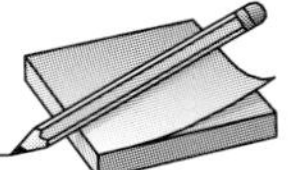

What Do You Want to Know?

1. Prepare at least ten questions you could ask at an interview. These should be designed to help you discover if the job and organization are aligned with your work preferences and qualifications.
2. Practice asking your questions.

In addition to asking questions, observe the facility and the people who work here. Does this "feel" like a place where you would want to work? Is it clean? Organized? Does it appear that safety precautions are followed? What is the pace? Are the people who work there courteous and helpful? How do they interact with patients? If your interview is with the person who would be your supervisor, do you think you would get along? Do you believe you would fit in?

It may not be possible for you to see anything other than the interviewer's office. In fact, at a large facility, your first interview may take place in the personnel office. You won't see the area where you would work. If this is the case, you will want to ask for a tour if you are offered a job. (More about this in Chapter 11.)

Leaving Graciously

The end of the interview gives you an opportunity to make a final impression, so make it a good one. It is important to be sensitive to signals the interviewer gives that it is time to wrap up. Failure to do so shows a lack of consideration for his or her time, and this is definitely not the parting message you want to leave. Some interviewers will make it obvious that the time is almost up by:

- Telling you directly
- Asking if you have any "final" questions
- Telling you that everything has been covered

Less obvious signs include looking at their watch, clock, appointment book, or papers on their desk; pushing their chair back; or saying that they have "taken enough of your time." Show respect for *their* time by moving along with the final steps of the interview:

1. Ask any final questions (limit these to a couple of the most important ones that haven't been answered).
2. Make a brief wrap-up statement.
3. Thank them for their time.
4. Inquire about what comes next.

If you are interested in the job, say so in the wrap-up statement. Tell the interviewer why: you believe you can make a contribution; you are impressed with the facility; your qualifications seem to fit the position very well. Express your excitement about the possibility of working there and state that you hope you are chosen for the position.

Whether you want the job or not, *always* thank the interviewer for his or her time. This applies even if the interview did not go well. Health care professionals and personnel staff are extremely busy. Let them know how much you appreciate being given the opportunity to present your qualifications.

Finally, if you aren't told about the next step in the application process, don't hesitate to ask. Inquire about when the hiring decision will be made. Find out if there is anything you need to send. If asked, give the interviewer your reference sheet. Be sure that you have the interviewer's last name, including the spelling and title. And be sure that he or she has your telephone number and any other information needed to contact you. Then smile, give a firm handshake, and leave as confidently as you entered, regardless of how you believe the interview went.

PRESCRIPTION FOR SUCCESS 10–14

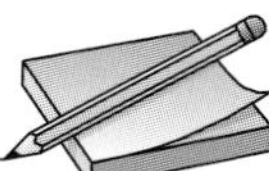

Wrapping It Up

1. Create several short summaries that express your interest in various jobs and statements about why you should be hired.
2. Practice your statements aloud, along with a "thank you" and questions about follow-up. (Note: the purpose is not to prepare a canned summary but to practice pulling a summary together.)

Some Final Thoughts

You wouldn't be nervous if you didn't care.—Robert Lock

You may be feeling a little—maybe extremely—overwhelmed at this point. "How can I remember all this *and* act natural *and* maintain eye contact *and* give good examples *and* . . ." It *is* a lot, and that's why it is essential to spend time learning about the interviewing process, preparing, and *practicing.* Take every opportunity to role-play. Make your practice sessions as realistic as possible.

When you inventoried your many skills, were you amazed at how much you can do now that you would never have attempted before beginning your educational program? You learned these skills by studying and practicing them—over and over. We have pointed out throughout this book how many "school success skills" are applied to the job search. If you have been working on developing these skills, this is your chance to use them for job success. You are almost certainly more qualified for the job search than you realize. And using the skills to *get* a job will reinforce your ability to use them once you are *on* the job.

A final note: it's okay to be nervous. It can even be a good thing, because it means you are not taking this experience for granted. Interviewers know you are nervous, and it tells them that this job is important to you and that you care about the outcome. This is a positive message to communicate.

SUMMARY OF KEY IDEAS

1. An interview is a sales opportunity, so consider the customer's needs.
2. Advance preparation is the key to a successful interview.
3. Practice will help you present your qualifications effectively.
4. First impressions are critical.
5. It's natural to be nervous.

POSITIVE SELF-TALK FOR THIS CHAPTER

1. I am well prepared for interviews.
2. I present myself and my qualifications effectively.
3. I answer questions clearly and confidently.
4. I make a positive impression.

BIBLIOGRAPHY

Drake, John. *The Perfect Interview: How to Get the Job You Really Want,* 3rd ed. New York: American Management Association, 1997.

Ferrett, Sharon. *Getting and Keeping the Job You Want.* Chicago: Irwin Mirror Press, 1996.

Lock, Robert D. *Job Search: Career Planning Guide, Book II,* 3rd ed. Pacific Grove, CA: Brooks/Cole Publishing Company, 1996.

11

After the Interview

OBJECTIVES

THE INFORMATION AND ACTIVITIES IN THIS CHAPTER CAN HELP YOU TO:

- ➢ Learn from every interview you attend.
- ➢ Write appropriate thank-you letters to interviewers.
- ➢ Know when and how to call and inquire about hiring decisions.
- ➢ Develop appropriate criteria for determining whether to accept a job offer.
- ➢ Calculate the total value of a compensation package.
- ➢ Accept and turn down job offers properly.
- ➢ Know how to deal with and learn from the experience if you are not selected for a job.

KEY TERMS

Benefits: Items of value provided by employers in addition to salary. They include insurance, tuition reimbursement, paid days off, and a uniform allowance.

Compensation: The payment an employer gives for work done. It include wages and other benefits that have monetary value.

401(K) retirement plan: A retirement plan offered by some employers. It gives you an opportunity to save and invest for the future. You choose an amount to be deducted from your wages each pay period. You pay no taxes on this money, which is then placed in an investment plan. Some employers match a certain percentage of the money you save. You cannot withdraw money from the plan, without paying a penalty, until you reach age fifty-nine and a half.

Reward Yourself

Celebrate all successes on the job-search journey.

Attending an interview is a success, whether or not you are hired for this particular job. You have qualifications that were worthy of the interviewer's time, you prepared well, and you met the challenge of presenting yourself one-on-one to a potential employer. Take a moment to reward yourself for completing this important step.

Maximize the Interview Experience

Nothing is a waste of time if you use the experience wisely.—Auguste Rodin

Making the most of every interview means that you see each one as an experience that provides opportunities to improve your presentation skills and learn more about the health care world. This knowledge will help you on future interviews and occasions such as performance evaluations. When you leave the interviewer's office, your reaction may be "Whew! That's over!" and the last thing you want to do is spend more time thinking about it. This is especially true if you believe it didn't go well. But this is precisely when you need to spend some time thinking about and evaluating the experience and your performance. Using an interview evaluation sheet will help you concentrate on the important factors that determine the success of an interview and create a plan for improvement. Make copies of the form provided in the exercise and keep a record of your interviews in your job search notebook.

PRESCRIPTION FOR SUCCESS 11–1

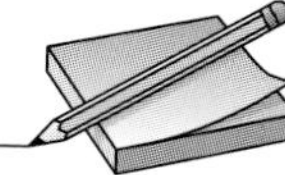

How Did I Do? Postinterview Self-Evaluation

Name of Organization ____________

Interviewer's Name ____________

Job Title ____________

Date of Interview ____________

____ I arrived on time

If not, what can I do to make sure that I'm not late for future interviews?__

____

____ I displayed good nonverbal communication skills

____ Smiled

____ Maintained good eye contact

____ Waited to be seated

____ Shook hands properly

If not, what do I need to improve? ____________________

____

____ I presented my qualifications effectively

____ Used examples to support my skills and qualities

____ Used my portfolio effectively

____ Accurately answered questions that tested my knowledge

____ Performed hands-on skills correctly

If not, how can I improve my presentation skills? ____________

____

Are there subjects and skills I need to review? ____________

____

PRESCRIPTION FOR SUCCESS 11–1 (*continued*)

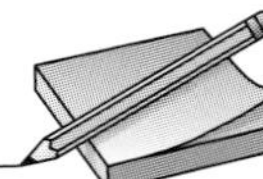

____ I was prepared to answer the interviewer's questions

____ Understood the content of the questions

____ Was able to compose my thoughts and organize good responses

____ Had correctly anticipated the types of questions that were asked

If not, what steps can I take to prepare to handle interview questions more effectively? ____________

____ I asked good questions

____ Was able to think of them as the interview progressed

____ Fit them in appropriately

____ Had appropriate questions prepared in advance

If not, how can I be better prepared to ask what I need to know? ____________

What things seemed to make a positive impression on the interviewer? ____________

What things seemed to make a negative impression? ____________

What would I do differently if I could do it over? ____________

What did I learn from this experience? ____________

(Questions adapted from Drake, 1997)

Consider sharing your self-evaluation with someone you trust. Sometimes we are too hard on ourselves and need a second point of view to help us see the real situation. Review the interview with your instructor, career services personnel, or mentor. You may have friends and family members who can provide insight and support. Create an improvement plan and practice so that you'll feel more confident at the next interview.

When seeking help or discussing interviews with others, it is best not to make negative remarks about the interviewer or the facility. This serves no purpose, unless you are seeking advice about whether to accept a job you have doubts about. A friend may have a friend who works there and your words, said "in confidence," may be passed along to the wrong party.

You may feel that you will receive a job offer. You very well might. But *don't* cancel or turn down other interviews *until you are formally hired.* You may have done a superb job and the facility plans to hire you. Then the next day, your soon-to-be supervisor is informed that there is a facilitywide hiring freeze. You don't want to be left out in the cold with no other options. You may even find something better before they make the offer. Stay actively involved in the search until you have a job.

Thank-You—Plus

Whether the interview went like a dream or a nightmare, *send a thank-you note.* This courtesy is something most job seekers don't do. Yet it is a simple action that can set you apart from the others. Suppose the employer interviewed nine people in two days, in addition to carrying on a normal work load. Tired? Very likely. Able to remember each candidate clearly and recall who said what? Maybe. But why take the chance of being lost in the crowd?

If you know for sure that you don't want the job, send a thank-you note anyway. Keep it simple, say something positive about the interview, and express your appreciation for the time taken to meet with you. *Do not* say that you are not interested in the job. See Figure 11–1 for an example.

Why, you might ask, would you write if you don't want to work there? There are at least three good reasons:

1. The employer may know someone else who is hiring. Impressed by your follow-up, he or she recommends you.
2. An opening for a job that you do want becomes available at this facility. You are remembered for your thoughtfulness.
3. At this time, when courtesy and consideration for others are disappearing, it is the right thing to do.

1642 Windhill Way
San Antonio, TX 78220
October 18, 2001

Nancy Henderson, Office Manager
Craigmore Pediatric Clinic
4979 Coffee Road
San Antonio, TX 78229

Dear Ms. Henderson:

Thank you so much for the time you spent with me yesterday. You have a busy schedule and I appreciate the time you took to describe the opening for a medical assistant at Craigmore Pediatric. The Clinic enjoys a good reputation in Craigmore for the services it provides children in the community and it was a pleasure to learn more about it.

Sincerely,
Karen Gonzalez
Karen Gonzalez

FIGURE 11–1 Simple thank-you letter.

PRESCRIPTION FOR SUCCESS 11–2

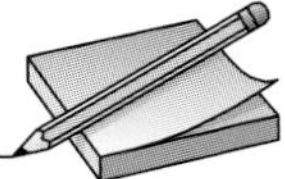

Thank You

1. Imagine a job for which you interviewed and have decided not to accept.
2. Write an appropriate thank-you note

If you want the job (see the next section for how-tos on making that decision), then take the time to write a thank-you-plus letter. The "plus" refers to a paragraph or two in which you do at least one of the following:

- Briefly summarize your qualifications in relation to the job as it was discussed in the interview.
- Point out specifically how you can make a positive contribution—again, based on specifics you learned.

Let the employer know that you want the job and hope to be the candidate selected. Include your full name and telephone number. See Figure 11–2 for an example of a thank-you-plus letter.

Thank-you notes should be sent no later than the day following the interview. Consider keeping a box of cards in the car and writing the note immediately after leaving the interview. Interviewers will be impressed when they receive your note the very next day.

PRESCRIPTION FOR SUCCESS 11–3

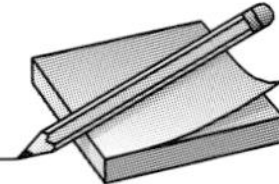

Thank-You—Plus

1. Imagine interviewing for a job that you decide you want.
2. Write a thank-you-plus letter, including a description of what you can contribute.

Alert Your References

If you left a reference sheet with the interviewer, call your references as soon as possible to tell them that they may receive a call. Of course, they already know that you have given their names out as references. (You *did* ask them, right?) Give them the job title, nature of the work, and type of facility. Add anything you learned about the type of candidate the employer is seeking. This gives your references an opportunity to stress those features that best support your bid for the job. Help them to help you by keeping them informed.

When to Call Back

Following up after an interview is a kind of balancing act: you don't want to be considered a pest by calling too soon and too frequently. On the other hand, you took the time to attend the interview and have a right to be informed when the hiring decision is made.

The best strategy is to wait until the day after you were told a decision would be made. Call and identify yourself and inquire about the decision. If none has been made, ask when you might expect to hear. It is essential that you use your best telephone manners. This is still part of the interview, and courtesy counts. Never express impatience about a delay. You want to show interest but not pressure the employer for a decision he or she is not ready to make. Sometimes the interviewer is deciding between two candidates and the decision may be influenced by your follow up.

1642 Windhill Way
San Antonio, TX 78220
October 18, 2001

Nancy Henderson, Office Manager
Craigmore Pediatric Clinic
4979 Coffee Road
San Antonio, TX 78229

Dear Ms. Henderson:

Thank you so much for the time you spent with me yesterday. You have a busy schedule and I appreciate the time you took to describe the opening for a medical assistant at Craigmore Pediatric. The Clinic enjoys a good reputation in San Antonio for the services it provides children in the community and it was a pleasure to learn more about it.

After visiting your facility and meeting the health professionals who work there, I sincerely believe that I could make a positive contribution to your facility. My ability to communicate in both English and Spanish would allow me to work with patients from various cultural backgrounds. My previous experience working in a daycare facility gave me a love for and understanding of children that enables me to work effectively with them. Finally, my organizational skills and knowledge of current insurance requirements will be of benefit in helping to develop the new billing system you described.

I am interested in this position and enthusiastic about working at Craigmore Pediatric. Please let me know if you need anything further from me. I can be reached at (210) 123-4567. I look forward to hearing from you.

Sincerely,

Karen Gonzalez

Karen Gonzalez

FIGURE 11–2 Thank-you-plus letter.

Is This the Job for You?

Very rarely are jobs offered on the spot during the first interview. If this *does* happen to you, it is a good idea to ask when a decision is needed and say that you are very interested (if you are) but need a little time to make a decision. There are exceptions, of course. You may have performed your clinical work at this site and know for sure that this is the place for you. In this case, the interview is more of a formality and it makes sense to accept the position immediately.

Interviewers will usually give you a time range during which a hiring decision will be made. You, too, need to make a decision: if this position is offered, will you accept it? Many factors will influence your decision. In Chapter 8 we discussed how the job market is affected by various economic and governmental conditions. When the unemployment rate is high, you probably can't be as choosy about the job you take. In fact, you may have very few choices, because there will be more candidates competing for a limited number of positions. You can be more selective when the unemployment rate is low. Of course, your location and specific occupation will influence the number of opportunities available to you. Some parts of the country are highly desirable places to live, and competition is intense. And some occupations are in either high or low demand, depending on current health care trends.

Here are some questions to guide your thinking about the specific job and facility in which you would be working:

1. Do the job duties match my skills and interests?
2. How closely do the job and facility match my work preferences?
3. Does the facility appear to follow safe and ethical practices?
4. Do I agree with the mission and values of the organization?
5. How well do I think I would fit in?
6. Are there opportunities to learn?
7. Will there be opportunities for advancement?
8. Can I commit to the required schedule?
9. Is the management style compatible with my work style?
10. How did the facility "feel"?

While you should consider these questions carefully, remember that the job that is "exactly what you want" probably doesn't exist. Finding the right job for you is a matter of finding a close match on the most important elements. You are starting a new career, and there are certain factors that will help your long-term success. Working with someone who is interested in teaching you, for example, may be a better choice than choosing a slightly higher-paying position that offers no opportunities for acquiring new skills. Many health care facilities make it a practice to promote from within. If there is a facility where you want to work, consider taking a job that gets you in the door.

Considering an Offer

A job offer may be extended in a telephone call, at a second or even third interview, or in a letter. Even if you feel quite sure that this is the right job, you must still be sure that you have all the information needed to make a final decision. It is essential that you understand:

- The *exact duties* you will be required to perform. If you haven't seen a written job description, ask for it now. If there is no written description, ask for a detailed oral explanation if this wasn't done in the interview.
- *Start date.* Be sure you are clear about the exact date and time you are to report for work.
- The *days and hours* you will work. Ask about the likelihood of required overtime and any change of hours or days that might take place in the future.
- Your *salary.* Earnings are expressed in various ways: hourly, weekly, biweekly, monthly, or annual rates. If you are quoted a rate that you aren't familiar with, you might want to convert it to one you know. For example, if you are accustomed to thinking in terms of amount per hour but are given a monthly salary, you may want to calculate the hourly equivalent. See Figure 11–3.
- *Orientation and/or training given.* This is especially important for recent graduates. Learning the customs and practices of the facility can make a big difference in your success. Letting the employer know that you are interested in learning as much as possible about the facility and the job communicates the message that you are motivated and interested in being prepared to do your best.

Calculating How Much You Will Earn

Basic Facts: Based on a forty-hour week: 1 year = 12 months = 52 weeks = 2080 work hours

If you are paid every 2 weeks, you will receive 26 paychecks per year.

Conversions Based on Annual Salary of $24,000.00

Monthly = $24,000/12 = $2000.00
Biweekly = $24,000/26 = $923.07
Weekly = $24,000/52 = $461.53
Hourly = $24,000/2028 = $11.53

Conversions Based on Hourly Rate of $11.00

Weekly = $11 x 40 = $440.00
Biweekly = $11 x 80 = $880.00
Monthy = $11 x 2080/12 = $1906.66
Annually = $11 x 2080 = $22,880.00

FIGURE 11–3 Calculating how much you will earn.

You may have received all this information at the interview(s). Don't hesitate, however, to ask about anything you don't fully understand. It is far better to take the time now rather than discover later that the job or working conditions were not what you expected. If you didn't have an opportunity to see any more than the interviewer's office, be sure to ask for a complete tour before deciding whether to accept the job.

UNDERSTANDING BENEFITS

Benefits can represent a significant portion of your **compensation.** Health insurance, for example, can cost hundreds of dollars per month for a family of four. If full family coverage is offered by the employer, this may be worth thousands of dollars each year. Find out if you must pay part of the cost of the premiums and what type of coverage is provided. Health insurance may not be available at the same rate if you don't belong to a group plan which is available through your employer. And many individuals find it difficult even to qualify on their own. This type of insurance is becoming an important benefit to consider when choosing where to work. In addition to medical insurance, there are various other types of insurance that can add value to the benefits package. These include dental, vision, life, and disability insurance.

If you are planning to continue your education, tuition benefits might be important to you. Some employers will cover all or part of educational expenses if the studies are related to your work and you receive a grade of C or better. Time off to take classes and workshops is an additional advantage. This benefit is especially helpful for health care professionals who are required to earn continuing education units on a regular basis.

Other benefits to consider when calculating your overall compensation include the number of paid vacation, holiday, and personal days offered and whether there is a retirement plan such as a **401(k) plan.**

When considering the compensation offered by an employer, think in terms of the total package. One job may offer a higher hourly rate but require you to pay part of your health insurance premium. You may end up financially ahead by accepting the lower salary. On the other hand, if you are included on your spouse's group plan, this would not be significant. Salary alone should not be the determining factor when deciding if a job "pays enough."

Let's look at an example: suppose you are offered Job A, which pays $24,000 and includes medical insurance, for which the employer pays $2700. The total value is of this package, then, is $26,700. Another employer offers you Job B at $27,000 in salary with no insurance benefits. You need insurance and plan to pay for it yourself with the extra salary you will earn. Assuming that everything else about the two jobs is equal, with which one would you come out ahead financially? Almost certainly Job A. Let's see why.

1. You will pay taxes on wages of $24,000 rather than $27,000. (Health insurance benefits are not taxed.)
2. The $2700 for medical insurance is the cost for a member of a group plan. If you buy insurance as an individual, it may cost you even more. (*And* you may have to qualify medically, which makes it more difficult to get.)

JOB A

$24,000 − $7200 (standard deduction + single exemption)
= $16,800 (taxable income)

$16,800 × 15% tax rate = $2520 (taxes)

$24,000 − $2520 = *$21,480 (amount of money you keep)*

JOB B

$27,000 − $7200 = $19,800 (taxable income)

$19,800 × 15% = $2970 (taxes)

$27,000 − $2970 = $24,030

$24,030 − $2700 (amount spent on health insurance)
= *$21,330 (amount of money you keep)*

The lesson here is to collect information and consider all aspects of the compensation plan. While this was just an example, it shows how important it is to do the math. If you are unsure about how to do these calculations, ask for help. Your long-term financial health depends on it.

Accepting an Offer

When you accept a job, express your appreciation and enthusiasm. In addition to responding orally, write a letter of acceptance. See Figure 11–4 for a sample letter.

When speaking with the employer, inquire about any necessary follow-up activities. It is also a good idea to disclose any future commitments or other factors that will impact your work. For example, if your son is scheduled for surgery next month and you know you will need to take several days off to care for him, let the employer know this during the hiring process. It is a sign of integrity to make important disclosures before the hiring is completed. There is usually no risk of losing the job by revealing reasonable, unavoidable future commitments. If the employer does refuse to accommodate you, it is better to learn now that this job lacks flexibility regarding family needs. You may want to reconsider your acceptance. (Be aware, however, that employers cannot grant repeated requests for days off due to family responsibilities. *Their* first responsibility must be to the patients they serve.)

You may want this job but need to negotiate some conditions. For example, suppose that the work hours are 8:00 a.m. to 5:00 p.m. You have a three-year-old child who cannot be left at day care before 7:45 a.m., and it takes at least twenty-five minutes to drive to work. It is better to ask if you can work from 8:30 a.m. to 5:30 p.m. than to take the position and arrive late every day. Many problems on the job can be avoided by discussing them openly in advance. (Again, you must also consider the employer's needs. Accommodations like this are not always possible if they disrupt the facility's schedule and patient flow.) And sometimes, having a "Plan B" will save the day—in this case, having someone reliable who can take your child to day care.

1642 Windhill Way
San Antonio, TX 78220
October 18, 2001

Nancy Henderson, Office Manager
Craigmore Pediatric Clinic
4979 Coffee Road
San Antonio, TX 78229

Dear Ms. Henderson:

I was very pleased to receive your telephone call this morning advising me that I have been chosen to fill the medical assistant position at Craigmore Pediatric. This letter confirms my response to accept your offer. I am very excited about joining your organization and look forward to reporting for work at 9:00 a.m. on November 6, 2001.

Thank you for placing your confidence in me. I will do my best to merit your support.

Sincerely,
Karen Gonzalez
Karen Gonzalez

FIGURE 11–4 Sample letter of acceptance.

PRESCRIPTION FOR SUCCESS 11–4

I'll Take It!

Write a letter of acceptance for a job in your field.

WHAT TO EXPECT

Once you are hired, employers can ask questions that were unacceptable during the hiring process. Information that cannot be used to make hiring decisions is often necessary for other personnel matters. Examples include the following:*

1. Provide proof of your age (ensure that you are of legal age to work).
2. Identify your race (for affirmative action statistics, if applicable in your state).
3. Supply a photograph (for identification).
4. State your marital status and number and ages of your children (for insurance).
5. Give the name and address of a relative (for notification in case of emergency).
6. Provide your Social Security number.

There may be mandatory health tests and immunizations. In addition, some employers require drug tests for all employees.

If you are asked to sign an employment contract, read it carefully first. As with all other employment issues, ask about anything you don't understand. Also, be sure to ask for a copy of anything that you sign.

Turning Down a Job Offer

After careful consideration, you may decide not to accept a job offer. It is not necessary to explain your reasons to the employer. Do express your appreciation and thanks for the opportunity, and *do* send a thank-you note. In addition to being an expression of courtesy, this leaves a positive impression on all employers. You may want to work at this facility in the future. See Figure 11–5 for a sample refusal letter.

PRESCRIPTION FOR SUCCESS 11–5

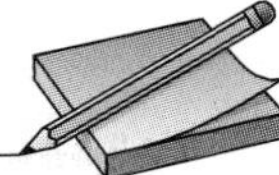

No, Thank You

Writer a sample refusal letter.

If You Don't Get the Job

Failure is a delay, but not a defeat. It is a temporary detour, not a dead-end street.
—William Arthur Ward

It can be difficult when you are not selected for a job that you really want. There are many reasons why applicants don't get hired. Some you can't change and must simply accept, such as the following:

- There was another applicant with more experience or skills that more closely met the employer's current needs.
- An employee in the organization decided to apply for the job.
- The employer believed that someone else was a better "match" for the organization in terms of work style, preferences, and so on.
- There were budget cuts or other unexpected events that prevented anyone from being hired at this time.

You may have lost this opportunity for reasons you *can* change. How do you know? First, do an honest review of your postinterview evaluation, school record, and resume. Are you presenting yourself in the best possible way? Second, look over the following list. These are the major reasons suggested by health care employers and career services personnel for students' failure to get hired. Do you recognize any areas that might apply to you?

1. Failure to sell themselves by clearly presenting their skills and qualifications
2. Too much interest in what's in it for them rather than what they can give
3. Unprofessional behavior, lack of courtesy

*Adapted from Lock, 1996

4. Lack of enthusiasm and interest in the job
5. Poor appearance
6. Poor communication skills
7. Unrealistic job expectations
8. Negative or critical attitude
9. Arrived late, brought children or the person who provided transportation, other demonstrations of poor organizational skills

You must be honest with yourself and commit to improving your attitude and/or job-search skills. If necessary, seek advice from your instructor, career services

1642 Windhill Way
San Antonio, TX 78220
October 18, 2001

Nancy Henderson, Office Manager
Craigmore Pediatric Clinic
4979 Coffee Road
San Antonio, TX 78229

Dear Ms. Henderson:

Thank you so much for your telephone call this morning advising me that I have been chosen to fill the medical assistant position at Craigmore Pediatric. I told you that I would give you a response within one day. After much careful consideration, I have decided to decline the offer at this time.

This was not an easy decision to make and I hope it does not exclude me from future consideration at Craigmore Pediatric. I am sincerely grateful for your time and consideration.

Sincerely,

Karen Gonzalez

Karen Gonzalez

FIGURE 11–5 Sample letter of refusal.

personnel, or mentor. Work on creating a winning attitude that will help you develop the interviewing skills it takes to get hired. Seek support from friends and family members if you are feeling down. They can help you keep your perspective and boost your self-confidence if it's a little low.

While you may not feel enthusiastic about writing a note to an employer who chooses another applicant, consider this: you may have come in a close second. The next opening may be yours! So take a few moments and demonstrate your high level of professionalism by thanking the employer and letting him or her know that you are still interested in working for the organization. See Figure 11–6 for a sample letter.

1642 Windhill Way
San Antonio, TX 78220
October 18, 2001

Nancy Henderson, Office Manager
Craigmore Pediatric Clinic
4979 Coffee Road
San Antonio, TX 78229

Dear Ms. Henderson:

Thank you for letting me know that you have chosen another candidate for the medical assistant position at Craigmore Pediatric. I am still very interested in working at Craigmore and hope you will consider me for future openings. I believe I can make a real contribution.

I am sincerely grateful for your time and consideration. I was treated professionally by everyone at Craigmore and have great respect for your organization.

Sincerely,

Karen Gonzalez

Karen Gonzalezv

FIGURE 11–6 Sample letter of response when you are not offered the position.

PRESCRIPTION FOR SUCCESS 11-6

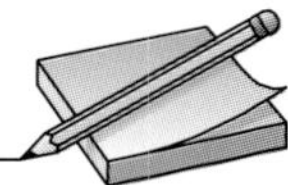

Thanks Anyway

Write a follow-up letter for a position that you wanted but for which you weren't chosen.

If you fail to get hired after attending a number of interviews, consider asking the employers for feedback. Some have a policy of only stating that another candidate was selected. Don't put employers on the spot by pressing for details if they refuse to be specific. Instead, ask someone at your school—an instructor or career services personnel—if he or she will call on your behalf. Employers are sometimes more willing to share reasons with school personnel to help them better assist students. Be willing to listen to any constructive criticism offered and to make any needed changes.

SUMMARY OF KEY IDEAS

1. Make it a point to learn something from every interview you attend.
2. Write thank-you notes to *everyone* who interviews you.
3. Consider *all* aspects of the job when deciding if it is the one for you.
4. Learn to accept defeat gracefully.

POSITIVE SELF-TALK FOR THIS CHAPTER

1. I am performing better at each interview I attend.
2. I am a considerate person and follow up all interviews with a thank-you note.
3. I can gracefully handle being selected or rejected for a job.

BIBLIOGRAPHY

Drake, John D. *The Perfect Interview: How to Get the Job You Really Want,* 2nd ed. New York: AMACOM, 1997.

Lock, Robert D. *Job Search,* 3rd ed. Pacific Grove, CA: Brooks/Cole Publishing Company, 1996.

Yena, Donna J. *Career Directions,* 3rd ed. Chicago: Irwin/Times Mirror, 1997.

12

Success on the Job

OBJECTIVES

THE INFORMATION AND ACTIVITIES IN THIS CHAPTER CAN HELP YOU TO:

- Set goals to help you succeed at a new job.
- Make a good impression when starting a job.
- Apply your study skills to learning a new job.
- Create a workplace guide to use for quick and easy reference.
- Apply the SCANS Competencies in the health care workplace.
- Avoid burnout on the job.
- Develop—and maintain—a positive relationship with your supervisor.
- Describe five competencies that will increase your value as a health care professional.
- List five laws and one regulatory agency that protect the rights of employees.
- Develop effective ways to deal with difficult situations at work.
- Understand the purpose of a grievance procedure.

KEY TERMS

Approval agency: An organization that sets standards for health care facilities. It requires that certain procedures be followed and reports filed periodically. On-site visits are conducted to ensure that all standards are being followed.

Burnout: A state of physical and emotional exhaustion related to conditions on the job.

Charting: Recording patient data in written or computerized form to document all aspects of the diagnosis and care. Charting ensures continuity of care and creates legal records should they be needed in court.

Code of Ethics: Standards of conduct created by professional organizations to guide members of the profession.

Coding: Matching identifying numbers—codes—to diagnoses and procedures for filing insurance claims. These codes are standardized and accepted by Medicare and Medicaid. There are three types of codes: Current Procedural Terminology (CPT), the Health Common Procedure Coding System (HCPCS), and the International Classification of Diseases 9th Revision Clinical Modification (ICD-9-CM).

Compliance reports: Reports submitted to approval agencies to demonstrate that standards are being followed.

Courtesy: More than saying "please" and "thank you," courtesy means treating others with kindness, consideration, and respect.

Cross-training: Learning to perform tasks in addition to those traditionally assigned to a given occupation. For example, a radiologic technician learning to perform venipuncture.

Employee manual: A written document that contains policies, rules, and guidelines that relate to employees. Examples of items included are vacations, holidays, overtime, personal and sick leave, absences, dress codes, and various employee responsibilities.

Grievance: In the workplace, a circumstance believed to be unjust and/or harmful to an employee and grounds for filing a formal complaint.

Integrity: The state of conducting oneself honestly, sincerely, and guided by high moral principles.

Morale: Group feelings of confidence, enthusiasm, and willingness to work hard to achieve common goals.

Scope of practice: Duties allowed to be performed in specific occupations. These are set by governmental or professional regulatory bodies.

Hit the Ground Running

Starting your first job in health care represents the achievement of a major goal. Enjoy the satisfaction of your achievement. At the same time, be aware that how you perform during the first months on the job will influence your future career success. You can help ensure this success by setting goals for this important period of your professional life.

The first few weeks at work are likely to be busy and stressful. There will be a lot to learn and many adjustments to make. Sometimes it may seem as if getting through each day is a major accomplishment. Be patient with yourself. Do your best, but remember that it takes time to learn a new job and develop a level of comfort. The purpose of setting goals for this period is not to add more stress, but to help keep you focused on what is most important. Aim to accomplish what will most contribute to your long-term success.

GOAL 1: SHIFT YOUR FOCUS

As a student, your main concern was your studies: mastering new material, learning new skills, completing assignments, and performing well on tests and evaluations. Your principal responsibility was to yourself and your personal progress.

As a health care professional, you must now shift your attention to the goals and needs of others: your employer, patients, and coworkers. You are accountable to people who are depending on what you do and how well you do it.

Important components of professionalism in health care are the ability to understand and willingness to attend to the needs of others. Being a professional includes determining what is most appropriate and needed to provide quality service. This is true whether you work in direct patient care or services that support the health care delivery system.

GOAL 2: MAKE A GOOD FIRST IMPRESSION

Each time you meet someone new or perform a task for the first time, you have an opportunity to make a first impression. The saying "You have only one chance to make a first impression" is worth thinking about. Why is it so important? Because people tend to make judgments about others very quickly and often on the basis of very little information. In the employment setting, information from first contacts will often be used by others to form opinions about the level of your professionalism and competence.

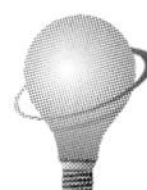

Take a Moment to Think

Think of someone who made a negative impression on you when you first met. Did your impression change after you got to know the person? Why and how? Did it take a long time to change?

As a recent graduate, you may not be 100% confident of your abilities. You may feel a little anxious about your performance. Keep in mind that no one expects you to know everything. However, there *are* two key factors under your control that influence first impressions: appearance and courtesy.

Most people are strongly influenced by visual impressions. If you look as if you know what you're doing, you are likely to be perceived that way. In Chapter 2 we discussed appropriate appearance for the health care professional. To review quickly, we said that the desired look is:

1. Conservative—out of consideration for patients.
2. Healthy—to provide an appropriate example.
3. Clean—for the safety and consideration of others.
4. Safe—for the benefit of self and others.

Review the appearance guidelines for interviews listed in Chapter 10. These apply to the workplace as well as the interview. There are, of course, variations in the styles of dress and grooming considered appropriate. Some facilities are more formal than others. What is proper in one is unacceptable in another. Follow the directions received during your interview or orientation. Read the written dress code. And remember, as a new employee, it is better to be more rather than less conservative.

Much more than simply using good manners, **courtesy** refers to being considerate and helpful. It means respecting the feelings of others and showing appreciation for the help you receive when you are new on the job. You are beginning to establish relationships with coworkers, and courtesy will go a long way toward ensuring that these are satisfactory.

GOAL 3: LEARN ALL YOU CAN ABOUT THE JOB

The first few weeks at a new job may be a bit overwhelming. Your educational program provided you with occupational knowledge and skills. But there will be a lot more to learn when you start your first job—*any* new job, in fact—because each facility has its own policies, rules, and procedures. Add to this the need to know the proper operation of equipment, location of supplies, and correct way to fill out forms and you have a full course to master: Job 101.

The good news is that you have what it takes to pass this course with flying colors. If you approach it with a "can do" attitude and apply the same skills that helped you succeed in school, you can learn and master your job systematically and effectively. Chapter 1 pointed out that "school skills" have valuable applications on the job. Let's see how you can use them now to succeed in your new environment.

Using Your Note-Taking Skills

Your supervisor and coworkers will be important sources of useful information. Just as you took notes in class, you can profit from taking notes on the job. They can serve as both learning aids and reference materials. Some note-taking situations will be formal, including structured orientation sessions and employee training programs. Informal situations in which note taking is useful include receiving explanations and demonstrations from your supervisor and fellow employees. There are several benefits to be gained from taking notes. It can help you to:

- Concentrate on what is being presented
- Reinforce what you hear by writing it down at the same time
- Create a record of information to study later
- Provide you with a reference so that you won't have to ask the same questions again

Notice that taking and using notes involves three different ways of learning: listening, writing, and reading. This variety will reinforce your learning and help you master the information.

Remember that a key factor in effective note taking is careful listening. This applies, of course, to all communication, whether you are taking notes or not. Clearing your mind of other thoughts, focusing on what the speaker is saying, and asking questions to clarify anything you don't understand will increase the productivity of your learning experiences.

Try to use an organizing scheme when taking notes: write down the key ideas, steps in a procedure, and/or important facts. Spend a few minutes after work editing your notes, if necessary, and reviewing the important points. Taking a few minutes each day to look them over and "rehearse" your job duties will give you confidence and make the time on the job more productive. (Review the section on note taking in Chapter 4.)

Asking Questions

The potential consequences of workplace errors make the ability to ask appropriate questions an essential professional skill. This applies to all types of health care employment situations:

- Direct patient care in which the physical safety of both you and the patient is at risk
- Use of equipment, chemicals, and other materials that can be hazardous if handled incorrectly
- Administrative responsibilities in which errors can jeopardize the facility's standing with a regulatory agency
- Coding and billing tasks in which errors can cause rejection of payment by insurance companies, Medicare, and other agencies

Knowing *when* to ask questions is important. Whenever possible, use resources, observe, and think through situations in an attempt to find the answer for yourself. If you cannot find the answer, there isn't time to do research, or the situation is urgent, don't hesitate to ask an appropriate person—someone who has the training and experience to know the answer or where to find it. In nonurgent situations, choose a time that is most convenient for the other person. And avoid asking questions about patients in the presence of anyone, including other patients, if the questions reveal confidential information. Remember that the patient's right to privacy is protected by law.

Creating a Workplace Reference Guide

When starting a job, it can be helpful to create a workplace reference guide. If you started a personal reference guide, as recommended in Chapter 6, you can add an on-the-job section. What should you include? Here are some items you might find useful:

1. Any materials given to you during orientation or training sessions
2. Notes taken during training sessions
3. The name and telephone number of the person to contact if you must be absent
4. Schedules: holidays, vacation, meetings, and weekly schedules if they vary
5. Facility staff directories and important phone numbers
6. Maps and floor plans if you work in a large facility
7. Notes from meetings attended
8. Printed instructions and other how-to information
9. Instructions about what to do in case of an emergency

There are several ways to organize your guide. If you work mostly at a desk or in one location, a standard-sized three-ring binder is a convenient place to store information. For jobs that involve moving about, such as in a hospital, a pocket-sized reference system that you can carry with you works well. Put important information on index cards, punch a hole in the corner of each card, and hook the cards together with a metal ring. Having everything in one place will be a big help when things get busy and you want to find something quickly.

Using Your Reading Skills

Reading is not limited to classroom-based learning. Printed materials are the source of important job-related information. The following examples highlight a few of the most common ones.

- **Employee manuals.** These generally contain policies and rules regarding employee conduct, holidays and vacations, the grievance procedure (discussed later in this chapter), and other topics related to the employer-employee relationship. Unfortunately, many people don't take the time to study the employee manual. While it may not be very exciting reading, it contains facts to help prevent problems and misunderstandings that cause the kind of excitement you *don't* want to happen on the job. If you don't receive an employee manual your first day on the job, be sure to ask for one.
- *Policy and procedure handbooks.* Facilities create manuals that provide standard instructions for routinely performed tasks. While it may not be necessary for you to read the entire manual, you should study the sections that apply to your job. Pay special attention to procedures to follow in emergencies. Knowing where to find this information quickly when needed has the potential to save lives.
- *Regulatory and* **approval agency** *standards.* Health care facilities are regulated by a variety of government and private agencies. Following the standards and rules set by these agencies is critical in determining the success—even the survival—of a facility. For example, reimbursement for Medicare patients requires the strict observance of certain guidelines. It is important that you know and understand all requirements that affect your job.
- *Instructions.* Techniques and equipment for today's jobs are more complex than ever. Being able to read and follow instructions (often called "documentation," especially when applied to computer software) is an important job skill. Examples include instructions for using equipment, performing laboratory tests, mailing special packages, and using computer software programs. The proper use of equipment and supplies is essential in health care because their misuse can result in serious consequences, including injury to the professional and/or patient.
- *Professional publications.* These include general health care newsletters and journals and those that apply to your specialty. They help you keep up-to-date in your field, which is essential in health care. (See the section entitled "Continue to Learn" later in this chapter.)

When reading technical material, apply the techniques for effective reading suggested in Chapter 4:

- Preview the material quickly.
- Ask questions that you will answer mentally as you read each section.
- Mark anything you don't understand.
- Periodically review the material.

Remember that repetition over time is the best way to learn. You can see the power of repetition in action by observing experienced professionals at work. Their self-confidence and ability to perform duties smoothly and effectively develop over time. The acquisition of knowledge is based on the same principle.

Using Your Observational Skills

There are important things you need to know about the workplace that no one will think to tell you. They are not written down anywhere and may not even be discussed. Everyone simply takes them for granted. These are the factors that make up the organizational culture, discussed in Chapter 7. Recall that it is composed of the customs and expectations of an organization and includes the

- Level of formality
- Amount of at-work socializing among employers
- Organizational values (what's really most important)
- Management styles
- Methods of communication

Learning the organizational culture and fitting in as a new employee depend on careful observation and asking the right questions. It can be a key factor in determining how well you fit in and work effectively with others. "Knowing the ropes" can also influence your job performance. It usually takes time to understand the organizational culture, but it is well worth the effort.

You may notice that some of the procedures and methods used at the facility are different from those you learned in school. As we discussed in Chapter 6, there is often no one right way to do a procedure. Experienced employees may have developed preferences or acceptable (in terms of safety and effectiveness) shortcuts. The facility may have specific reasons for using a different method. Use the method that is most comfortable for you *and* meets facility requirements. Never suggest that another employee is wrong because he or she is not doing something the way you learned in school. The only exception is if you believe that a law or safety measure is being broken. Under these circumstances, speak first with the employee. Then, if necessary, speak with the supervisor. And don't feel pressured, because you are new, to perform a task in a way that you know to be incorrect or unsafe.

Taking the Time to Learn

Taking the time to learn your job well will pay off in the future. Applying your study skills at work will help you increase your confidence and decrease your frustration. And you will build a foundation for progressing in your career and assuming increased responsibilities. For those who wish to climb the career ladder in their occupational area, it will provide a solid base for advanced formal studies.

GOAL 4: SEEK SATISFACTION IN YOUR WORK

Many of your waking hours are spent at the workplace. If you are to live a quality life, it makes sense that your work should be a source of satisfaction. This doesn't mean finding the "perfect job." In fact, it is unlikely that such a thing exists. It does mean approaching work with a positive attitude and focusing on those aspects that give you the opportunity to

- Perform meaningful work
- Make a positive contribution to the well-being of others
- Work in an interesting environment
- Continue to learn

Satisfaction is self-perpetuating. This means that health care professionals who project a positive attitude and like their work create satisfaction in those who receive their services. Performance levels and efficiency are also raised, further increasing the professional's sense of satisfaction. A win-win situation is created in which everyone benefits.

To keep yourself on the right track, ask yourself these questions as you work:

- Who is benefiting from the tasks I am performing now?
- What contributions am I making to the well-being of others?
- What can I learn today?
- Are there positive aspects of my work that I am overlooking?

PRESCRIPTION FOR SUCCESS 12-1

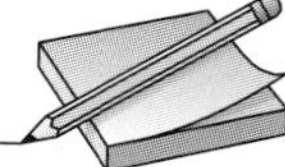

Increasing Your Job Satisfaction

1. What were your reasons for choosing a career in health care?

____

____

2. In what ways do you think you will receive satisfaction from your work?

____

____

3. What actions will you take to ensure that your work is fulfilling?

____

____

Checklist for Success on the Job: Revisiting the SCANS Report

The SCANS Report, introduced in Chapter 1, is a valuable tool for the new employee. As you recall, this report summarizes the opinions of thousands of employers about desirable employee characteristics. What better way is there to learn how to achieve success on the job than to go directly to the source—the employers themselves? You have completed several exercises that were based on the SCANS Competencies. Now we'll review the Competencies and see how they can be applied in the health care workplace.

BELIEVE IN SELF-WORTH

Positive feelings about oneself are essential to enhancing the life force in self and others.—Mattie Collins

Belief in self-worth means that you value yourself and your actions. You consider both to be important and deserving of respect. This enables you to recognize that you and your work truly make a difference. These beliefs provide the foundation for all the other SCANS Competencies, because they generate the self-confidence necessary to ask questions, learn new skills, and build positive relationships with others.

PRESCRIPTION FOR SUCCESS 12–2

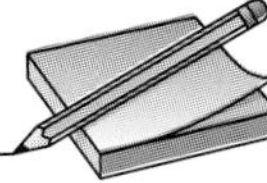

I Have Value

1. List five things that you like about yourself.
2. List five accomplishments that give you pride.
3. List five things that will make you an outstanding employee.

MANAGE YOURSELF

Managing your personal habits effectively enables you to serve others better. How does this work? We discussed the major components of self-management in Chapter 3:

- Personal organization
- Time management
- Good health habits
- Stress reduction techniques

Failure to maintain control in these areas can negatively impact your work in a number of ways:

- Arriving late can disrupt the schedules of patients and coworkers.
- Running out of energy before the work day is over can delay the completion of important tasks.
- Repeatedly calling in sick due to stress-related illnesses forces coworkers to fill in for you, disrupts schedules, and/or leaves tasks undone.
- Failure to prioritize tasks can result in missing important deadlines.
- Feeling tired can reduce your ability to concentrate and complete work assignments accurately.

As you can see, your personal habits are no longer just personal—they impact other people, too. Efficient use of time, for example, is especially critical in today's managed care systems. The inability to maintain schedules and complete tasks in a timely way can be a serious liability on the job. This book has repeatedly pointed out that once you commit yourself to serving others, as you have done by choosing a career in health care, you owe it to your profession to offer your best efforts. And this requires good self-management.

This does not mean, however, that your life should be entirely devoted to work. In fact, just the opposite is true. You need to take time out to attend to your own needs. The key is to achieve a balance between your needs and those of others in your life: patients, employer, coworkers, family members, and friends. If you continually ignore your own needs, you can deplete your physical, mental, and emotional resources. The result will be that you have nothing left to give others.

PRESCRIPTION FOR SUCCESS 12-3

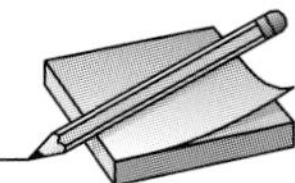

Are You Ready?

1. What are your backup plans for transportation, child care, and/or any personal responsibilities that could interfere with your job?
2. What organizational strategies have you developed to help balance your professional and personal lives?
3. Do your self-management skills need improvement?
4. If yes, what plans do you have to work on them?

Burnout

Burnout is a work-related condition that involves physical and emotional exhaustion. People suffering from burnout often have a feeling of hopelessness. They believe that their efforts have no purpose.

Burnout is a growing problem among health care professionals because of the responsibilities required by the work and the increasing emphasis on efficiency and cost control. Signs of burnout include extreme fatigue, irritability, frequent illnesses, and a feeling of discouragement.

There are several conditions that can lead to burnout:

- Continual job stress caused by factors such as constantly changing schedules; lack of feedback about work performance; lack of recognition for accomplishments
- More tasks assigned than can be accomplished during work hours
- Long work hours and inadequate time for rest
- A feeling of never getting caught up on tasks
- Continual pressure to meet tight deadlines and complete demanding assignments
- Lack of feedback or praise about work efforts

Consistent use of good self-management techniques provides protection against burnout.

- Develop organizational and time management techniques that work for you to avoid feeling constantly rushed and to make time for rest and recreation. (Review Chapter 3 for suggestions.)
- Practice the good health habits described in Chapter 3.
- Get enough sleep. Increasing your efficiency during waking hours can make up for extra time spent sleeping and resting.
- Make sure you are clear about your job tasks. Ask for a written job description if you don't have one. Talk with your supervisor about his or her expectations.
- Don't feel that you have to do everything yourself. Ask others for help when appropriate and needed. This includes family members and coworkers.
- Know your own limits. Don't take on more than you can manage physically and mentally.
- Develop interests outside of work.
- Seek satisfaction within yourself. Don't depend on recognition from others. Reward yourself for your achievements.

Self-Management on the Job

At the workplace, self-management means the ability to work without constant supervision. Supervisors don't have time to monitor employees continually. You can increase your value as an employee by identifying what needs to be done and staying with tasks until they are completed. Working without reminders will help you achieve a reputation as an excellent employee. In the event that you complete your work and have extra time, look for something else to do or ask for an additional assignment. There is no such thing as "free time" on the job, and you owe it to your employer to stay busy and productive.

It is more likely that you will experience the opposite problem: too much to do in too little time. In this case, learn to prioritize tasks so that the essential ones always get completed. If you are unsure about priorities, ask your supervisor for direction.

DEMONSTRATE INTEGRITY AND HONESTY

Integrity refers to having sound moral principles and being sincere and honest. Let's look at some examples of workplace behavior that demonstrate integrity:

- *Admit when a mistake is made.* Covering up errors in the health care environment can have serious consequences. For example, if lab results are reported for the wrong patient, a false diagnosis can cause ineffective—or even harmful—treatment to be prescribed.
- *Conduct yourself ethically.* This means conforming to established standards for moral and correct behavior. In addition to ethical standards that apply to society as a whole, each health care profession has a **Code of Ethics** that serves as a guide for proper conduct. Box 12–1 contains a Code of Ethics developed for medical assistants by the American Association of Medical Assistants (AAMA). (Note: The American Medical Technologists also have a code for medical assistants.) You should become familiar with the code for your profession.
- *Be loyal to your employer.* As long as you are being paid by an employer, it is your obligation to demonstrate loyalty. Examples of ways to show loyalty include:
  - Dedicating your time on the job exclusively to work. Personal tasks and telephone calls should be limited to the lunch hour or break time.
  - Never taking anything that belongs to the employer. Even small items, such as pens, add up when every employee thinks "This is so small that it won't make any difference." Taking something, however modest, is theft. Don't

BOX 12–1. CODE OF ETHICS FOR MEDICAL ASSISTANTS

The Code of Ethics of AAMA shall set forth principles of ethical and moral conduct as they relate to the medical profession and the particular practice of medical assisting.

Members of AAMA dedicated to the conscientious pursuit of their profession, and thus desiring to merit the high regard of the entire medical profession and the respect of the general public which they serve, do pledge themselves to strive always to:

A. render service with full respect for the dignity of humanity;
B. respect confidential information obtained through employment unless legally authorized or required by responsible performance of duty to divulge such information;
C. uphold the honor and high principles of the profession and accept its disciplines;
D. seek to continually improve the knowledge and skills of medical assistants for the benefit of patients and professional colleagues;
E. participate in additional service activities aimed toward improving the health and well-being of the community.

contribute to the rising cost of health care by increasing your employer's expenses.

- Speaking badly about your employer. This serves no purpose other than lowering employee **morale.** If overheard by patients, it can create doubts in their minds about the quality of care they are receiving. Seek solutions by discussing legitimate concerns directly with your supervisor.
- Complaining about your job, working conditions, and so on. Again, this does nothing to resolve the problem. Seek positive solutions through action or by speaking with someone who has the power to address the issue.

PRESCRIPTION FOR SUCCESS 12-4

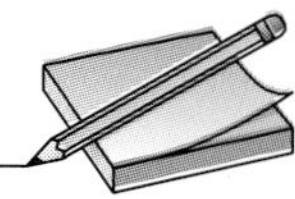

The Code as Your Guide

1. If you don't already have one, get a copy of the Code of Ethics for your profession.
2. Read the code and describe how it addresses the following issues:
   A. Integrity
   B. Human dignity
   C. Loyalty
   D. Honesty and sincerity
   E. Responsibility to patients
   F. Lifelong learning
   G. Community service

BE RESPONSIBLE

Being responsible is an important component of self-management. Employees who can be depended on to do what is expected—and then some—are worth their weight in gold. Today's health care environment puts many demands on employers. For example, they must provide high-quality services for patients, meet administrative deadlines, comply with a variety of regulations, and control operating costs. This is why it is essential that they can depend on you. Acting responsibly means that you:

- Complete all tasks. This includes returning equipment and supplies to their proper places for the next person who needs them.
- Strive for accuracy. Examples of the many health care tasks in which accuracy is critical include patient **charting,** medical **coding** and billing, filling out **compliance reports** and lab reports, preparing sterile fields, and providing patient education.
- Help out when needed, even when it's not your job. The unexpected must be anticipated in health care. Coworkers are sometimes absent, emergencies occur, and situations can quickly change from routine to urgent. A career in health care requires that you are willing to do what it takes to get the job done.
- Be on time. This includes arriving at work each day, returning promptly from lunch and breaks, and getting to meetings and appointments on time. One of the major complaints of patients is that they have to wait. They feel that their time is not respected. Sometimes this cannot be helped, but avoid being the cause. Don't let it happen because you were personally late. Absences should occur only for real emergencies. Have backup plans for transportation and child care.

- Follow through with everything you are directed or have offered to do. If you cannot perform a task or need assistance, let your supervisor know so that the task can be reassigned or help recruited. Don't allow work to go undone because you couldn't get to it yourself.

PRESCRIPTION FOR SUCCESS 12-5

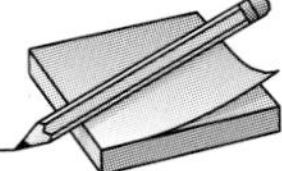

Consider the Consequences

A medical assistant who works in a busy pediatric office fails to autoclave the instruments as assigned. As a result, the physician cannot perform minor elective surgery that has been scheduled for a young patient. Discuss the possible impact on the following:

1. Patient
2. Parents
3. Physician
4. Medical assistant

DEMONSTRATE EMPATHY

Empathy, described in Chapter 7, means attempting to see the world through the eyes of others. Health care is a people business, and understanding the feelings and experiences of others—patients, supervisors, and coworkers—is essential. Empathy means remaining professional while caring about the other person. Patients who have experienced an illness or injury sometimes feel as if they have lost control of their lives. The empathy expressed by caregivers and other support personnel can be a critical component of their recovery. Empathy is also important in relationships with supervisors and coworkers. Mutual understanding promotes effective working relationships.

Each of us will interpret a given set of circumstances differently. This interpretation is shaped by factors such as cultural background, education, religious beliefs, and previous experiences, which lead us to make certain assumptions about the world. Difficulties and misunderstandings arise because most of us take our assumptions for granted and don't see them as only one possibility out of many. Our view makes sense to us and provides our basis for dealing with life. We believe it to be the right way, and it may not occur to us to question it. But the fact is, what is obvious to us is not necessarily obvious to others.

It takes awareness and effort to see around our assumptions, but that's what it takes to be empathetic. Let's review the suggestions from Chapter 7 for developing empathy:

- Listen carefully to what the other person is saying. We must know their view before we can begin to understand, and we can't know until we listen.
- Don't judge what you hear. You are gathering information to help you *understand* the other person—not to decide if he or she is right or wrong.
- Ask questions or give feedback to ensure that you have received the other person's message as it was intended.

An important point to keep in mind is that it's not necessary to agree with the beliefs of others. You must simply be aware of them and how they influence the perceptions and actions of others. In some cases, providing appropriate care requires that you try to persuade others to change ideas that are damaging to health. For example, a patient's cultural beliefs may cause him to adopt certain habits he believes to be beneficial when in fact they are potentially harmful. In this case, being empathetic does not mean *accepting* his beliefs. It *does* mean respecting him by learning why he holds these beliefs. Through this understanding, you increase the chance of convincing him that he can benefit from your suggestions.

WORK WITH OTHERS

Application of the people skills discussed in Chapter 7 and earlier in this chapter will help you establish positive relationships with coworkers. Getting along with others is one of the most talked-about yet taken-for-granted workplace necessities. Failure to work well with others is a major cause of employee dismissal, because it reduces the health care facility's capability to provide quality service. How well you develop your people skills, then, will greatly influence your future.

Quality health care requires the cooperation of many specialized individuals. And new members, in response to medical advances and increasingly complex delivery systems, continue to join the team. Whatever your particular occupation, you will be working with a variety of people who will bring different personalities, work styles, personal goals, and skill levels to the job. Your challenge will be to work in harmony with them all.

Working with Your Supervisor

How well you get along with your supervisor can make the difference between looking forward to each work day or dreading the thought of showing up. This relationship influences promotions, raises, and the quality of work assignments. Indeed, it is a critical factor in determining both job success and work life quality. But many people don't take the time or make the effort to get to know this important person. Use the information in this section to avoid missing what can be a career-enhancing opportunity.

Just as instructors have their own teaching and classroom management styles, described in Chapter 7, supervisors are characterized by a variety of management styles. These are shaped by the supervisor's basic beliefs about employees. Table 12–1 illustrates a variety of supervisory assumptions and corresponding behaviors. These are not mutually exclusive. That is, a supervisor may hold several of the beliefs listed. Keep in mind that there is no one right way to manage in all situations. There are advantages and disadvantages to each. Certain styles are more appropriate than others in specific situations and work settings. Here are a few examples:

- Being friendly with employees is not positive if it results in too much down time spent socializing. There is also the danger that some employees will believe there is favoritism if the supervisor is more friendly—or perceived to be—to some employees than to others.
- There are brilliant people who seem to be very disorganized. They may have numerous projects going and don't take the time to tidy up. Don't lose the chance to learn from them because you judged them negatively by their appearance.
- Inviting employee input and encouraging creativity is beneficial in some work settings. But in others, such as the emergency room, it's not appropriate. Employees must work as directed. Procedures must be strictly followed. Lives here depend on doing work the right way—and quickly.

Your work style may not match that of your employer. This is not uncommon. Mature employees see these differences as challenges rather than obstacles. There are a number of constructive ways to work effectively in spite of these differences:

- Keep communication open. One of the worst things you can do is avoid someone with whom you disagree or have difficulty. Cutting off contact is likely to increase distance and decrease understanding.
- Follow the chain of command. This means speaking with your supervisor *before* going to the next level with concerns and complaints. Failure to follow the proper order can result in dismissal.
- Be empathetic. Your supervisor may have pressures and problems which explain his or her actions.

TABLE 12–1 ***Common Supervisor Beliefs and Actions***

Supervisor's Belief	Supervisor's Actions
"Employees need close supervision."	Closely supervises your work. Frequently checks on you and wants frequent progress reports.
"Employees work best on their own" OR "I just don't have time to watch over them."	Doesn't pay much attention to your activities/work unless something goes wrong.
"It is best not to become friends with employees."	Keeps communication businesslike and mainly focused on work-related issues.
"Employees can be friends, too."	Conversation is warm and friendly. Interested in your family and other aspects of your personal life. Birthdays and holidays are celebrated at the workplace.
"I just can't seem to get organized" OR "I like order, but I'm much too busy."	Loses reports you've turned in. Forgets scheduled meetings. Doesn't give you promised follow-up. (Caution: don't assume that because your supervisor is disorganized, he or she will tolerate your disorganization—completing assignments late, etc.)
"I can only function if there is order."	Rarely misses deadlines and expects you to meet them, too. Keeps lists, calendars, and orderly files.
"It is best to be direct when communicating with others."	Lets employees know how they are doing. Offers suggestions and criticism as needed. Employees know where they stand.
"It is hard for me to be direct with employees. I don't really know what to say. I may hurt their feelings. It's important to avoid confrontation."	Will not discuss employee problems with the person who is making errors, causing problems, etc. (Caution: may speak with others behind the employee's back, depriving him or her of the opportunity to resolve the problem.)
"It's easier and faster to make all the decisions on my own."	Employees are not consulted about policy changes, future plans, budgets, etc.
"Better-quality decisions result when employees participate in making them."	Employees are asked for opinions and decisions may be made as a group. (Caution: group decision making can bog down and result in little being accomplished.)
"I need to know all the details."	Requires detailed plans for projects, including deadlines, what supplies you will use, etc. Wants to know all the factors that have led to a problem before seeking a resolution.
"Just give me the big picture. That's all I need to know."	Only wants to know the expected outcome. How you get there is up to you.
"We've got to work by the book and follow the rules."	Procedures and tasks must be done exactly as outlined by the supervisor or the procedure manual.
"Employee creativity should be encouraged."	Encourages employees to find new, more efficient ways of completing work. (Caution: health care safety practices and compliance requirements cannot be disregarded. Be aware that some areas don't allow too much creativity.)
"I'm the expert, and employees should follow my instructions precisely. I expect them to ask a lot of questions."	Requires work to be done as directed. Deviations are not allowed.

- Ask questions to learn your supervisor's priorities and find out what is most important. If the following questions weren't answered in the job interview, ask them now:
  - What is the mission of this organization and/or department?
  - What are your expectations of me?
  - What do you most value in an employee?
  - How can I best contribute to the success of the organization and/or facility?
  - How often would you like me to report to you?
  - What is the best time to report to you, ask questions, and receive progress reports about my work?
- Let the supervisor know how you work best. This can be a positive conversation: "I really want to be able to do my best work for the radiology department. I find that when my work is constantly being checked, I get nervous and tend to make more errors. Could we work out another way that my progress can be monitored?"
- Ask for clarification if you are unclear about your job duties or exactly what is expected of you.
- Deal with interpersonal problems directly. If you are having problems with your supervisor, talk with him or her *first.* It is all too common for employees to badmouth their supervisors and discuss problems with everyone *except* the one person who can actually do something to resolve them: the supervisor. In fact, complaining usually results in everything *but* resolution. It may actually create new problems: lowered morale among coworkers who hear your complaints, lost work time, decrease in the quality of service to patients, and worsened relations with the supervisor who hears about the grumbling through the grapevine.
- Realize that the bottom line is this: you must work with your supervisor, and this means adapting to his or her style. Do your best to make the situation positive. Focus on learning as much as possible from both the supervisor and the situation.

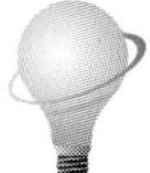

Take a Moment to Think

1. What types of supervisors have you worked for in the past?
2. How did you get along?
3. Did you learn any strategies that you can apply at future jobs?

USE REASONING

Reasoning means drawing logical conclusions. Simply stated, it involves deciding if something makes sense. Let's look at a couple of examples:

- Mr. Cardenas is scheduled for a lab test that requires him to follow certain procedures the day before. Because he doesn't understand English, it wouldn't make sense to give him a written instruction sheet in English. He will need directions in Spanish in order to ensure that he is properly prepared for the test.
- Mrs. Lonewolf, a cardiac (heart) patient, complains to nursing assistant Doris Anderson that she feels warm and sweaty. Doris does not think through the situation but takes the statement at face value: the patient needs to be cooled off. She responds by opening the window and leaving the room. In actuality, Mrs. Lonewolf is having a heart attack.

Health care professionals must keep their minds in gear, continually observing and thinking as they perform their duties. Your daily work can never be performed automatically. You must continually ask yourself questions, think about the significance of what you see, and use this information to determine the most appropriate action to take. Be on the lookout for cause-and-effect relationships. In the example of

Mrs. Lonewolf, Doris failed to recognize the connection between the symptoms reported and the patient's history of heart disease. As a health care professional, you cannot cruise along in neutral. Your work is too important, and the potential consequences of failing to apply reasoning are too serious.

THINK CREATIVELY

Creativity means seeing things in new ways. It means coming up with better ways of doing things: more caring, less painful, faster, more economical, and/or more effective. In health care work, creativity needs to have a purpose and be directed toward making an improvement.

If you come up with a new idea, be *sure* to get the approval of your supervisor before making any changes. This is especially important when you are new on the job and have not accumulated the experience necessary to predict the outcome of changes reliably. "Improving" the patient record filing system with a method you believe to be more efficient may not be appreciated by your coworkers! Even more important, it may be that certain procedures, while they seem unnecessarily time-consuming, are required by regulators or have safety implications.

SOLVE PROBLEMS AND MAKE DECISIONS

The problem-solving method introduced in Chapter 6 can be used at the workplace. To review quickly, it consists of the following six steps:

1. Define the problem.
2. Gather information.
3. Brainstorm alternative solutions.
4. Consider possible results and consequences.
5. Choose a solution and act on it.
6. Evaluate the results and revise as needed.

Good problem-solving skills involve the application of both reasoning and creativity:

- Examine what you believe to be the problem. Try to see it in different lights. Mentally walk around the problem, looking at it from all sides. Be sure that you are not defining the problem in terms of the symptoms rather than the problem itself. (Recall the case in Chapter 6 of Kathy, who believed her problem to be low grades in pharmacology when it was actually a lack of math skills.)
- Brainstorm solutions. Create as many as possible, from the seemingly sensible to the apparently crazy. Good problem solving is often the result of an original approach. It requires you to see new possibilities.
- Look for connections between circumstances and ideas.

While creativity generates ideas, reasoning enables you to put them together in ways that work. It also helps you to test potential outcomes mentally. Use it to check "What would happen if . . ." scenarios for the possibilities you have brainstormed. Reasoning helps you ask the right questions:

- Based on what I know, could this solution work? Why or why not?
- Do all the pieces fit together?
- Does it make sense?

Effective solutions are the result of using creativity to generate new ideas and applying reasoning to test them. Creativity is the artist and reasoning is the critic.

Before you approach your supervisor with a problem, think it through. Do your best to come up with solutions to suggest. This demonstrates your initiative and willingness to take an active part in the problem-solving process. It is important to distinguish between knowing when it is appropriate to ask questions and when to find solutions on your own.

CONTINUE TO LEARN

The need to learn is important in all fields today, but it is doubly so in health care. This field is in a state of continual change brought about by medical discoveries, transformations in the delivery system and methods of payment, government regulations, and technological innovations. Outdated knowledge and skills can be useless. You've got to keep up to remain effective. There are many ways to do this:

- Attend the meetings and learning activities sponsored by your professional organization.
- Read journals and publications devoted to your field, as well as books and articles about the general field of health care.
- Take courses at local schools and colleges.
- Observe and ask questions at work.
- Request information from organizations, like the American Heart Association, that publish free educational literature. Most also have informative Internet sites.
- Join newsgroups on the Internet, as described in Chapter 8.
- Use the Internet to explore topics of interest. (Remember to check the reliability of Internet sources, as explained in Chapter 4.)
- Check the availability of resources at your workplace: library, reference books, journals, people with expertise and special interests.

PRESCRIPTION FOR SUCCESS 12-6

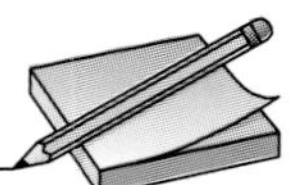

What's Available?

1. Does your professional organization have a local chapter? ________________
2. What types of learning activities does it sponsor? ________________
3. Which journals are available in your field? ________________
   Where are they available?
   ___ Subscription
   ___ Part of professional membership
   ___ Library
   ___ Health care facility
4. What types of classes are available in your area?
5. Choose a topic of interest in health care and conduct an Internet search for information. How many sites did you locate?

Increase Your Value as a Health Care Professional

In addition to the SCANS Competencies, there are specific competencies especially important for the health care professional. Adding these to your checklist of competencies will help move you into the class of "superemployee."

PRACTICE COST CONTROL

Cost control is a major concern in health care today. The United States spends more of its total income on health care than any other nation. Unfortunately, this doesn't always result in better overall outcomes. There are several countries, for example, in which people live longer and have a lower infant mortality rate (number of babies who die at birth).

How can you help control costs? There are a number of ways. They may seem insignificant, but if practiced by everyone, they can make a difference:

- Work carefully and thoughtfully so that tasks don't have to be repeated by you or anyone else. When you are being paid, time is a resource with monetary value.

- Don't waste supplies. Use what is needed and no more.
- Learn how to use supplies correctly. For example, follow the instructions when using lab test kits.
- Take care of equipment. Follow directions, use it carefully, and report any problems promptly.
- Never take supplies or use services for your personal use. A few "short" long-distance calls for personal business or runs through the copy machine add up quickly.
- Use work time for work. Your salary is a major employer expense.

ADAPT TO CHANGING CONDITIONS

Change is to be expected in most health care environments. Adapting to change—and doing so willingly and agreeably—is an essential job skill. We have mentioned the continuing changes in health care. Other factors that require flexibility include responding to patient emergencies and ensuring that all responsibilities are covered when employees are absent. Here are a few everyday examples that demonstrate the need for flexibility:

- A dental assistant learning to assist the dentist with new laser equipment that has replaced traditional drills
- A medical insurance biller keeping informed and using revised reporting methods required for Medicare reimbursement
- An emergency medical technician agreeing to change her work schedule to cover for a fellow worker who is ill
- The members of a clinic staff learning to work with a new supervisor and under new policies that accompanied an ownership change
- A nurse developing relationships with new coworkers after the hospital reorganizes departments and staff to create a team approach to patient care
- A lab technician applying new Occupational Safety and Health Administration (OSHA) requirements to the handling of chemicals and biological waste
- A medical assistant learning a new medical office management software program

Change can be viewed as an opportunity to learn and avoid boredom on the job—or as an inconvenience that requires you to "grin and bear it." The approach you choose will influence how much satisfaction you gain from your work.

PRESCRIPTION FOR SUCCESS 12–7

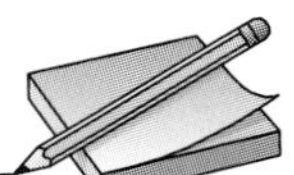

What's in the Future?

1. Review the information you gathered in completing Prescription for Success 1–4. What can you do to prepare for anticipated changes in your field?
2. If you did not do the exercise, it would be helpful to do it now.

BE WILLING TO CROSS-TRAIN

Learning tasks that are usually—or used to be—performed by professionals outside your specific occupational area are known as **cross-training.** Job duties are not separated as distinctly by occupation as they once were. Certain tasks that were only performed by the nurse, for example, may now be expected of other professionals. The movement toward the expansion of responsibilities has been encouraged by the major goals driving health care today: increase the quality of patient care while controlling costs.

Learning additional skills will add to your value as an employee. In some cases, it will even determine your success in securing the job that you want. Having opportunities to learn new skills on the job should be viewed as a benefit, not an imposition. Take advantage of them. You are learning new skills that will enhance your career and being paid at the same time!

One word of caution: check the **scope of practice** for your professional level. Some skills require you to be licensed or certified before they can be legally performed. Be sure that you know and respect your limits.

PRESCRIPTION FOR SUCCESS 12–8

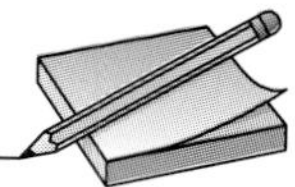

You Mean There's More?

1. Review the scope of practice for your occupation.
2. What additional skills would be appropriate for you to learn in the future? Sources of information include your instructors, employer, mentor, and professional organization.

____

____

SERVE AS A ROLE MODEL FOR WELLNESS

Personal habits are now recognized as having a major impact on health. In a dual effort to help people live healthier lives and avoid the expense of preventable medical problems, health care providers are placing more emphasis on promoting wellness. This is in contrast to the traditional focus on treating disease and injury. A growing number of patients want to take a more active role in the management of their health.

As a health care professional, you can encourage this positive trend in several important ways:

- Become an advocate of good health by promoting the benefits of healthy living.
- Serve as an example of healthy lifestyle choices, as discussed in Chapter 1. Are you a good "advertisement" for the industry you represent?
- Teach patients, as appropriate for your profession, about prevention and good habits.

RESPECT CONFIDENTIALITY

The health care professional has an ethical and legal responsibility to respect patient confidentiality. As mentioned in Chapters 1 and 7, this includes both oral and written communications. You must be willing to monitor your work habits and conversation to ensure that this important patient right is constantly guarded. Here are some suggestions to help you avoid unintentional "leaks" during the busy workday:

- Avoid discussing patient issues with anyone other than health care professionals who are directly involved in the care of the patient.
- Limit allowable discussion to locations where you won't be overheard.
- When speaking with patients about personal matters, do so in a voice that they, but not everyone else, can hear.
- Take care when speaking to and about patients on the telephone so that you are not overheard by others in the area.
- Leave patient-related matters at the workplace. While it is natural to want to share your work with family and friends, any reference to patients and "interesting cases" is inappropriate.
- Clear computer screens containing patient records when you leave the computer.
- Don't leave paperwork or files containing patient information on reception counters and other areas where they can be viewed by unauthorized people.

Confidentiality must be safeguarded for both the patient's sake and yours. Serious or habitual disregard of this principle can be a cause for dismissal of health care personnel. Box 12–2 contains statements from professional organizations about this very important issue.

In addition to patient confidentiality, health care professionals have an obligation to guard the privacy of the facility where they work. Engaging in conversation about problems at work is a popular activity. But airing what you consider to be the facility's "dirty laundry" does nothing to help the situation. In fact, it can have the opposite effect by damaging its reputation and undermining patient confidence. Problems must be addressed at the source if positive changes are to be made.

A final note regarding privacy is to respect your own. This means that personal problems don't belong at work and should not be discussed there. It is not the responsibility of coworkers to listen to and spend time advising you about personal affairs. Remember that your focus should be on work activities.

PRESCRIPTION FOR SUCCESS 12–9

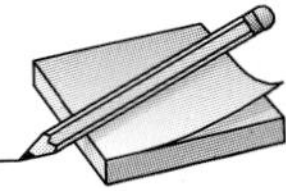

Focus on Confidentiality

1. Does the Code of Ethics for your profession include a statement about patient confidentiality?
2. List at least five techniques you would use in your occupation to guard patient confidentiality.

____

____

BOX 12–2. CONFIDENTIALITY: A SERIOUS MATTER

Excerpts from Documents That Guide Professional Conduct

American Hospital Association's Patient's Bill of Rights:

(5) The patient has the right to every consideration of privacy. Case discussion, consultation, examination, and treatment should be conducted so as to protect each patient's privacy.

(6) The patient has the right to expect that all communications and records pertaining to his/her care will be treated as confidential by the hospital, except in cases such as suspected abuse and public health hazards when reporting is permitted or required by law. The patient has the right to expect that the hospital will emphasize the confidentiality of this information when it releases it to any other parties entitled to review information in these records.

(Used with permission of the American Hospital Association.)

American Medical Association Code of Ethics:

(4) A physician shall respect the rights of patients, of colleagues, and of other health professionals, and shall safeguard patient confidences within the constraint of the law.

(Used with permission of the American Medical Association.)

Your Legal Rights

It may seem that, as an employee, you have an endless lists of "shoulds" and "must dos." In fact, there are safeguards to protect your rights on the job. These range from laws to prevent discrimination to agencies charged with ensuring your physical safety. You should be aware of the major laws described in this section. Ask your employer for information or check the library or the Internet for further resources.

FAMILY MEDICAL LEAVE ACT (FMLA)

This federal legislation was passed in 1993 to make it easier for employees to take time off to attend to health and family matters. There are certain eligibility requirements:

- You must be a public employee or work for an employer who has at least fifty employees.
- You must have worked for at least 12 months and at least 1250 hours during the 12 months immediately before taking the leave.
- The purpose of the leave must be to take care of serious personal health problems or those of a spouse, parent, or child, or for the birth or adoption of a child.

Employees who take a leave under the act must be given their previous job or the equivalent at the same pay upon their return. The employer is not required to pay the employee during the leave, but benefits such as medical insurance must stay in effect.

EQUAL PAY ACT

This act was passed in 1963 as an amendment to the Fair Labor Standards Act, the federal regulation of wages, hours, and working conditions. Its purpose is to protect workers from pay discrimination based on gender. Although the act protects both men and women, it is women who have traditionally been prohibited from performing certain jobs and have been paid less for the same work. Therefore, most equal pay complaints are filed by women.

For a successful claim, the jobs in question must be proven to be equal. This means that they are similar in skill, effort, and responsibility. Also, claims of unequal pay can only apply to employees in the same workplace. In other words, a medical assistant can't file a claim because the physician at another office pays a higher wage to medical assistants. She could, however, file a claim if a male medical assistant in the same office is paid more for performing similar work. The Equal Pay Act covers all categories of employees, including executives and managers.

CIVIL RIGHTS ACT OF 1964

This important legislation was passed to protect the rights and opportunities of all Americans. Title VII of the act prohibits the denial of employment opportunities on the basis of race, color, religion, sex, or national origin. Once hired, employees cannot be treated differently based on these factors.

Sexual harassment is classified as a form of discrimination and is, therefore, illegal under Title VII. It refers to unwelcome and unwanted sexual attention. Sexual harassment can take many forms, ranging in severity from telling dirty jokes to rape. It does not prohibit behavior that is mutually agreeable to employees such as flirting and dating. (These behaviors are not recommended, however, as workplace romances that go sour can become workplace nightmares for the people involved.)

Because some people find any reference to sexual matters offensive, it is best to play it safe by avoiding any speech or behavior that is sexual in nature. This is especially important when you are new on the job. It takes time to get to know people and the organizational culture. People respond differently, and it is best to avoid anything that might be misinterpreted. For example, remarks you intend as compliments, such as references to any part of the body, may be misinterpreted.

An important point to keep in mind is that the victim of sexual harassment does not have to be directly involved. Consider the example of two hospital employees who have become friends and regularly share jokes of a sexual nature. They find them amusing and stress-reducing. A third person, who works in the same department, finds them extremely offensive. She asks them to stop, but they consider her to be prissy and unreasonable. The third person may have a legitimate claim of sexual harassment.

You are in the beginning stages of establishing your reputation as a health care professional. Do everything possible to get a good start and avoid any behavior that might be interpreted as harassment.

At the same time, you need to know what to do if you become the victim. Most experts recommend that the first step of defense should be to speak directly with the harasser and request an immediate stop to the behavior you find objectionable. It is best not to let it go, hoping that the problem will go away, because this can send the message that the person's actions are acceptable. As a result, the actions are likely to continue and may even get worse.

When speaking with the harasser, focus on the objectionable behavior. State exactly what you find unacceptable and tell him or her to stop. You should keep a dated, written record of all events connected with the incident(s), including when you spoke to the harasser. If the behavior continues, report it to the appropriate person. This may be your supervisor or a specific person who has been appointed to deal with discrimination issues at your organization. Follow the proper procedures for filing a complaint. It is best to seek a resolution within the organization. If this does not occur, however, a complaint can be filed with the Equal Employment Opportunity Commission. This must be done within 180 days of the incident.

AMERICANS WITH DISABILITIES ACT (ADA)

This act protects the right of disabled workers to secure and maintain employment. A disability may be mental or physical and affects one or more of an individual's major life activities. The act requires employers to make "reasonable accommodations" for disabled employees who have the necessary qualifications to perform the job. A reasonable accommodation refers to both the financial impact on the employer and how the modifications affect the ability of the organization to function. Examples of reasonable accommodations are to provide a specially designed desk and chair for an employee with a back injury or an adaptive computer keyboard for an administrative worker who has the use of only one hand. Ramps, wheelchair access to work areas, and phone equipment for the hearing impaired are other examples of accommodations that might be considered reasonable under the act.

FEDERAL AGE DISCRIMINATION ACT (FADA)

Passed in 1967, this act protects workers over the age of forty from discrimination in the workplace. Employers who have more than twenty employees are subject to this act. The following actions are prohibited if they occur only as the result of an employee's age:

- Refusal to hire
- Dismissal
- Layoff
- Denial of a promotion
- Limits placed on wages and other benefits

Complaints about possible age discrimination, not resolved at the workplace, can be filed with the Equal Employment Opportunity Commission.

OCCUPATIONAL SAFETY AND HEALTH ACT (OSHA)

This 1970 act requires employers to provide safe workplaces. The act is comprehensive and contains a wide variety of provisions to protect workers by:

- Ensuring that equipment is safe and in operating order.
- Keeping the environment free of toxic and potentially harmful wastes, chemicals, and other materials.

- Providing employee with training about the safe handling of chemicals, equipment, and other materials that are potentially hazardous as a result of improper use.
- Offering hepatitis B vaccines free of charge to employees who are at risk of contracting the disease.
- Requiring that Standard Precautions be followed in the handling of blood and other body fluids.
- Providing protective equipment, such as gloves and protective eyewear, to employees who are exposed to blood-borne pathogens
- Disposing of medical waste properly.
- Having Material Safety Data Sheets (MSDSs) for all products used in the workplace. These sheets list every ingredient, as well as precautions and clean-up instructions in case of spills.

While OSHA requirements are intended to protect workers, they also carry a burden of responsibility for employees. You will be required to follow certain OSHA policies and procedures on the job. It is essential that you become familiar with those that affect your occupational duties because failure to comply can have serious consequences for you and the facility where you work.

PRESCRIPTION FOR SUCCESS 12–10

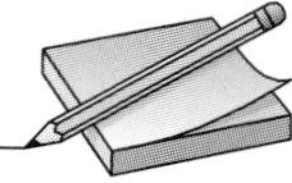

Where Can I Learn More?

Use the Internet, library references, or class notes to review and/or learn more about OSHA regulations in health care.

1. Which ones apply to your field?
2. What related skills and knowledge are you expected to have?
3. How can you help ensure that your facility complies with the regulations?

Focus on the Goal

In spite of your best efforts, difficulties may arise on the job. These can range from the annoying to the intolerable. The ability to handle them effectively is a major job and life skill. Some problems can be handled with your own resources. Others require the assistance of others to resolve.

In Chapter 2 we introduced Stephen Covey's advice to "Begin with the end in mind." Slightly modifying this sentence gives us words to keep in mind when faced with a serious problem at work: "Act with the end in mind." This means that you approach problems with the intention of finding solutions that will enhance rather than jeopardize your career. Choose actions that are appropriate for the situation and that will build your professional reputation. Some situations must simply be tolerated. For example, simple patience may be required when working with people who have annoying habits. Actions such as refusing to work with them and/or complaining to others behind their back may hurt you professionally. On the other hand, resigning from a workplace in which illegal actions are taking place—and not being corrected—may be the most appropriate action. Your professional goals should be the guiding force for all your actions.

Dedicate your efforts to finding *solutions* to difficult situations. It's easy to wear yourself out worrying or complaining about a problem, leaving little energy left over for actually dealing with it. Be clear about the resolutions you hope to achieve and look for ways to achieve them.

If you have a mentor, he or she may be a good source of advice for dealing with workplace issues. Talking them over with someone experienced in the field can help you gain perspective and see potential solutions that may not have occurred to you. Take care, however, to protect the confidentiality of the facility if your mentor does not work there.

Here are some examples of workplace problems that occur in health care settings:

1. You are asked to perform duties that fall outside your scope of practice, tasks for which you were not trained, or tasks that are illegal.

Fortunately, this problem is rare. Unfortunately, it does happen occasionally and places the health care professional in a difficult situation. The best advice in these cases is *don't*. Even if you are pressured by your supervisor, or assured that it is okay and "everyone does it," this is too big a risk to take. Once lost, your professional trustworthiness is very difficult to re-earn. Furthermore, illegal acts can result in fines and/or imprisonment.

2. You find it difficult to get along with your supervisor.

First, take an honest look at your own behavior to see if there is something you are doing—or not doing—to contribute to the problem. Speak privately and frankly with your supervisor about how important your job is to you. Tell him or her that you want to have a good working relationship. Ask if there is anything you need to do to improve your performance.

Identify your supervisor's priorities and communication style. Use mirroring, the technique discussed in Chapter 10, to match your communication styles. Not all supervisors have good communication skills. Listen carefully, and use feedback to increase the quality of communication and the likelihood of mutual understanding.

Make an effort to find out what is important to your supervisor. Review Table 12–1. Are your actions in conflict with his or her management style? Is the management style in conflict with your preferred way of working? Do you have different assumptions about the right way to do the work? This can result in major misunderstandings. Each person seems uncooperative and difficult to the other. We must become aware of the assumptions and expectations of the other person before we can attempt to meet them.

When trying to communicate with your supervisor, keep in mind that your purpose is to promote mutual understanding and get the information needed to perform your job effectively. It is *not* to prove that you are right or to tell your supervisor off, actions that will most likely make the situation worse. Find a way to relieve your stress, but don't vent your frustration at your supervisor.

3. Low employee morale. Your coworkers are unhappy and complain a lot. You'd like to get along with everyone and be part of the group, but the conversation and atmosphere are getting you down.

This can be a tough situation because it's unlikely that you can change the opinion of the group. And being a newcomer, you want to fit in, but not at the expense of joining in the complaint sessions. Complaints that are justified are resolved through action, not endless discussion that wastes time, drains energy, and generally leads nowhere. Apply your communication and problem-solving skills to try to find solutions. And do your best to avoid participating in complaint sessions. It's a negative note on which to start a new career.

4. There's too much to do and you can't finish all your work.

Start by reviewing your work habits: are you taking too much time to complete each task? Are there some tasks that you are still learning? Are you practicing good time management skills? You may be able to draw on the experience of your supervisor and/or coworkers to help you increase your efficiency. Talk with your supervisor about prioritizing your work. If you can't complete everything, which tasks are the most critical? What help is available? The time crunch is a growing problem in health care as professionals are being required to do more work in less time. Learning to maximize your efficiency will serve you well.

Work can be very satisfying in spite of problems like these. At best, problems provide opportunities for professional growth. Some situations, however, cannot be resolved or require compromises that you are not willing to make. You may choose to leave and seek employment elsewhere, a topic that is discussed in Chapter 13. In the meantime, it is critical that you do everything possible to maintain your professionalism and build a good reputation as a competent and cooperative employee.

PRESCRIPTION FOR SUCCESS 12–11

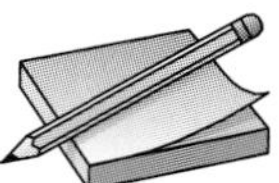

Handling the Tough Ones

Role-play the following situation with a classmate. He or she plays the part of your supervisor. You are newly hired and have been trying your best to complete what you understand to be your assignments. However, you only received a one-hour orientation to the job and are not clear about your duties, the policies at the facility, and exactly what you are expected to do. You haven't been able to locate all the supplies and resources you need and aren't sure how to operate the computer system. Your supervisor is always rushed. You now have fifteen minutes to talk with him. What would you say?

GRIEVANCE PROCEDURE

A **grievance** procedure is a written policy that gives employees a formalized, structured method to resolve workplace issues that they do not believe have been satisfactorily resolved by their supervisor. Common grievance issues include fair treatment, discrimination, and disciplinary actions.

Organizations develop their own procedures, which consist of specific steps to take to file a grievance. This procedure is usually described in the employee handbook or in a policy and procedure manual. If you belong to a labor union, ask your representative how to file a grievance. It is important to follow the directions and meet any deadlines outlined in the policy.

Grievances should be filed only when:

- You have made a sincere attempt to handle the issue at a lower level
- The issue is serious
- You are willing to follow a formal process.

Used appropriately, the grievance procedure can be an effective and fair means of resolving employee issues in an organization.

SUMMARY OF KEY IDEAS

1. Your first job sets the groundwork for your future career success.
2. Your study skills can serve as useful employment skills.
3. The SCANS Competencies are a guide to workplace success.
4. Learning to work well with your supervisor is worth the effort.
5. Employees have rights that are protected by law.

POSITIVE SELF-TALK FOR THIS CHAPTER

1. I am a confident and competent health care professional.
2. My job brings me great satisfaction.

3. I have the skills to deal with various kinds of workplace issues.
4. I work well with others.
5. My health care career is off to a good start.

BIBLIOGRAPHY

Flight, Myrtle. *Law, Liability, and Ethics for Medical Office Professionals,* 3rd ed. Albany, NY: Delmar Publishers, 1998.

Yena, Donna J. *Career Directions.* Chicago: Irwin/Times Mirror, 1997.

13

Navigating Your Career

OBJECTIVES

THE INFORMATION AND ACTIVITIES IN THIS CHAPTER CAN HELP YOU TO:

- Gain maximum benefit from performance reviews.
- Explain why it is important to maintain your professional network throughout your career.
- Describe the continuing education requirements for your career, if applicable, and list ways to earn them.
- Increase your chances of earning a promotion.
- Describe the characteristics of a successful supervisor.
- Use self-questioning and a decision matrix to choose the right job.
- Know the proper actions to take when leaving a job voluntarily.
- Understand how to survive and learn from the experience of being fired from a job.
- Add variety to your work and keep it interesting.

KEY TERMS

Decision matrix: A table created to help you decide among alternatives. You compare and rate alternatives by assigning scores based on predetermined criteria.

Job shadow: Spending time with a professional during typical work days to observe the kinds of tasks performed, the environment in which the work takes place, and so on. This is a good way to learn about job titles that interest you.

Step-up program: An educational program in which credits and/or experience earned for one occupational level can be applied for credit when studying for a higher level.

Staying on Course

Only he who keeps his eye fixed on the far horizon will find his right road.—Dag Hammarskjold

You're on your way! You have launched your health care career and should be enjoying the results of your efforts. But maintaining a successful career is like traveling successfully by ship. Without plotting and paying attention to your course, you can end up drifting aimlessly for years. Even worse, inattention can result in collisions that can sink your ship.

MONITORING YOUR POSITION: PERFORMANCE REVIEWS

Many people believe that performance reviews (work evaluations) are the responsibility of supervisors. This is not true. In fact, *you* should be conducting regular self-evaluations to monitor your progress and keep yourself on course. You should review your performance periodically using your job description and the facility's evaluation form as guides. See Figure 13–1 for a sample evaluation form. Honest self-evaluations are like an internal quality control system. They enable you to:

- Ask appropriate questions
- Seek necessary help from your supervisor
- Identify skills that need improving
- Know when to locate additional resources and information

Self-awareness empowers you to be proactive and in control. You don't wait for others to suggest needed improvements, but continually review your performance and set your own goals. Keep a list of what you do on the job to help you with both self- and formal evaluations.

Your supervisor is, of course, a valuable source of information and feedback about your progress. Take the initiative to maximize the value of your formal performance evaluations. More than one-sided progress reports, these meetings should be an opportunity for you to:

- Review the supervisor's expectations and determine whether you are meeting them.
- Ask questions:
  - Which tasks am I performing well?
  - Which tasks need improvement?
  - Do you have suggestions for improvements?
  - Can you recommend sources that might help me?
  - How can I increase my value to the team/department/facility?
- Request information. If you are unsure about certain job duties, rules, policies, or procedures, use this opportunity to ask.
- Ask for clarification. If it is unclear why you received a low rating, ask for examples that demonstrate how you do not meet the criteria, performed poorly, and so on.
- Offer explanations, but don't make excuses. If you feel you have a good reason for performance on which you were rated poorly or believe there has been a misunderstanding, it is perfectly acceptable to give an explanation. For example, if it turns out that you were given incorrect instructions about how to perform a procedure, take this opportunity to let your supervisor know and ask for help.
- Help your supervisor help you. In the spirit of developing a positive relationship and increasing your value to the facility, tell your supervisor how he or she can assist you. Examples include providing additional information about the job, explaining rules, giving you regular feedback about your work, or directing you to sources of additional training and information.
- Set goals. Work together to set goals for job improvement and/or enrichment.

Withhold criticism and complaints during the review. This is not the appropriate time to present your list of complaints about the workplace. You will come across as defensive. Do not become angry. Suggestions can best be presented at another time.

Wellness Plus Physicians Group
Employee Performance Review

Name: ____________________ Position: ____________________

Hire Date: ____________________ Date of last Performance Evaluation: ____________________

Supervisor: ____________________

Rating Scale: 1 = Excellent 2 = Very Good 3 = Satisfactory 4 = Needs some improvement 5 = Needs much improvement

Item	Rating	Comments
A. Quality of work performed	1 2 3 4 5	
B. Use of judgement	1 2 3 4 5	
C. Dependability	1 2 3 4 5	
D. Cooperation with others	1 2 3 4 5	
E. Appearance and hygiene	1 2 3 4 5	
F. Attendance and punctuality	1 2 3 4 5	
G. Time management	1 2 3 4 5	
H. Proper use of equipment and supplies	1 2 3 4 5	
I. Ability to work independently	1 2 3 4 5	

(1)

FIGURE 13–1 Sample performance review, page 1.

Wellness + Physicians Group
Employee Performance Review

Rating Scale: 1 = Excellent 2 = Very Good 3 = Satisfactory 4 = Needs some improvement 5 = Needs much improvement

J. Communication skills
Rating 1 2 3 4 5
Comments:

K. Willingness to take direction and suggestions
Rating 1 2 3 4 5
Comments:

L. Ability to adapt to change
Rating 1 2 3 4 5
Comments:

Employee's greatest strengths: ______

Progress in meeting goals from last review: ______

New goals for improvement: ______

Plan for acheiving goals: ______

Overall evaluation of this employee: ______

Reviewed By: ______
Date: ______

Employee signature ______
Date: ______
(Signature does not necessarily mean agreement)

(2)

FIGURE 13–1 (*Continued*). Sample performance review, page 2.

Formal performance evaluations, when approached as opportunities rather than something to be endured, can be constructive experiences. Combined with self-evaluations, they can help keep your career on course.

PRESCRIPTION FOR SUCCESS 13-1

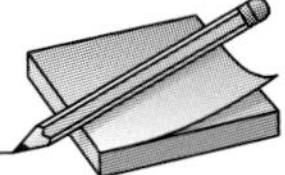

Make Reviews Work for You

Role-play the following situations with a classmate who takes the role of your supervisor.

1. Explain that you failed to follow certain safety procedures because you weren't told about them when you were hired.
2. Discuss three goals you want to achieve by your next formal evaluation.

KEEPING CURRENT

In Chapter 12 we discussed the importance of staying current in your field by pursuing a variety of learning opportunities. In some professions, earning a certain number of continuing education units (CEUs) or participating in continuing professional education (CPE) is mandatory for renewing your license or certification. The required numbers are set by licensing boards, state regulatory agencies, and/or professional organizations. It is important that you know exactly what is required for your profession.

There are a variety of ways to earn these credits:

- Classes at local colleges and universities
- Workshops sponsored by your employer, another health care facility, or your professional organization
- Written assignments that are offered through correspondence courses or in your professional journal
- Distance education classes offered over the Internet

The agency or organization that requires the units, not the education provider, determines which units will be accepted. Before participating in any learning activity for credit, make sure it will be accepted by the appropriate agency. Request documentation that you attended and/or completed the work necessary to earn the credits. You may be required to submit proof along with your renewal application. Some employers provide training allowances to help employees stay current.

PRESCRIPTION FOR SUCCESS 13-2

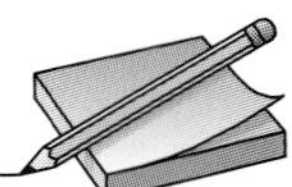

Getting Those Units

Identify ways you can earn the CEUs necessary for your profession. Create a table to organize the information.

Learning Activity	*Sponsor*	*Requirements*	*Units and Cost*
Workshops			
College classes			
Distance learning			
Reading assignments			
Hands-on activities			
Professional conferences			
Others			

STAYING CONNECTED

Once you are employed, maintain and expand your network. *Stay in touch* with your instructors, career services staff, classmates, mentors, and professionals who assisted you during your training or job search. It is important to stay connected because:

- Others professionals can help you keep up-to-date in your field by sharing knowledge, ideas, and sources of information.
- They can be good sources of information if you want to change jobs.
- Others may need *your* assistance, and networking should be a two-way street.
- It's fun to have friends in the profession. Seeing them at meetings, workshops, and conferences adds to the enjoyment of having a career.
- You can encourage each other during difficult times.

BECOMING A LEADER IN YOUR PROFESSION

Achieving excellence on the job is the first step toward becoming a leader in your profession. As you gain experience, there are other actions you can take to both enhance your career and increase your contributions to your employer, profession, and the general health care field:

- Participate actively in your professional organization. Join committees, run for office, give presentations, and attend the annual conference.
- Help new employees get started. Volunteer to orient, train, and act as a mentor.
- Become a clinical supervisor at your facility. Help students acquire the on-site experience they need to complete their education.
- Teach seminars and workshops for your professional organization, facility, or local schools and colleges.
- Write articles for professional journals.
- Support legislation that promotes health care issues.
- Promote wellness and public access to health care.

EARNING A PROMOTION

Earning a promotion is a satisfying reward for your hard work. Note the use of the word *"earning."* You must demonstrate that you have what it takes to take on more responsibility, *earning* the confidence of those doing the promoting. If earning promotions is on your list of career goals, there are a number of ways to increase your chances:

- Be 100% dependable. Develop a reputation for being on time, on task, and following through on all tasks.
- Demonstrate leadership skills. Help and encourage others, be a productive and cooperative team member, and develop excellent communication skills.
- Strive for excellence. Set high personal and professional standards. Continually develop your skills and acquire new ones.
- Increase your value to the organization. Take on additional responsibilities, and volunteer for committees and special projects. Make positive contributions to the organization.
- Advertise your interest. Let your supervisor know you are interested in a promotion. Find out about the necessary qualifications and develop a plan for acquiring any that you are lacking.
- Sell yourself. If you must formally apply for the new position, be prepared. Review your accomplishments and select examples of work that demonstrate why you are qualified for the new position. Don't assume that the interviewer—even if this is your own supervisor—is aware of all your qualifications.

Becoming the Supervisor

The purpose of management is to maximize people's strengths and make their weaknesses irrelevant.—Peter Drucker

Receiving a promotion is something you can be proud of. Enjoy the good feelings that come with having attained a significant accomplishment. At the same time, recognize and be willing to accept the increased responsibilities that are almost certainly included. If you are promoted to a supervisory position, you are now accountable not only for your own work, but that of others as well. A special challenge occurs if former coworkers now report to you. This is sometimes an awkward situation, especially if you are friends outside the workplace. You may feel uncomfortable telling them what to do. On the other hand, you can build on these positive relationships to develop a team that pulls together to accomplish group goals. Your priority now must be to ensure that assigned work is completed satisfactorily. True friends will understand and support these efforts. Do take care that all employees are treated equally and fairly, regardless of previous relationships.

Being a successful supervisor may mean adding some new skills to the ones that helped you earn the new position. For example, building productive teams, organizing work schedules, and running effective meetings require different skills than those needed to be a good dental assistant, medical transcriptionist, or laboratory technician. If your future goals include becoming a supervisor, prepare ahead by acquiring the necessary knowledge through taking classes and/or self-study on topics such as:

- Personnel management
- Motivation
- Public speaking
- Budgeting
- Evaluation techniques
- Long-range planning

Successful supervisors have good people skills. They inspire others to do their best. There are many ways to accomplish this:

- Set a positive tone for the group. Promote the mission of the organization. Emphasize the value of the work. Be enthusiastic and share your enthusiasm with others.
- Keep the group focused on accomplishing worthy goals: delivering high-quality patient care, performing work accurately, and supporting the efforts of the medical staff.
- Give continuous, appropriate feedback. Encourage the employees' best efforts with public praise. Help them improve by giving constructive criticism in private. Employees deserve the opportunity to make needed changes, and this is possible only if they know what the problems are.
- Recognize and build on each employee's strengths and weakness, whenever possible, by assigning appropriate tasks.
- Clearly communicate your expectations. Assumptions are dangerous: what is obvious to you may be "clear as mud" to others.
- Delegate appropriately. Too much and employees will resent you. Too little and you will find yourself worn out and/or unable to complete your work.

PRESCRIPTION FOR SUCCESS 13–3

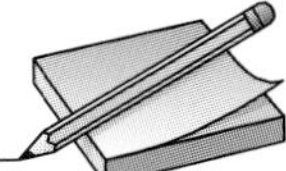

What Has Helped You Succeed?

Think about your previous supervisors.

1. Would you describe any of them as excellent supervisors?
2. If yes, describe what made them excellent. If not, describe why not.
3. List the qualities you consider most important in a supervisor.
4. Research the promotional opportunities that are available in your field.
   A. Is additional training necessary?
   B. Do these promotions usually include supervisory responsibilities?
   C. Is being promoted a goal for you?
   D. If yes, what can you do in your first job to start working toward this goal?

Deciding to Leave a Job

Making the decision to leave a job should be done thoughtfully. It is important that you are clear about why you want to leave. Take time to review the situation carefully and identify the real problems. If you are unhappy at work, changing jobs may not be the answer. For example, if your own work habits are at the root of your dissatisfaction, working elsewhere will not necessarily be an improvement. Our personal baggage, consisting of our attitudes, habits, and abilities, goes along with us. Some people spend years jumping from one job to another and never finding the right one. They fail to realize that the changes need to come from within themselves.

Review your current job by answering the following questions as honestly as possible:

- How might I be contributing to my own dissatisfaction?
- Do I have difficulty communicating effectively?
- Does it take me longer than others to complete assigned tasks?
- What can I do to improve my performance?
- Have I asked for assistance?
- Have I spoken with my supervisor about my dissatisfaction?
- Do I need additional skills?
- Are my expectations about work realistic?
- Would requesting a transfer or promotion resolve the problem?
- Do I have the experience and training for the job I really want?

You may discover that you are capable of transforming your job into one that is acceptable. Once identified, some problems can be resolved by changing your attitude, developing a plan, seeking help, and applying your best efforts. On the other hand, some factors are simply out of your control. Your best efforts may not be enough to overcome poor management, disorganization, lack of adequate resources, and low integrity. An example is being repeatedly told to perform tasks that are beyond your level of training and experience or scope of practice. Before making the decision to leave a job, consider filing a grievance, described in Chapter 12, if you feel you are being treated unfairly or illegally. When all efforts at resolution fail or if the facility is simply unable to accommodate your needs, finding employment elsewhere may be in your best professional interest.

PRESCRIPTION FOR SUCCESS 13-4

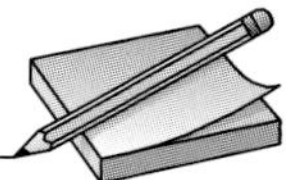

Scope of Practice

1. Does your profession have a published scope of practice?
2. Who defines the occupational roles for your career?
3. Who determines the duties you can perform?
4. What, specifically, are these duties?
5. What, specifically, are you prohibited from doing?

SEEKING NEW OPPORTUNITIES

You may like your job but still feel the need to make a change. This can happen as you gain work experience, discover areas of particular interest, and want more opportunities for professional growth. Changes can be necessary steps on the road to achieving your long-term personal and career goals when:

- You are ready—and qualified—for more challenge and responsibility, but opportunities are limited due to the size or organizational structure of the facility.
- You want to spend more time working in a particular occupational area.
- You need assistance paying for additional training, and the facility's budget does not include funding for this purpose.

- You want to spend more time with your family, and the required work schedules do not permit this.
- Your duties are limited, and you want a chance to apply more of your training.
- You would like to work with a different patient population or health care specialty.

Sometimes opportunities simply present themselves. For example, a friend tells you about an opening in the clinic where she "just loves working." Or a facility with an excellent reputation in your field may announce a promising position. You may find yourself in the position of having to make a choice between the known—your current job—and the unknown—a new job that might be better.

USING A DECISION MATRIX

When you are faced with choosing among alternatives, a **decision matrix** helps you compare how they meet your requirements. The matrix is a table consisting of intersecting squares in which you record ratings and scores for each alternative. Create this effective tool by following these steps:

1. List all the job characteristics that are important to you. Review the list provided in Prescription for Success 8–3 and see Table 13–1. Add any others that apply to you.
2. On a piece of paper, prepare a table with a row for each of the characteristics and a column for each job under consideration.
3. Rate each characteristic by number:
   1 = Not important
   2 = Somewhat important
   3 = Very important
   Write the corresponding number next to each characteristic.
4. Rank each job as you believe it will meet your needs:
   1 = Unlikely or unknown
   2 = Very likely
   Write the numbers in the top of the square.
   The new job(s) may require some research: good interview questions, talking with people who work at the facility, and reviewing the organization's web pages and published information.
5. Multiply the number assigned to each characteristic by that assigned to each job. Write the result in the center of the intersecting square.
6. Add the columns. The job with the highest score is most likely to meet your needs.

Create a matrix form, including your list of characteristics, before you interview for a new job. This gives you a means of planning questions to get the exact information you'll need to make an informed decision.

If going through this process seems to be too much trouble, consider the trouble that can result from making poor career decisions. Where you spend the majority of your waking hours impacts the quality of your life. Taking sufficient time to research, review, and properly manage your career will pay off. Using a decision matrix enables you to identify what matters most to you and measure to what degree your professional needs are being met.

The decision matrix is also a useful tool for periodically reviewing your level of job satisfaction. Instead of comparing two or more jobs, rate the one you have every few months and compare the results over time. How well does it continue to meet your needs? Have your preferences changed over time? Clearly identifying sources of dissatisfaction makes it much easier to find solutions, whether that means seeking changes in the job you have or looking for another one. Saying "I'm bored here" is not very informative. Saying "I only perform three tasks over and over each day" is more useful information. You can request more assignments at your present job or look for a job that offers a wider variety of tasks.

TABLE 13–1 ***Sample Decision Matrix for Choosing a Job***

Characteristic	Ratings (1, 2, 3)	Current Job	Proposed Job
Population served	2	1 2 × 1 = 2	3 2 × 3 = 6
Geographic location	1	2 1 × 2 = 2	1 1 × 1 = 1
Specialty	1	2 1 × 2 = 2	3 1 × 3 = 3
Independence given employees	3	1 3 × 1 = 3	2 3 × 2 = 6
Work pace	1	2 1 × 2 = 2	2 1 × 2 = 2
Variety of duties	2	2 2 × 2 = 4	3 2 × 3 = 6
Training opportunities	3	1 3 × 1 = 3	2 3 × 2 = 6
Reputation of facility	3	2 3 × 2 = 6	3 3 × 3 = 9
Opportunities for advancement	2	1 2 × 1 = 2	2 2 × 2 = 4
Challenge	2	2 2 × 2 = 4	2 2 × 2 = 4
Responsibility	2	2 2 × 2 = 4	2 2 × 2 = 4
Cooperativeness of coworkers	2	2 2 × 2 = 4	2 2 × 2 = 4
Work and mission align with my values	3	2 3 × 2 = 6	2 3 × 2 = 6
Orientation to health care (emphasis on wellness, acceptance of alternative therapies)	3	1 3 × 1 = 3	1 3 × 1 = 3
Pay	2	1 2 × 1 = 2	2 2 × 2 = 4
Benefits (insurance, vacation, etc.)	2	2 2 × 2 = 4	2 2 × 2 = 4
Work schedule	1	2 1 × 2 = 2	1 1 × 1 = 1
Contribution to society	2	2 2 × 2 = 4	2 2 × 2 = 4
Total scores		59	77

Finally, using the matrix allows you to see if your preferences align with your personal qualities and abilities. For example, if you rate "opportunities for advancement" as "very important" and "independence," "challenge," and "responsibility" as "not important, " your goals are not realistic. Wants must be balanced with willingness to perform.

You can apply the decision matrix to other areas of your life. Some examples include choosing the:

- Most practical car to buy
- Most appropriate medical insurance plan for your family

- Best school to attend for your advanced training
- Most desirable house to buy or rent

Try the decision matrix next time you must choose between alternatives. Use the left column to list the features most important to you. Then assign rating numbers and compare the alternatives. This method helps you keep focused on what's most important to you in the long run. Your values will be directing your decisions.

PRESCRIPTION FOR SUCCESS 13–5

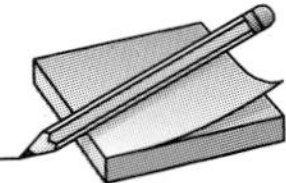

What's Important to Me?

Create your own job-search decision matrix tool.

1. Select from the job characteristics listed in Table 13–1.
2. Add any others that are important to you.

Create and use a decision matrix to assist in making a decision in your personal life.

1. Describe the results.
2. Did you find the process helpful?

Preparing to Change Jobs

Most employment experts recommend that you don't resign from a job until you have a firm offer for another one. It is the general belief that you are considered to be more employable if you are currently working. Perhaps more important, you are in a better position financially to look around and find a suitable position. This is especially true if the job market is tight and few positions are available.

You may decide, however, that you need time to reenergize and reorganize. Difficulties at work can take all your attention and leave you with little energy to look for another job. In this case, plan to have at least two months of living expenses put aside. (Actually, it is good personal management to *always* have at least two months of living expenses available in case of an emergency, even if you aren't planning to leave your job.)

Develop a network of support among friends and family members. Even leaving a job voluntarily can be stressful. Call on people who endorse your decision and can offer encouragement during your job search and transition.

Long-term career success requires that you establish a stable work record. A pattern of frequent job changes can discourage employers from hiring you. They want employees to stay for a reasonable period of time because hiring and training expenses represent a substantial investment. On the other hand, remaining too long in a position that drains your enthusiasm and stifles your progress is not a sound career decision. Consider your mission, personal values, and long-term goals when deciding whether to change jobs.

LEAVING ON A POSITIVE NOTE

Regardless of the circumstances, make your departure as gracious as possible. "It's a small world" certainly applies to employment, including health care. Employers meet at professional meetings, seminars, and country clubs. Even if you didn't like your last supervisor, he or she may play golf with someone you would *love* to work for. Keep the relationship as positive as possible.

- Give sufficient notice. Two weeks is considered the minimum.
- Write a letter of resignation in which you thank the employer for the opportunities extended. It's not a good idea to include complaints in the letter. See Figure 13–2 for a sample letter of resignation.

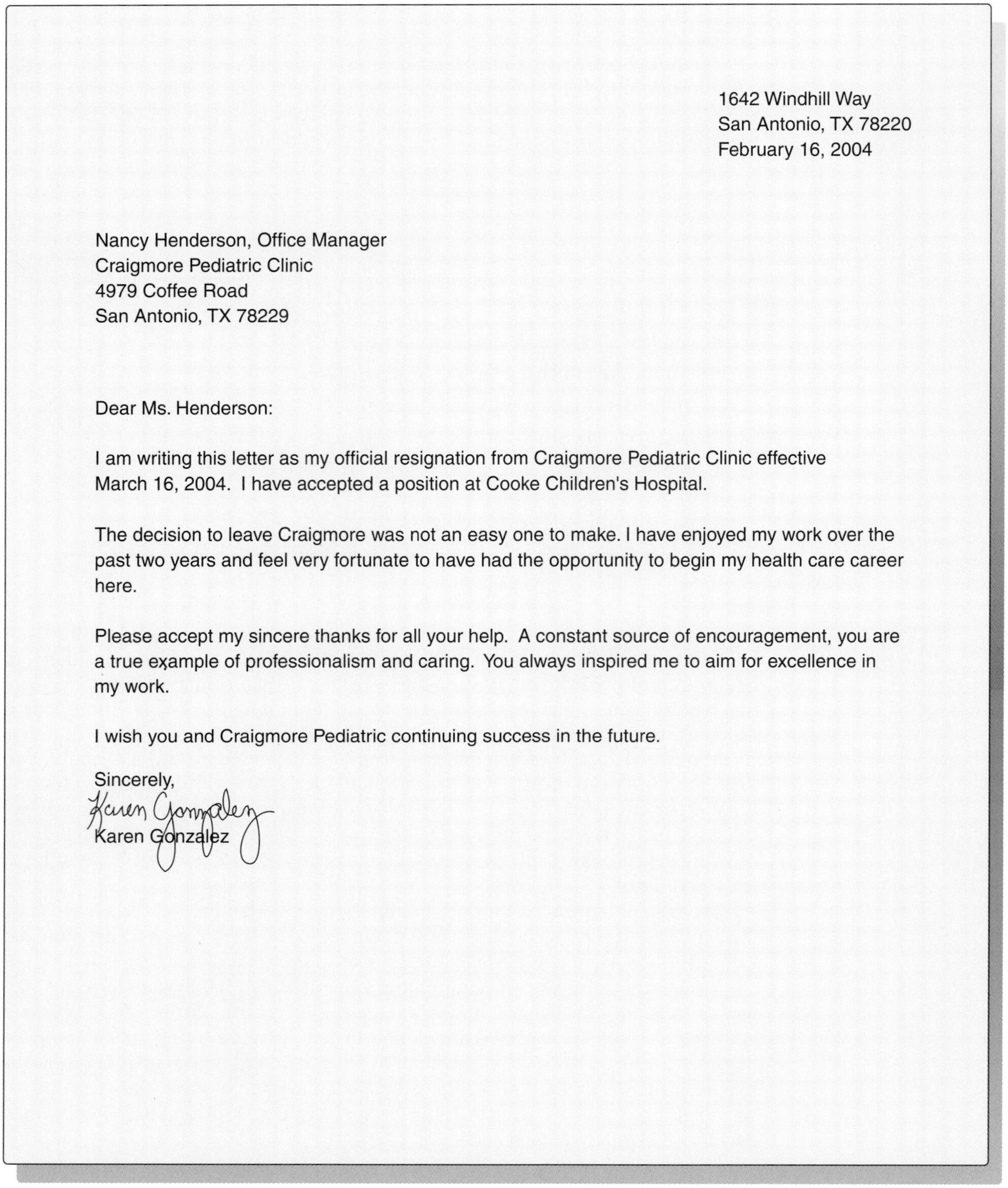

1642 Windhill Way
San Antonio, TX 78220
February 16, 2004

Nancy Henderson, Office Manager
Craigmore Pediatric Clinic
4979 Coffee Road
San Antonio, TX 78229

Dear Ms. Henderson:

I am writing this letter as my official resignation from Craigmore Pediatric Clinic effective March 16, 2004. I have accepted a position at Cooke Children's Hospital.

The decision to leave Craigmore was not an easy one to make. I have enjoyed my work over the past two years and feel very fortunate to have had the opportunity to begin my health care career here.

Please accept my sincere thanks for all your help. A constant source of encouragement, you are a true example of professionalism and caring. You always inspired me to aim for excellence in my work.

I wish you and Craigmore Pediatric continuing success in the future.

Sincerely,

Karen Gonzalez

Karen Gonzalez

FIGURE 13–2 Sample letter of resignation.

- Submit your resignation to your supervisor *before* discussing it with anyone else at work.
- Pursue job leads and attend interviews on your *own* time, not that of your current employer.
- Be willing to help train your replacement.

- Refrain from complaining and informing your employer and coworkers about everything you find wrong with the workplace.
- Put forth your best efforts through your last day. Finish all tasks and leave your work area, equipment, and files in order.

During your last days on the job, you may find it difficult to focus fully and maintain a positive attitude. Situations like these are true tests of professionalism. Doing your best and completing your obligations under any circumstances will help you build your reputation as a dependable health care professional. You are, in a sense, buying insurance for a successful future.

If you have enjoyed working with your supervisor, let him or her know. A thank-you note, separate from the letter of resignation, is a nice gesture. Express your appreciation for the supervisor's help. You may work with this person in the future. Add him or her to your network of contacts and stay in touch.

PRESCRIPTION FOR SUCCESS 13-6

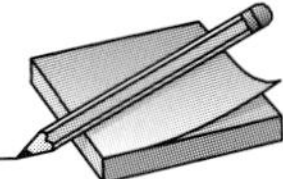

Put It in Words

Write a letter of resignation for a job that you have enjoyed. You are leaving to work in a larger facility where you have been offered a position with more responsibilities at higher pay.

HITTING ROUGH WATERS: WHAT TO DO IF YOU'RE FIRED

Men's best successes come after their disappointments.—Henry Ward Beecher

Being fired from a job is like being tossed off a ship into high seas. The water is cold and the waves are scary. You may wonder if you'll survive. But not only can you survive being fired, you can use the experience to grow personally and professionally.

Your first concern, however, is to stay afloat. Thrashing about by becoming angry and defensive and lashing out at your supervisor will only make matters worse and put your career in danger of drowning. When you receive the news that you are being fired, it is recommended that you:

- Ask for an explanation of the reasons for the decision. It is likely that you've already been advised about problems regarding your performance. Ask about anything you don't understand or believed had been corrected.
- Listen carefully and ask for feedback when necessary. This may be difficult under the circumstances, but it is critical that the communication be as clear as possible.
- Request an opportunity to explain your side of the situation if you believe there has been a misunderstanding. Don't insist, however, if you are told that the decision is final. It will only hurt your case to argue, yell, or use abusive language.
- Ask your supervisor for suggestions about what you can do to prevent this from happening at a future job.
- Don't bring out your list of what is wrong with the workplace, supervisor, coworkers, and so on. This gives the appearance of making excuses and acting defensively. Keep focused on learning why this decision was made about you.

Be aware that in today's legal climate, many employers have dismissal policies that may seem harsh. For example, your supervisor may not be allowed to give you details about how the decision to dismiss you was made. You may be asked to gather your things, under supervision, and leave the workplace immediately. Keep in mind that these policies apply to all employees who are dismissed, not just you. Don't feel that you have been targeted or are necessarily considered to be dishonest. Do your best to maintain your composure and not make an already difficult situation worse.

Getting to Shore

Success seems to be largely a matter of hanging on after others have let go.—William Feather

Life preservers come in many forms: friends, family, mentors, instructors, and other school personnel. Use them wisely. Their role is to provide encouragement, emotional support, and honest feedback; it is not to listen to endless complaints and harrowing stories about the job and how you were mistreated.

Bring your personal resources to the rescue efforts. Rebuild your confidence by reviewing your strengths, achievements, and positive traits. Losing a job need not drown your chances for long-term success. You can get to shore by deciding to learn from the experience and taking the actions necessary to move on with your career.

Start the process by looking at yourself honestly. Recognizing the need for self-improvement is empowering because *you* can take responsibility for making changes that will affect your future. Blaming others, or denying that you are at fault in any way, puts change out of your control. It's like saying, "I'm doomed, because I have to depend on others to save me. There's nothing I can do."

Accepting responsibility means asking some hard questions. Their purpose is to help you learn from the experience of being fired so that you can prevent it from happening again. Whatever the problems, you must be willing to face them and commit to finding solutions. Table 13–2 contains examples of questions and actions based on specific problems.

Getting Back on Course

Turn your stumbling blocks into stepping stones.—Anonymous

When looking for another job, you may be worried about telling potential employers that you were fired from your last one. First of all, you don't have to volunteer this information if you are not asked. But if you are, be truthful. State that it didn't work out and that you were let go. It's not necessary to explain the situation in detail. Do *not* blame or criticize your previous employer. *Do* explain what you have learned from the situation and what you have done to ensure that it won't happen again. This demonstrates your honesty and ability to learn from mistakes, important qualities in the workplace. Let the employer know that you are committed to getting your career back on course and want to begin by making a positive contribution to his or her organization. Once you are reemployed, there are ways you can avoid getting back into rough waters:

- Do your best to keep communication open with your supervisor.
- Learn to recognize warning signs and address problems immediately. Don't try to deny or cover them up. This only makes the situation worse.
- Ask for help before you get into trouble.
- Request regular feedback from your supervisor about your performance.
- Be conscientious about performing regular self-evaluations.

Many people who lose their jobs manage to bounce back and achieve career success. You can, too, if you use the experience as an opportunity to learn and grow, not as an excuse for future failure.

TABLE 13–2 ***Learning from Experience***

Reason Given for Dismissal	Types of Questions to Ask Yourself	Suggested Actions
Poor work performance	Do I lack the skills? Am I simply careless? Do I work too quickly? Do I care about the quality of my work? Am I aware of my poor performance? Do I ask for help when I'm not sure about something? Am I willing to work on improving my skills?	Contact your school for refresher training. Review textbooks, notes, and tests. In the future, ask your supervisor for help if you are having difficulty. Don't ignore problems. Never try to cover up poor performance. It will become obvious, and is not fair to those who depend on your work.
Excessive absences	Am I failing to make work a top priority? Am I practicing good health habits? Getting enough rest? Are there health problems I need to take care of? Do I need to improve my personal organization skills to prevent frequent personal emergencies?	Commit to making work a top priority. Develop good health habits and seek professional help if necessary. Develop backup plans for child care, transportation, etc. Re-define "emergency." Work to become accident-proof rather than accident-prone. Seek help in resolving personal and/or family problems.
Violation of facility rules and/or failure to follow directions	Do I know the rules but choose to disregard them? Why? Do I misunderstand directions? How can I learn what rules are in force?	Review the importance of following rules for maintaining personal and patient safety and legal and regulatory requirements. Ask for explanations of rules or directions you don't understand. Read policies and procedures manuals and any others sources of facility rules.
Inability to get along with others/poor interpersonal skills	Is there a pattern to my relationships with others? Do I fail to listen? Do I insist on being right and/or having my own way? Am I willing to do my share of the work?	Review the principles of good communication. Take a communications and/or interpersonal relations class. Request honest feedback from someone you trust. Seek counseling to help you examine and improve your relationships with others.
Poor attitude, lack of professionalism	In what ways is my behavior unprofessional? Is my concept of "professionalism" different from the employer's? Am I willing to change? Can I put patient and employer needs before my own preferences? What contributes to my poor attitude? What can I do to change?	Think about your reasons for choosing a career in health care to see if your conduct is aligned with them. Review the purpose and components of professionalism. Observe successful health care professionals. Seek help from a mentor.
Failure to follow safe techniques	Do I know the proper techniques? Do I understand the importance of using safe techniques? Do I understand the negative consequences of using improper techniques?	Review textbooks and notes from class and skills lab. Take refresher courses that include skills training.

Note: If, after conducting your self-evaluation, you sincerely believe that your dismissal was unjust, unfair, and/or based on factors that were not related to your job performance (discrimination), you may decide to seek legal advice. You must be prepared to demonstrate that your performance was satisfactory and show how you were treated unfairly.

Enriching Your Career

The health care field offers many employment opportunities. There are dozens of ways to add interest and variety to your career. Your training may qualify you to work in a variety of settings. For example, here are just some of the environments in which registered nurses work:

Hospitals
Long-term care facilities
Schools
Prisons
Shelters for the homeless
Mobile vans that provide medical care to migrant farm workers
Private homes
International settings, such as the Peace Corps or religious missions

Some professions offer great flexibility in locations and schedules. Certain occupational areas allow you to choose between working for one employer or for an agency that sends you on a variety of assignments that range from one day to six months or longer. Those who enjoy a change of scenery can accept short-term assignments at locations around the country—or even around the world.

The nature of health care delivery today enables professionals to apply their skills in a variety of ways. Your profession may allow you to accept new challenges and gain enriching experiences. Continuing with our nursing example, let's look at the types of jobs available for registered nurses who have the necessary qualifications:

- Direct patient care in many specialty areas
- Education of both patients and other health care personnel
- Management and administration
- Case management (coordinating and monitoring the care of individual patients with complex health problems)
- Quality review (checking patient records for accuracy and completeness of documentation and treatment outcomes)
- Oversight of performance improvement (comparing a facility's performance in specific areas, such as infection control, to health care industry standards)

PRESCRIPTION FOR SUCCESS 13-7

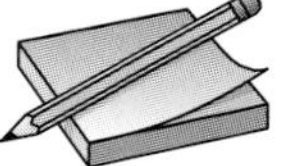

Find Out More

Research the work settings and types of jobs that are available in your occupational area.

1. How many can you find?
2. What qualifications are necessary for each?
3. Which ones look most interesting to you?

CAREER LADDERING

The concept of career laddering was introduced in Chapter 1. A career ladder consists of all the job titles within an occupational area that require various levels of education, skills, and responsibility. See Figure 13-3 for three health care examples.

Being successful does not necessarily mean climbing the ladder. In fact, aiming to do your best at your chosen level is a worthy goal. Gaining experience, perfecting your skills, and staying current are activities that can provide long-term satisfaction.

It is important to understand that the nature of the work varies among the levels. What is most appealing to you may not be at a higher level. For example, in the field of occupational therapy, the certified occupational therapist assistant generally spends more time working with patients than does the therapist, who often spends more time performing patient assessments, writing treatment plans, and performing administrative tasks. The conditions under which you work and the nature of the tasks may be different as well. In another example, the dental assistant works closely

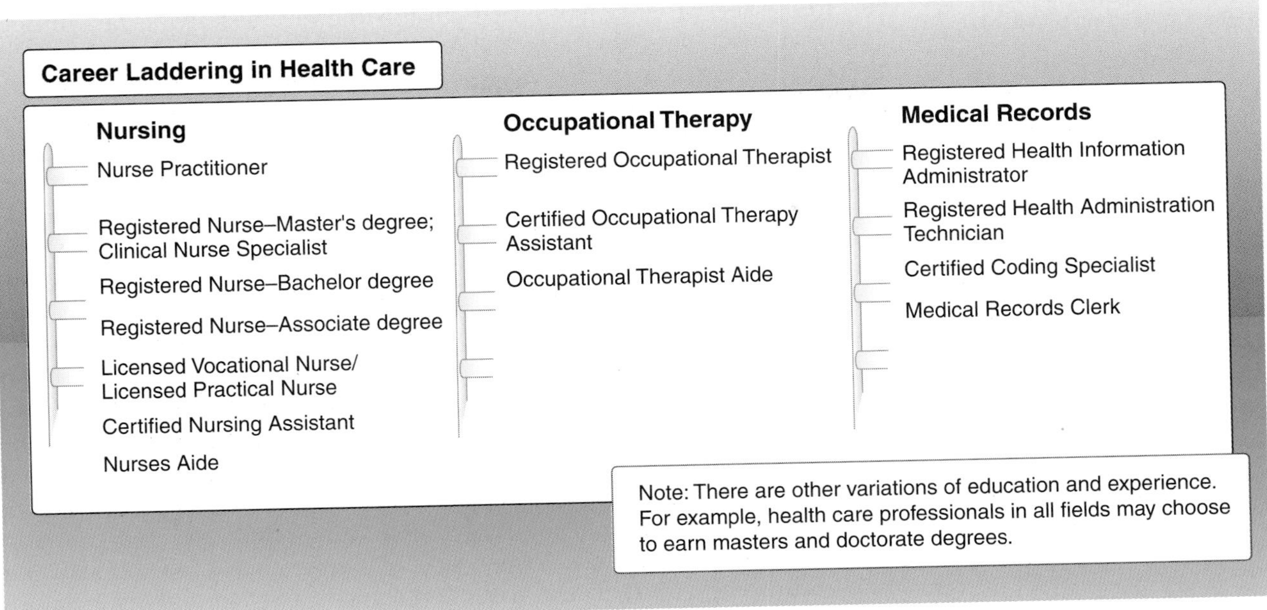

Career Laddering in Health Care
Nursing
Nurse Practitioner
Registered Nurse–Master's degree; Clinical Nurse Specialist
Registered Nurse–Bachelor degree
Registered Nurse–Associate degree
Licensed Vocational Nurse/ Licensed Practical Nurse
Certified Nursing Assistant
Nurses Aide
Occupational Therapy
Registered Occupational Therapist
Certified Occupational Therapy Assistant
Occupational Therapist Aide
Medical Records
Registered Health Information Administrator
Registered Health Administration Technician
Certified Coding Specialist
Medical Records Clerk
Note: There are other variations of education and experience. For example, health care professionals in all fields may choose to earn masters and doctorate degrees.

FIGURE 13–3 Career laddering in health care.

with the dentist, helping with a variety of procedures. The hygienist, on the other hand, primarily works alone with patients and performs similar work with each.

Positions that have more supervisory responsibilities may limit the time spent performing lab tests, getting to know patients, giving treatments, or doing other tasks that you enjoy. Before deciding to pursue additional training to move up the ladder, thoroughly investigate the job title that interests you:

- Observe people at work who have that position.
- Interview them about their duties and responsibilities.
- If you are not working closely with professionals at the targeted level, ask permission to **job shadow** in another department or facility.
- Read about the job title (see the bibliography at the end of the chapter).
- Request information from the appropriate professional organization.
- Review a sample curriculum and course descriptions.
- Obtain job descriptions.

Some schools have designed **step-up programs** that allow students to apply the courses taken for one occupational level to the next level. For example, there are programs that grant academic credits and waive certain courses for licensed practical nurses/licensed vocational nurses who enroll in registered nurse programs. Step-up programs are not available at all schools. They may also be selective about the schools from which they accept credits. Be sure to inquire about the transfer of credit policy when deciding where to pursue advanced training.

PRESCRIPTION FOR SUCCESS 13–8

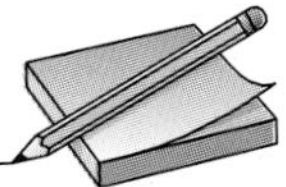

Your Occupational Ladder

Investigate career laddering in your occupational field.

1. What are the specific job titles on each rung of the ladder?
2. What are the educational requirements for each?
3. What are the licensing requirements for each?
4. Describe the differences in skill level and responsibility among the levels.
5. How do the tasks differ?

DEVELOPING A NEW CAREER

Many health care professionals have skills that can be transferred from one occupational area to another. After acquiring work experience, you may decide to choose another type of work in which you apply your health care background. Additional training or self-directed learning may be necessary to supplement your knowledge and skills.

The following examples illustrate careers that are open to people with health care backgrounds:

- Sales: medical and pharmaceutical products
- Instructor or program director: vocational schools, colleges, and universities
- Legal assistant: for attorneys who specialize in health care cases
- Consultant: providing advice to individuals and organizations in your areas of expertise
- Writer: reports, articles, proposals, textbooks, and patient education materials

THE HEALTH CARE ENTREPRENEUR

An entrepreneur is someone who organizes and manages a business. Starting a business or working on your own may appeal to you. Being the boss is an attractive idea: setting your own schedule, being accountable only to yourself, and enjoying the benefits of your work. There is another side, of course: having to work many hours, doing all the work yourself, and assuming responsibility for any financial losses. Not everyone is cut out for self-employment. Certain characteristics have been identified as desirable for successful entrepreneurs. Ask yourself if you are:

1. *Competitive.* Do you see yourself as a winner? Are you willing to put in the necessary effort to be one?
2. *Professionally competent.* Are you skilled and experienced in the area you wish to pursue? Are your skills up-to-date?
3. *Persistent.* Can you keep trying, even after experiencing failure?
4. *Willing to take risks.* Are you comfortable taking a chance with your time? Your income?
5. *Self-disciplined.* Do you stay with tasks until they are completed? Meet deadlines? Can you stay focused on work when there is something more enjoyable to do?
6. *Self-confident.* Do you believe in yourself and your ability to succeed?
7. *A problem solver and decision maker.* Are you comfortable making decisions on your own? Do you follow through with action once decisions are made?
8. *Financially prepared.* Do you have enough money to support yourself until you develop an income?
9. *Organized.* Do you organize your time well? Can you attend to more than one thing at a time?
10. *Informed about laws and regulations.* Are you familiar with the laws that affect the area of health care in which you work? Do you understand the tax implications for people who work for themselves?

Health care lends itself to a number of home-based and small businesses. The following are just a few examples:

- Health care and nutritional product sales
- Medical report transcription
- Coding and billing services
- Consulting
- Provision of residential care

A key success factor is choosing a product or service for which there is a market. Even a good idea will fail if there aren't enough customers. Conducting market research is the first step when considering a business idea.

There are many sources of assistance for those who are interested in starting a small business or working on their own. Local chambers of commerce, the Small Business Administration, and SCORE, a volunteer group of retired business people, offer a variety of services ranging from free advice to reasonably priced classes to market research data. Colleges, universities, and adult education programs offer useful classes. Learn all you can before making the decision to venture out on your own.

Smooth Sailing Managed wisely, your career can be a continual source of satisfaction. Choosing to work in health care ensures that what you do each day will be of benefit to others. Monitor your performance, watch for opportunities, and enjoy the gratification that comes from staying on course and arriving at your planned destinations.

SUMMARY OF KEY IDEAS

1. Careers must be managed to stay on course.
2. Take responsibility for your performance evaluations.
3. Staying connected and current increases both your career success and your enjoyment.
4. Promotions are not given; they are earned.
5. Getting fired from a job is not the end of a career.
6. Never burn your bridges when leaving a job.

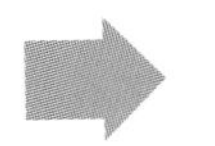

POSITIVE SELF-TALK FOR THIS CHAPTER

1. I am successfully managing my career.
2. I continually strive to improve my work and stay on course.
3. I am able to make wise decisions about the direction of my career.
4. I effectively use self-management tools like performance evaluations, decision matrices, and self-questioning.
5. I get great satisfaction from my work.

BIBLIOGRAPHY

Anderson, Shirley A. and Karen Jody Smith. *Delmar's Handbook for Health Information Careers.* Albany, NY: Delmar Publishers, 1997.

Levitt, Julie Griffin. *Your Career: How to Make It Happen.* Cincinnati: South-Western Educational Publishing, 1996.

McCutcheon, Maureen. *Exploring Health Careers,* 2nd ed. Albany, NY: Delmar Publishers, 1998.

Occupational Outlook Handbook. Indianapolis: JIST Works, Inc., 1998.

Swanson, Barbara. *Careers in Health Care.* Lincolnwood, IL: VGM Career Horizons, 1994.

Appendix

Professional Organizations for Health Care Occupations

OCCUPATION	ORGANIZATION	CONTACT INFORMATION
Cardiovascular Technologist	Alliance of Cardiovascular Professionals	910 Charles Street Fredericksburg, VA 22401
Dental Assistant	American Dental Assistants' Association	666 N. Lake Shore Drive Suite 1130 Chicago, IL 60611
Dental Hygienist	American Dental Hygienists' Association	444 N. Michigan Avenue Suite 3400 Chicago, IL 60611 www.adha.org
Dental Laboratory Technician	National Association of Dental Laboratories	8201 Greensboro Drive Suite 300 McLean, VA 22102 www.nadl.org
Diagnostic Medical Sonographer	Society of Diagnostic Medical Sonographers	12770 Coit Road Suite 708 Dallas, TX 75251
Emergency Medical Technician	National Association of Emergency Medical Technicians	408 Monroe Street Clinton, MS 39056 www.naemt.org
Health Information Technician	American Health Information Management Association	919 N. Michigan Avenue Suite 1400 Chicago, IL 60611 www.ahima.org
Medical Assistant	American Association of Medical Assistants	20 N. Wacker Drive Suite 1575 Chicago, IL 60606 www.aama-ntl.org

	American Medical Technologists' Association	710 Higgins Road Park Ridge, IL 60068 www.amt1.com
Medical Insurance Coder	American Academy of Procedural Coders	309 West 700 South Salt Lake City, UT 84101 www.aapcnatl.org
	American Health Information Management	919 N. Michigan Avenue Suite 1400 Chicago, IL 60611 www.ahima.org
Medical Laboratory Assistant/Medical Laboratory Technician	American Medical Technologists' Association	710 Higgins Road Park Ridge, IL 60068 www.amt1.com
	American Society for Clinical Laboratory Science	7910 Woodmont Avenue Suite 530 Bethesda, MD 20814 www.ascls.org
Medical Transcriptionist	American Association for Medical Transcription	3460 Oakdale Road Suite M Modesto, CA 95355 www.aamt.org
Occupational Therapy Assistant	American Occupational Therapy Association	4720 Montgomery Lane PO Box 31220 Bethesda, MD 20824 www.aota.org
Ophthalmic Laboratory Technician	Commission on Opticianry Accreditation	7023 Little River Turnpike Suite 207 Annandale, VA 22003 www.coaccreditation.com
Ophthalmic Medical Assistant	Association of Technical Personnel in Ophthalmology	PO Box 25036 St. Paul, MN 55125 www.atpo.com
Pharmacy Assistant/Technician	American Pharmaceutical Association	2215 Constitution Avenue NW Washington, DC 20037 www.aphanet.org
Phlebotomist	American Medical Technologists' Association	710 Higgins Road Park Ridge, IL 60068 www.amt1.com
Physical Therapist Assistant	American Physical Therapy Association	1111 North Fairfax Street Alexandria, VA 22314 www.apta.org
Physician Assistant	American Academy of Physician Assistants	950 N. Washington Street Alexandria, VA 22314 www.aapa.org
Practical/Vocational Nurse	National Association for Practical Nurse Education and Service, Inc.	1400 Spring Street Suite 330 Silver Springs, MD 20910 www.aoa.dhhs.gov/aoa/dir/130.html
Psychiatric/Mental Health Technician	American Association of Psychiatric Technicians	336 Johnson Road Suite 2 Michigan City, IN 46360
Radiographer/Radiologic Technologist	American Society of Radiologic Technologists	15000 Central Avenue SE Albuquerque, NM 87123 www.asrt.org

Registered Nurse	National League for Nursing	350 Hudson Street New York, NY 10014 www.nln.org
	American Nurses' Association	600 Maryland Avenue SW Suite 100 West Washington, DC 20024 www.ana.org
Respiratory Therapist	American Association for Respiratory Care	11030 Ables Lane Dallas, TX 75229 www.aarc.org
Surgical Technologist	Association of Surgical Technologists	7108-C S. Alton Way Englewood, CO 80112 www.ast.org

Index

Note: Page numbers in *italics* indicate figures; those followed by t indicate tables; those followed by b indicate boxed material.

SPECTRUM®

Word Problems
Grade 7

Published by Spectrum®
an imprint of Carson-Dellosa Publishing LLC
Greensboro, NC

Spectrum® is an imprint of Carson-Dellosa Publishing.

Send all inquiries to:
Carson-Dellosa Publishing
P.O. Box 35665
Greensboro, NC 27425 USA

Printed in the USA

ISBN 1-6244-2733-2

01-336137811

Table of Contents Grade 7

Table of Contents, continued

Chapter 9 Geometry

Chapter 10 Perimeter, Area, and Volume

Chapter 11 Variables, Expressions, and Equations

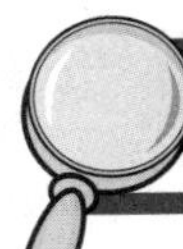

Check What You Know

Whole Numbers

Read the problem carefully and solve. Show your work under each question.

Parville has a population of 8,124 children and 32,492 adults, for a total population of 40,616 people. Somerset has a total population of 358,412 people.

1. What is the difference between the number of adults and the number of children in Parville?

   ________ people

2. What is the total population of Parville and Somerset?

   ________ people

3. There is an average of 5 school textbooks per child in Parville. How many textbooks are there in total?

   ________ textbooks

4. Parville surveys every 15th person in the town to see if there is support for a new library. How many people are surveyed?

   ________ people

5. In Parville, every 4th child plays a sport. How many children play a sport?

   ________ children

6. A new company moves into Parville, which brings 1,945 new residents. Assuming no one moves out, what is the total population of Parville now?

   ________ people

NAME ____________________

Lesson 1.1 Adding and Subtracting through 6 Digits

Read the problem carefully and solve. Show your work under each question.

A national appliance store chain keeps track of the appliances it sells each year. Last year, the store sold 102,039 microwave ovens, 87,382 stoves, 45,392 refrigerators, 128,905 toaster ovens, and 72,682 blenders.

Helpful Hint

When two digits add up to more than 10, rename the digits and carry, if necessary. For example:

$$\begin{array}{r} {\scriptstyle 1} \\ 37 \\ +\,65 \\ \hline 2 \end{array}$$

$7 + 5 = 12$

Rename 12 as "1 ten and 2 ones."

1. What is the total number of toaster ovens and blenders sold last year?

   ________ toaster ovens and blenders

2. How many more microwave ovens were sold than refrigerators?

   ________ more microwaves were sold

3. How many of the appliances sold were not microwave ovens?

   ________ appliances sold were not microwave ovens

4. What is the total number of stoves and refrigerators the appliance store sold last year?

   ________ stoves and refrigerators

5. How many more toaster ovens were sold than stoves?

   ________ more toaster ovens were sold

NAME ______________________

Lesson 1.2 Multiplying through 4 Digits

Read the problem carefully and solve. Show your work under each question.

José manages the shipping department of a calculator manufacturing company. He ships calculators in 3 different types of boxes. A small box can hold 46 calculators, a medium box can hold 354 calculators, and a large box can hold 1,178 calculators.

Helpful Hint

When multiplying by a two-digit number (the bottom number), remember to put a zero in the ones place before you multiply the digit in the tens place of the bottom number by each digit in the top number.

1. If José ships 32 small boxes of calculators, how many calculators does he ship altogether?

   ________ calculators

2. José ships 54 large boxes of calculators in one month. What is the total number of calculators shipped in that month?

   ________ calculators

3. In another month, José ships 67 medium boxes of calculators. How many calculators does he ship in that month?

   ________ calculators

4. A large school district orders 112 medium boxes of calculators. How many calculators will the school district receive?

   ________ calculators

5. José receives an order for 125 large boxes of calculators to be shipped overseas. How many individual calculators will that order contain?

   ________ calculators

NAME ____________________

Lesson 1.3 Dividing by 1 and 2 Digits

Read the problem carefully and solve. Show your work under each question.

A school district has 325 administrators, 2,462 teachers, and 43,920 students.

Helpful Hint

When dividing with whole numbers, you may find that the numbers do not divide evenly. The amount left is called a **remainder**.

1. The school superintendent decides to send every 4th teacher to a professional development workshop. How many teachers go to the workshop? What is the remainder?

   ________ teachers

   remainder ________

2. During an administrative meeting, the district administrators are divided into groups of 5. How many administrators are in each group?

   ________ administrators

3. The school district has an event that includes every student in the district. The students take buses to this event and each bus holds 60 students. Assuming no students are absent, how many buses will be used to bus the students to the event?

   ________ buses

4. During a professional development day for the teachers, the teachers are placed into groups of 40. Next, any remaining teachers will be added to a group. How many groups are there and how many remaining teachers need to be added to a group?

   ________ group

   ________ teachers need to be added to a group

5. If 30 students are in each class, at any given time during the school day, how many classes are in session in the district?

   ________ classes

NAME ______________________

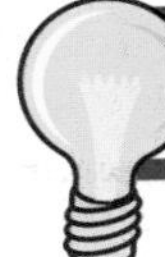

Check What You Learned

Whole Numbers

Read the problem carefully and solve. Show your work under each question.

Students from five different high schools collected cans of food to donate to a food bank. The table below shows the number of cans of food collected in one year at each school.

School	Kent	Midway	Rockville	Langley	Roxbury
# of Cans	9,058	28,250	36,424	100,264	94,550

1. What is the total number of cans collected at Midway and Roxbury schools?

   ________ cans

2. What is the difference between the number of cans collected at Rockville High School and at Midway High School?

   ________ cans

3. What is the total number of cans collected at Langley and Roxbury high schools?

   ________ cans

4. If Kent High School collects 3 times as many cans of food next year than listed in the table, how many cans will that total?

   ________ cans

5. The cans collected at Midway High School are put into boxes with 25 cans in each box. How many boxes are used?

   ________ boxes

6. Half of the cans collected at Kent High School are cans of vegetables. How many cans of vegetables are there altogether?

   ________ cans of vegetables

CHAPTER 1 POSTTEST

NAME ______________________

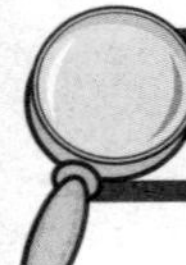

Check What You Know

Fractions

Read the problem carefully and solve. Show your work under each question.

Carlos is redesigning his dining room. The room measures $8\frac{1}{4}$ feet by $10\frac{1}{2}$ feet. He has several pieces of furniture that he plans to put in the room.

1. Carlos has two buffet tables. One table is $\frac{2}{3}$ yard wide and the other is $\frac{3}{4}$ yard wide. He wants to add the lengths of tables, so he finds the LCM for the denominators. What is the LCM of 3 and 4?

   ____

2. Use the least common multiple to compare the widths of the buffet tables. What is the width of the wider table?

   ________ ________ yard

3. If he places the two buffet tables side-by-side along the wall, what will be the total length of the tables? Show your answer in simplest form.

   ________ yards

4. Carlos's dining table measures $6\frac{1}{2}$ feet in length, including a $1\frac{3}{4}$-foot leaf. If he removes the leaf, how long will the table be?

   ________ feet

5. Carlos wants to know the area of the dining room. What is the total area in square feet?

   ________ square feet

6. Carlos uses $2\frac{1}{2}$ cups of cleaning fluid to clean 6 chairs. If he uses the same amount of fluid on each chair, how much cleaning fluid is used on each chair?

   ________ cup

NAME ______________________________

Lesson 2.1 Reducing to Simplest Form

Read the problem carefully and solve. Show your work under each question.

The Fun Wheel at a carnival is divided into 60 equal sections. Five of the sections are green, 8 are blue, 9 are purple, 16 are orange, and 22 are yellow. Players choose a color and then spin the wheel. If the wheel stops on the color chosen, they win a prize based on that color.

Helpful Hint

To reduce a fraction to **simplest form**, divide both the numerator and denominator by their greatest common factor.

1. Lamont chooses yellow and there is a $\frac{22}{60}$ chance that the Fun Wheel will stop on yellow. Write $\frac{22}{60}$ in simplest form.

   ____

2. Anton chooses blue. There is an $\frac{8}{60}$ chance that the Fun Wheel will stop on blue. Write $\frac{8}{60}$ in simplest form.

   ____

3. Amira thinks that there is a $1\frac{9}{60}$ chance that the Fun Wheel will stop on purple. Explain why this is impossible.

   ____

   ____

   ____

4. Connor does not know what the likelihood is that the Fun Wheel will stop on orange. What is the likelihood that the wheel will stop on orange? Write your answer in simplest form.

   ____

5. Robert wants the Fun Wheel to stop on green. What is the probability that the wheel will stop on green? Write your answer in simplest form.

   ____

NAME ____________________

Lesson 2.2 Finding Common Denominators

Read the problem carefully and solve. Show your work under each question.

Mr. Johnston gives each student the same puzzle. He records how long it takes each student to complete the puzzle in fractions of an hour.

Marlene	Kareem	Bianca	Paul
$\frac{5}{6}$ hour	$\frac{2}{3}$ hour	$\frac{5}{12}$ hour	$\frac{5}{8}$ hour

Helpful Hint

To find a common denominator for two or more fractions, find the **least common multiple (LCM)** of the denominators. The least common multiple is the smallest multiple of both numbers.

1. Mr. Johnston wants to compare the time it took Marlene and Bianca to complete the puzzle. Rename their times using the least common multiple for the denominator.

   Marlene ________

   Bianca ________

2. Who completed the puzzle faster, Paul or Kareem?

   ____

3. Use the least common multiple to compare Marlene and Paul's times for completing the puzzle. Use >, <, or =.

   ____

4. Mr. Johnston wants to compare all four students' times for completing the puzzle. What is the least common multiple of all the fractions in the table?

   ____

5. Which student completed the puzzle with the second fastest time?

   ____

NAME ____________________

Lesson 2.3 Renaming Fractions and Mixed Numerals

Read the problem carefully and solve. Show your work under each question.

Natalie and Inez play a game. They each write three improper fractions and three mixed numerals on a piece of paper. They switch papers and rename the improper fractions as mixed numerals and the mixed numerals as improper fractions. They each get a point for every fraction and mixed numeral they rename correctly.

Helpful Hint

To rename a mixed numeral, multiply the whole number by the denominator and add the numerator to the product. This is the numerator of the renamed fraction. The denominator stays the same.

1. Inez has to rename $\frac{25}{7}$ as a mixed numeral. Write the correct mixed numeral.

   ____

2. Natalie rewrites $\frac{15}{4}$ as a mixed numeral. What is the mixed numeral she writes?

   ____

3. Inez has to rename the mixed numeral $4\frac{5}{8}$. Write the correct improper fraction on the line below.

   ____

4. Natalie writes $2\frac{2}{9}$ as an improper fraction. What fraction does she write?

   ____

5. Inez has to rename the mixed numeral $6\frac{3}{5}$. Write the correct improper fraction on the line below.

   ____

NAME ____________________

Lesson 2.4 Adding and Subtracting Fractions and Mixed Numerals

Read the problem carefully and solve. Show your work under each question.

Jared buys food for a party. He buys $\frac{5}{8}$ pound of roast beef, $\frac{6}{7}$ pound of ham, $\frac{3}{4}$ pound of chicken salad, $2\frac{2}{5}$ pounds of corned beef, $3\frac{2}{3}$ pounds of turkey, $1\frac{3}{4}$ pounds of havarti cheese, and $1\frac{1}{3}$ pounds of cheddar cheese.

Helpful Hint

To rename a mixed numeral, multiply the whole number by the denominator and add the numerator to the product. This is the numerator of the renamed fraction. The denominator stays the same.

1. How many pounds of roast beef and ham did Jared buy altogether?

   ________ pounds

2. What is the difference between the amount of chicken salad Jared bought and the amount of roast beef he bought?

   ________ pound

3. How many more pounds of turkey than corned beef did Jared buy?

   ________ pounds

4. How many total pounds of ham and corned beef did Jared buy?

   ________ pounds

5. How many more pounds of havarti cheese than cheddar cheese did Jared buy?

   ________ pound

NAME ____________________

Lesson 2.5 Multiplying Fractions and Mixed Numerals

Read the problem carefully and solve. Show your work under each question.

Trey buys five different types of coffee beans. He buys $\frac{1}{2}$ pound of vanilla, $\frac{8}{9}$ pound of Columbian, $2\frac{1}{4}$ pounds of mild blend, $1\frac{1}{2}$ pounds of dark roast, and $3\frac{2}{3}$ pounds of hazelnut.

Helpful Hint

When multiplying mixed numerals, first rename the numbers as fractions. Then, reduce to simplest form, multiply the numerators and denominators, and simplify.

1. Trey ran out of mild blend too quickly. Next time, he will buy $1\frac{1}{2}$ times as much mild blend. How much mild blend will he buy next time?

   ________ pounds

2. The next time Trey buys coffee, he will multiply his order of dark roast by $2\frac{2}{3}$. How many pounds of dark roast will he order?

   ________ pounds

3. Next time, Trey will multiply his order of hazelnut coffee beans by 2. How many pounds of hazelnut coffee will he buy?

   ________ pounds

4. Trey sends $\frac{1}{2}$ the amount of vanilla coffee beans to his mother. How many pounds of vanilla coffee beans does he send?

   ________ pound

5. On his next visit to the store, Trey buys $\frac{1}{4}$ of the amount of Columbian coffee beans that he bought last time. How many pounds of Columbian coffee beans does he buy?

   ________ pound

NAME ______________________

Lesson 2.6 Reciprocals

Read the problem carefully and solve. Show your work under each question.

Mrs. Anderson wrote the following list numbers on the whiteboard. Then, she assigned each student one of the numbers.

$\frac{15}{19}$ 45 $4\frac{5}{7}$ $\frac{4}{9}$ $3\frac{2}{9}$

Helpful Hint

Reciprocals are any two numbers with a product of 1. Rename a mixed numeral as a fraction to find the reciprocal.

1. Aaron was given $\frac{15}{19}$. What is its reciprocal?

   ______

2. Brooke has to write the reciprocal of 45. What does she write?

   ______

3. Jan was assigned the number $4\frac{5}{7}$. What is its reciprocal?

   ______

4. Camden writes the reciprocal of $\frac{4}{9}$. What does he write?

   ______

5. Hunter writes the reciprocal of $3\frac{2}{9}$. What does he write?

   ______

NAME ______________________________

Lesson 2.7 Dividing Fractions and Mixed Numerals

Read the problem carefully and solve. Show your work under each question.

Emilio is cooking a roast turkey with stuffing for dinner. He uses a recipe given to him by his grandmother, but he plans to make some modifications to the recipe. The modifications he plans to make are explained in each question below.

Helpful Hint

To divide by a fraction, multiply by its reciprocal. If a problem has mixed numbers, rename them as fractions before you divide.

1. The recipe calls for 4 tablespoons of butter. Emilio wants to divide the amount of butter by $1\frac{3}{4}$. How much butter will he use?

   ________ tablespoons

2. The recipe calls for $2\frac{3}{4}$ teaspoons of salt. Emilio plans to divide this amount by $1\frac{1}{2}$. How much salt will he use?

   ________ teaspoons

3. The recipe calls for $6\frac{1}{2}$ cups of flour, but Emilio plans to divide this amount by $\frac{3}{4}$ because he is serving fewer people. How much flour will he use?

   ________ cups

4. The recipe calls for $1\frac{3}{4}$ cups of onion, but Emilio doesn't like onions. He plans to divide this amount by 2. How many cups of onion will he use?

   ________ cup

5. The recipe calls for $2\frac{1}{2}$ cups of celery, but one of Emilio's guests doesn't like celery, so he divides this amount by 2. How many cups of celery will he use?

   ________ cups

NAME ____________________

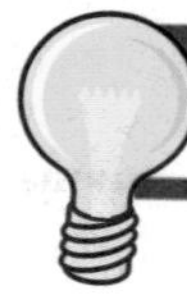

Check What You Learned

Fractions

Read the problem carefully and solve. Show your work under each question.

Demitri rents a new office space. The room measures $10\frac{3}{8}$ feet by $14\frac{3}{4}$ feet. He has several pieces of furniture that he plans to put in the office, as well as some decorative molding.

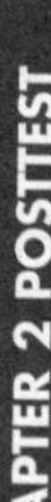

1. Demitri has two tables with different lengths. One is $\frac{7}{10}$ meter long and the other is $\frac{4}{5}$ meter long. He plans to put the tables together, so he finds the least common multiple of 5 and 10. What is the LCM?

   ____

2. Demitri compares the lengths of the tables using <, >, or =. Write a statement that compares the lengths of the tables.

   ____

3. Demitri puts the tables side-by-side to make one long table. What is the length of the tables together?

   ________ meters

4. Demitri buys a piece of molding that is $3\frac{5}{8}$ meters long. He cuts a piece $2\frac{1}{2}$ meters long to put on a wall. What is the length of the left over molding?

   ________ meters

5. Carlos wants to know the area of Demitri's office. What is the area of the office?

   ________ square feet

6. Demitri buys $12\frac{1}{3}$ yards of fabric to make 4 curtains. If he uses the same amount of fabric for each curtain, how much fabric does he use for each curtain?

   ________ yards

NAME ____________________

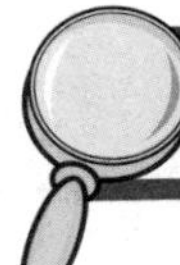

Check What You Know

Decimals

Read the problem carefully and solve. Show your work under each question.

Mischa works at an electronics store. She is in charge of ordering items and tracking sales.

1. If 15 TVs are sold for $324.99 each, what are the total sales for the TVs?

   ____

2. This year, the store sold $3\frac{3}{8}$ times more headphones than last year. Mischa needs to convert this number into a decimal for calculating inventory. What is $3\frac{3}{8}$ written as a decimal?

   ____

3. Mischa calculates that $556.50 in cameras was sold at the store. Using your answer for Question 1, what is the difference between the total sales for the TVs and the total sales for the cameras?

   ____

4. If $85.50 in earphones is sold and $590.88 in speakers is sold, what are the total sales for earphones and speakers?

   ____

5. A box of cameras weighs 16.055 pounds. If each camera weighs 1.235 pounds, how many cameras are in each box?

   ________ cameras

6. Mischa calculated that the store has 2.25 times more sales at night than during the day. If the sales during one day are $865.60, how much does Mischa expect the sales to be that night?

   ____

NAME ____________________

Lesson 3.1 Converting Decimals and Fractions

Read the problem carefully and solve. Show your work under each question.

Kenyon is organizing his CD collection into a CD tower. He is separating the CDs into different music categories.

Helpful Hint

To convert a decimal to a fraction, say the decimal out loud. To convert 0.75, say "seventy-five hundredths." This will help you write the fraction $\frac{75}{100}$, which simplifies to $\frac{3}{4}$.

1. While organizing his CDs, Kenyon realizes that $\frac{5}{40}$ of his CDs are from jazz artists. Write this fraction in decimal form.

   ____

2. Kenyon has $1\frac{3}{4}$ the amount of CDs that he had last year. What is $1\frac{3}{4}$ written as a decimal?

   ____

3. While organizing his CDs, Kenyon realizes that $\frac{57}{200}$ of his CDs are from alternative rock bands. Write this fraction in decimal form.

   ____

4. Kenyon calculated that 0.14 of his CDs are from hip-hop artists. Convert this decimal to a fraction.

   ____

5. The CD tower weighs 3.375 pounds. Convert 3.375 to a mixed numeral.

   ____

NAME ____________________

Lesson 3.2 Adding Decimals

Read the problem carefully and solve. Show your work under each question.

Elena is training for a race and using a pedometer to track the distances on runs. The decimals below show the number of kilometers she ran during 8 training runs.

Day 1	Day 4	Day 7	Day 10	Day 13	Day 17	Day 20	Day 23
5.38	7.935	2.45	10.56	8.425	15.048	17.5	6.2

Helpful Hint

When adding and subtracting decimals, keep the decimal points aligned. If the decimals have a different number of digits, add zeros as placeholders.

1. Elena ran the farthest during days 17 and 20. How many total kilometers did she run on these two days?

________ kilometers

2. How many total kilometers did Elena run on days 1 and 4?

________ kilometers

3. How many total kilometers did Elena run on the three shortest runs?

________ kilometers

4. How many total kilometers did Elena run on days 7, 10, and 13?

________ kilometers

5. Find the total number of kilometers Elena ran during her last three training runs.

________ kilometers

NAME ______________________________

Lesson 3.3 Subtracting Decimals

Read the problem carefully and solve. Show your work under each question.

John has six containers with the volume written on the side of each container. The table below shows the number of ounces each container holds.

Container 1	Container 2	Container 3	Container 4	Container 5	Container 6
35.52 oz.	16.25 oz.	24.825 oz.	20.485 oz.	32.6 oz.	14.46 oz.

Helpful Hint

Before you subtract decimals, be sure to align the decimal points. Subtract the decimals as you would whole numbers. Align the decimal point in the answer with the decimal points above.

1. What is the difference between the number of ounces containers 1 and 2 hold?

   ________ ounces

2. How many more ounces can container 5 hold than container 6?

   ________ ounces

3. What is the difference between the number of ounces containers 3 and 2 hold?

   ________ ounces

4. What is the difference of the volumes of the largest container and the smallest container?

   ________ ounces

5. How many more ounces can container 1 hold than container 5?

   ________ ounces

NAME ____________________

Lesson 3.4 Multiplying Decimals

Read the problem carefully and solve. Show your work under each question.

Kyle is reading some of the nutrition labels for the food in his cabinet. He wants to determine the amount of the food he eats.

Helpful Hint

When multiplying decimals, count the number of decimal places in each factor. The sum of the decimal places tells you how many digits should be to the right of the decimal point in the product.

1. The cereal Kyle eats contains 8.1 ounces per serving. If he eats 1.75 servings, how many total ounces of cereal does he eat?

   ________ ounces

2. The beans Kyle eats contain 8.5 grams of protein per serving. If he eats 2.15 servings, how many total grams of protein does he eat?

   ________ grams

3. Kyle has 5 containers of almonds. Each container has 9.5 ounces of almonds. How many total ounces of almonds does he have?

   ________ ounces

4. One serving of salad dressing has 2.5 grams of fat. How many grams of fat are in 0.75 serving?

   ________ grams

5. If Kyle eats 1.7 servings of rice, and each serving contains 14.5 grams of carbohydrates, how many total grams of carbohydrates does Kyle eat?

   ________ grams

NAME ___________________________

Lesson 3.5 Dividing Decimals by Whole Numbers

Read the problem carefully and solve. Show your work under each question.

Sara's mom takes her shopping to buy some clothes.

Helpful Hint

When dividing a decimal by a whole number, place the decimal point in the quotient directly above the decimal point in the dividend.

Example: $5\overline{)10.55}$ = 2.11

1. Sara spends $56.60 on 4 shirts that each cost the same amount. What is the price of each shirt?

   ____

2. Sara spends $65.98 for 2 pairs of shoes. If each pair costs the same, what does each pair of shoes cost?

   ____

3. Sara buys a package of 12 pairs of socks. If the package costs $23.76, what is the cost per pair of socks?

   ____

4. Sara buys 3 of the same type of dress, but in different colors. If she spends a total of $80.34, how much does each dress cost?

   ____

5. Sara wants to ship 2 pairs of her new pants to her cousin. She weighs the pants at the shipping store. The weight of both pairs of pants is 2.3568 pounds. How much does one pair weigh?

   ________ pounds

NAME ______________________

Lesson 3.6 Dividing Whole Numbers by Decimals

Read the problem carefully and solve. Show your work under each question.

Arianna works at a restaurant. She is separating large amounts of food into servings for cooking.

Helpful Hint

Multiply the divisor and the dividend by the same power of 10 to change the divisor to a whole number.

Example: $0.25\overline{)10.5} \longrightarrow 25\overline{)1050}$

Multiply by 100

1. Arianna has 48 pounds of potatoes. Each serving of potatoes is 1.2 pounds. How many servings are in 48 pounds?

   ________ servings

2. There are 12 pounds of shrimp. If Arianna divides the shrimp into 0.25-pound portions, how many portions will she have?

   ________ portions

3. Arianna is making patties from 21 pounds of ground beef. If each patty weighs 0.35 pound, how many patties will there be?

   ________ beef patties

4. There are 51 pounds of salmon. If Arianna divides the salmon into 0.3-pound portions, how many portions will she have?

   ________ portions

5. Arianna weighs a bag of salt that she will divide evenly into 6 smaller bags. If the bag weighs 6.8052 pounds, how much will each smaller bag weigh?

   ________ pounds

NAME ______________________

Lesson 3.7 Dividing Decimals by Decimals

Read the problem carefully and solve. Show your work under each question.

Lee is a farmer who sells his produce to local grocery stores. Today, he has 22.5 pounds of broccoli, 8.4 pounds of lettuce, 6.8 pounds of green peppers, 1.8 pounds of basil, and 38.25 pounds of tomatoes.

Helpful Hint

To divide a decimal by a decimal, multiply the divisor and the dividend by the same power of 10 to change the divisor to a whole number.

1. Lee divides the broccoli into 0.75-pound portions. How many portions does he have?

   ________ portions

2. Lettuce is sold in bags that weigh 0.2 pound each. How many bags of lettuce will be filled with Lee's lettuce?

   ________ bags

3. Lee divides the green peppers into 0.4-pound portions. How many portions does he have?

   ________ portions

4. Basil is divided into 0.06-pound packets. How many packets will be filled with Lee's basil?

   ________ packets

5. The grocer gives Lee bags for packing his vegetables. The total weight of the bags is 9.2442 pounds. If each bag weighs 0.035 pound, how many bags are there? Give your answer as a decimal and also as the nearest whole number.

   ________ about ________ bags

NAME ____________________

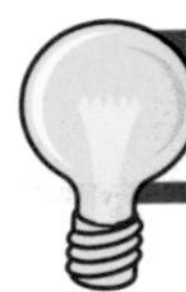

Check What You Learned

Decimals

Read the problem carefully and solve. Show your work under each question.

Anna works at her father's kitchen supply store. A set of pots and pans sells for $229.59. A set of glasses sells for $74.10. A frying pan sells for $38.98.

1. If Anna sells 12 sets of pots and pans, what are her total sales for pots and pans?

   ____

2. If a set of glasses contains 6 glasses, what is the price per glass?

   ____

3. Anna sells 5 frying pans. What is the difference between her total sales for the frying pans and 12 sets of glasses?

   ____

4. On one day, Anna sells one set of glasses and $459.18 in sets of pots and pans. What are her total sales for the day?

   ____

5. A box of frying pans from the supplier weighs 38.88 pounds. If each pan weighs 3.24 pounds, how many pans are in the box?

   ____

6. Anna sold 2.56 times more in the winter than in the summer. Write 2.56 as a fraction.

   ____

NAME ______________________

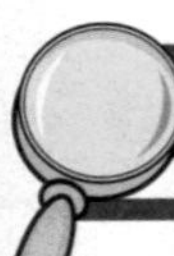

Check What You Know

Finding Percents

Read the problem carefully and solve. Show your work under each question.

Chrissie works at a fabric store. She orders fabric once a month.

1. Chrissie orders 25% of her fabric from the same vendor each month. Write 25% as a decimal.

   ____

2. She orders $1\frac{3}{4}$ yards of blue fabric and 1.7 yards of red fabric. Compare $1\frac{3}{4}$ and 1.7 using <, >, or =.

   ____

3. Chrissie orders 30% more fabric in December. Write 30% as a fraction in simplest form.

   ____

4. Write the following numbers in order from least to greatest.
   0.35, 34%, $\frac{1}{3}$

   ____

5. In January, $\frac{3}{25}$ of the fabric she ordered was textured. Write $\frac{3}{25}$ as a percent.

   ____

6. In March, Chrissie orders 40 yards of fabric. 15% of the order was for lining fabric. How many yards of lining fabric did Chrissie order?

   ________ yards

NAME ________________

Lesson 4.1 Understanding Percents

Read the problem carefully and solve. Show your work under each question.

Mrs. Adams gave a science test to her class last week. The following are test scores for five of her students:

78% 80% 65% 94% 88%

Helpful Hint

Any percent can be written as a fraction with a denominator of 100. Percents can also be written as decimals by removing the percent symbol and dividing the number by 100 (the decimal point moves 2 places to the left).

25% $\frac{25}{100}$ 0.25

1. Javier scored 78% on the test. Write this percent as a fraction in simplest form and as a decimal.

   ________ and ________

2. Carly scored 80% on the test. Write this percent as a fraction in simplest form and as a decimal.

   ________ and ________

3. Andrew received a 65% on the test. Write this percent as a fraction in simplest form and as a decimal.

   ________ and ________

4. Rebecca scored 94% on the test. Write this percent as a fraction in simplest form and as a decimal.

   ________ and ________

5. Emilio scored 88% on the test. Write this percent as a fraction in simplest form and as a decimal.

   ________ and ________

NAME ______________________________

Lesson 4.2 Comparing and Ordering Percents, Fractions, and Decimals

Read the problem carefully and solve. Show your work under each question.

Clarke invests his money in a variety of ways. The portions of his total investment are: 40% in mutual finds, $\frac{1}{4}$ in bonds, 0.15 in stocks, and 20% in real estate. He also owns 3.68 shares of a computer store and $3\frac{4}{5}$ shares of a restaurant.

Helpful Hint

When comparing fractions, decimals, and percents, remember the meaning of each symbol.

> greater than
< less than
= equal to

1. Compare Clarke's investment portions of 40% in mutual funds to $\frac{1}{4}$ in bonds. Use <, >, or =.

____

2. Compare Clarke's 3.68 shares in the computer store to the $3\frac{4}{5}$ shares in the restaurant. Use <, >, or =.

____

3. Compare Clarke's $\frac{1}{4}$ investment in bonds to his 0.15 investment in stocks. Use <, >, or =.

____

4. Order the following from least to greatest: 40%, $3\frac{4}{5}$, 3.68

____

5. Order the following from least to greatest: $\frac{11}{10}$, $1\frac{1}{4}$, 1.111, 105%.

____

NAME ____________________

Lesson 4.3 Percent to Fraction and Fraction to Percent

Read the problem carefully and solve. Show your work under each question.

Byron paints shells he collected. He paints 8% of the shells yellow, $\frac{7}{20}$ of the shells purple, 22% of the shells blue, $\frac{1}{4}$ of the shells green, and 10% of the shells red.

Helpful Hint

Percent to fraction:

$40\% = 40 \times \frac{1}{100} = \frac{40}{100} = \frac{2}{5}$

Fraction to percent:

$\frac{1}{4} \times \frac{25}{25} = \frac{25}{100} = 25\%$

1. What is 8% written as a fraction in simplest form?

   ____

2. What is $\frac{7}{20}$ written as a percent?

   ____

3. What is 22% written as a fraction in simplest form?

   ____

4. What is $\frac{1}{2}$ written as a percent?

   ____

5. Byron wants to sell the shells and make a profit of 125%. What is 125% written as a fraction in lowest terms?

   ____

NAME ____________________

Lesson 4.4 Percent to Decimal and Decimal to Percent

Read the problem carefully and solve. Show your work under each question.

Kennan grows many different kinds of plants in his backyard. He has a tomato plant, a sunflower, a rose bush, a daisy, and a hosta. He keeps a record of their growth over time.

Helpful Hint

Percent to decimal:
25% = 25 x 0.01 = 0.25

Decimal to percent:
0.73 = 0.73 x 100 = 73%

1. Kennan's tomato plant grew 12% in one week. Write 12% as a decimal.

   ____

2. The sunflower had a growth rate of 0.58 in one month. Write 0.58 as a percent.

   ____

3. Kennan's rose bush had a growth rate of 0.06 in one week. Write 0.06 as a percent.

   ____

4. The daisy grew 2% in one week. Write 2% as a decimal.

   ____

5. Kennan recorded that the hosta grew 62% in one month. Write 62% as a decimal.

   ____

NAME ______________________

Lesson 4.5 Finding the Percent of a Number

Read the problem carefully and solve. Show your work under each question.

Jai loves to read. He owns 60 books. The different types of books he owns are action, mystery, sports, literature, and non-fiction.

Helpful Hint

To find a percent of a number, express the percent as a fraction or a decimal and multiply.

1. Of the books Jai owns, 15% are action books. How many action books does he own?

   ____

2. The percentage of Jai's books that are mystery is 20%. How many mystery books does he own?

   ____

3. Sports books make up 10% of the books Jai owns. How many sports books does he own?

   ____

4. Of Jai's books, 30% are classic literature books. How many classic literature books does he own?

   ____

5. There are 600 poetry books at the library. Of the poetry books, $8\frac{1}{2}$% are for children. How many poetry books at the library are for children?

   ____

NAME ______________________

Lesson 4.6 Simple Interest

Read the problem carefully and solve. Show your work under each question.

Five people each have an amount of money they plan to deposit in saving accounts with simple interest rates.

Helpful Hint

Simple interest (I) is determined by multiplying the amount of money (principal, or p) by the rate of interest (r) by the number of years (time or t).

$$I = prt$$

Remember to substitute the number of years into the simple interest formula. The total amount in the account is the interest earned plus the initial deposit.

1. Abe has $550 to deposit at a rate of 3%. What is the interest earned after one year?

   $________

2. Jessi can get a $1,500 loan at 3% for $\frac{1}{4}$ year. What is the total amount of money that will be paid back to the bank?

   $________

3. Heath has $418 and deposits it at an interest rate of 2%. What is the interest after one year? How much will he have in the account after $5\frac{1}{2}$ years?

   $________, $________

4. Pablo deposits $825.50 at an interest rate of 4%. What is the interest earned after one year?

   $________

5. Kami deposits $1,140 at an interest rate of 6%. What is the interest earned after one year? How much money will she have in the account after 4 years?

   $________, $________

NAME ___________________

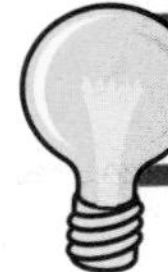

Check What You Learned

Finding Percents

Read the problem carefully and solve. Show your work under each question.

Bill's family owns a hardware store. He orders supplies for the store each month.

1. Bill orders 14% of the paint for the store from one supplier. Write 14% as a decimal.

   ____

2. Bill orders nails in two lengths, $\frac{5}{8}$ inches and 0.62 inches. Compare these lengths using <, >, or =.

   ____

3. Bill orders 135% more kitchen supplies this month than he ordered last month. Write 135% as a fraction in simplest form.

   ____

4. Write the following numbers in order from least to greatest: 0.44, 4%, $\frac{3}{4}$

   ____

5. Bill needs to determine which parts of his inventory take up the most space. Four items are represented by $\frac{11}{8}$, $1\frac{1}{4}$, 1.3, $13\frac{1}{2}$%. Order these amounts from least to greatest.

   ____

6. In July, Bill orders 150 cans of paint. 28% of the order was for white paint. How many cans of white paint did he order?

   ________ cans

CHAPTER 4 POSTTEST

NAME ______________________________

Mid-Test Chapters 1–4

Read the problem carefully and solve. Show your work under each question.

Company A sold 683,400 golf balls last year. Company B sold 872,300 golf balls last year. Company A sells golf balls in packs of 3 and Company B sells golf balls in packs of 4. In one month, Blair uses $3\frac{2}{3}$ packs of golf balls from Company A and $2\frac{1}{2}$ packs of golf balls from company B.

1. How many golf balls did companies A and B sell altogether last year?

____

2. How many more golf balls did Company B sell than Company A?

____

3. Company A plans to sell 4 times as many golf balls this year than it did last year. How many golf balls does it plan to sell this year?

____

4. How many packs of golf balls did Company A sell?

____

5. How many golf balls did Blair use from Company A in the month?

____

6. Blair used $3\frac{2}{3}$ packs of Company A golf balls per month. If he used $29\frac{1}{3}$ packs of golf balls, how many months did this cover?

________ months

NAME ______________________

Mid-Test Chapters 1–4

Read the problem carefully and solve. Show your work under each question.

Crystal is making bread at her bakery job. She has 15.6 pounds of white dough and 22.4 pounds of wheat dough.

1. How many total pounds of dough does Crystal have?

_______ pounds

2. How many more pounds of wheat dough does she have than white dough?

_______ pounds

3. Crystal makes mini baguettes with the white dough. If each baguette weighs 0.3 pound, how many baguettes can she make?

_______ baguettes

4. Crystal needs to record the amount of dough she uses every day. The amounts she uses need to be recorded as fractions. How much dough for wheat bread does Crystal have, written as an improper fraction in simplest form?

____

5. For her next batch, Crystal orders 2.55 times as many pounds of wheat dough than she has now. How many pounds of wheat dough does she order?

_______ pounds

6. Last week, Crystal used 51.761 pounds of dough to make biscuits. If it takes 0.0955 pound of dough per biscuit, how many biscuits did Crystal make?

_______ biscuits

NAME ____________________

Mid-Test Chapters 1–4

Read the problem carefully and solve. Show your work under each question.

Ken wants to invest $8,000 he has saved over the last few years. He distributes his money into different types of investments.

1. Ken deposits $360 into a savings account with a simple interest rate of $6\frac{1}{4}$%. How much money will he have after 1 year?

   ____

2. How much money will be in Ken's savings account after $3\frac{1}{2}$ years?

   ____

3. Ken invests $1,200 into a fund with a simple interest rate of 5%. How much will be in the account after 9 months?

   ____

4. Ken invested $2,300 in a 3-year CD with a simple interest rate. After 3 years, Ken had $2,472.50. What was the interest rate?

   ____

5. Ken invested $19\frac{3}{4}$% of his $8,000 in ownership of a store. How much did he invest?

   ____

6. Ken's cousin India also invested some money. India's total investments were 115% of Ken's $8,000 investment. How much money did India invest?

   ____

NAME ____________________

Mid-Test Chapters 1–4

Read the problem carefully and solve. Show your work under each question.

Ava works for a house-painting company. She uses scale drawings to buy paint for the houses and to plan the work.

1. Ava finds that 3 out of every 5 houses the company paints are white. If they paint 20 houses, how many are white?

   ____

2. It took 8 quarts of paint to paint 2 sides of a garage. If the 3rd side is the same size as each of the first 2 sides, how much paint will it take to paint 3 sides of the garage?

   ________ quarts

3. Two windows on the house have 18 total panes of glass. How many panes of glass are there for 7 windows?

   ____

4. A scale drawing of one house has a scale of 2 inches = 3 feet. The drawing of the house is 18 inches high. What is the actual height of the house?

   ________ feet

5. The scale drawing on another house has a scale of 4 inches = 16 feet. If the actual house is 36 feet high, how tall is the drawing of the house?

   ________ inches

6. On a map with a scale of 3 inches = 9 miles, Ava's house is 10 inches from her workplace. How many miles does Ava live from her workplace?

   ________ miles

NAME ______________________________

Check What You Know

Ratio and Proportion

Read the problem carefully and solve. Show your work under each question.

William is a real estate developer. He plans to build a mall.

1. Four out of 100 parking spaces in the lot will be near elevators. If there are 1,225 parking spaces in all, how many spaces will be near elevators?

   ____

2. One out of every 4 exits will be an emergency exit. If there are 88 exits at the mall, how many are emergency exits?

   ____

3. William wants 2 out of every 3 stores in the mall to be clothing stores. If there are 150 stores in the mall, how many stores will be clothing stores?

   ____

4. In the food court area of the mall, 1 out of every 4 restaurants will be for healthy-choice foods. If there are 3 healthy-choice restaurants in the food court, how many restaurants are there in all?

   ____

5. A scale drawing for a store in the mall has a ratio of 2 inches = 5 feet. If the width of the store on the drawing is 8 inches, what is the width of the actual store?

   ________ feet

6. A scale drawing for a window in the mall has a ratio of 2 inches = 4 feet. If the width of the window on the drawing is 3 inches, what is the width of the actual window?

   ________ feet

NAME ______________________

Lesson 5.1 Ratio and Proportion

Read the problem carefully and solve. Show your work under each question.

Mrs. Ryan writes several ratios on the whiteboard. Students are asked to write or identify equal ratios. Ratios that are equal are proportions and represented by an equal sign.

Helpful Hint

A proportion is a statement that two ratios are equal. In a proportion, the cross products of the terms are equal.

1. The ratios $\frac{4}{7}$ and $\frac{16}{28}$ are written on the whiteboard. Are the ratios equal?

   ____

2. The ratios $\frac{3}{5}$ and $\frac{15}{30}$ are written on the whiteboard. Are the ratios equal?

   ____

3. The ratios $\frac{2}{4}$ and $\frac{3}{6}$ are written on the whiteboard. Do the ratios form a proportion?

   ____

4. The ratios $\frac{16}{9}$ and $\frac{48}{27}$ are written on the whiteboard. Do the ratios form a proportion?

   ____

5. The ratios $\frac{4}{24}$ and $\frac{?}{30}$ are written on the whiteboard. Which number can be inserted to make the ratios equal?

   ____

NAME ______________________

Lesson 5.2 Solving Proportion Problems

Read the problem carefully and solve. Show your work under each question.

Mr. Dolby is in charge of ordering supplies for his school. Each month, he takes inventory of the supplies.

Helpful Hint

To set up a proportion problem, use a variable to represent the missing number. Then, cross-multiply and solve for the variable.

1. There are 64 pencils in 4 boxes. How many additional pencils will there be when Mr. Dolby orders 8 more boxes?

   ____

2. Mr. Dolby finds that 3 out of every 8 highlighters are yellow. If there are 64 highlighters in all, how many of them are yellow?

   ____

3. There are 96 reams of paper in 12 boxes of paper. How many reams of paper are there in 16 boxes of paper?

   ____

4. There are 90 pens in 5 boxes. Mr. Dolby needs 216 more pens. How many boxes will he order?

   ____

5. There are 42 notebooks in 3 boxes. If there are 7 boxes of notebooks, how many notebooks are there in all?

   ____

NAME ___________________________

Lesson 5.3 Proportions and Scale Drawings

Read the problem carefully and solve. Show your work under each question.

Denise works for the city planning department. She is an architect. Denise often uses scale drawings to represent buildings, parks, bridges, and other real objects in the city.

Helpful Hint

Remember to keep the units in the same parts of the proportion. For example, if yards are the denominator of the first ratio, then yards should be in the denominator of the other ratio.

1. A map of the city uses a scale of 2 inches = 8 miles. If the city is 24 miles wide, how wide is the city on the map?

   ________ inches

2. A bridge is 68 feet long. A scale drawing of the bridge has a ratio of 1 inch = 17 feet. How long is the drawing of the bridge?

   ________ inches

3. A scale drawing of a city park uses a scale of 3 inches = 9 feet. If the width of the park on the drawing is 9 inches, how wide is the actual park?

   ________ feet

4. A scale drawing of the new city hall building uses a scale of 2 inches = 7 feet. If the height of the building on the drawing is 36 inches, how tall is the actual building?

   ________ feet

5. A library is 75 feet long. A scale drawing of the library has a ratio of 3 inches = 15 feet. How long is the library in the drawing?

   ________ inches

NAME ____________________

Lesson 5.4 Proportions and Unit Rate

Read the problem carefully and solve. Show your work under each question.

The graph to the right represents the price of bananas at one store.

The graph shows that 4 pounds of bananas is $1.00. Therefore, 1 pound of bananas is $0.25, which is the constant rate of proportionality, or unit rate, for the graph. Any point on the line will yield this constant of proportionality.

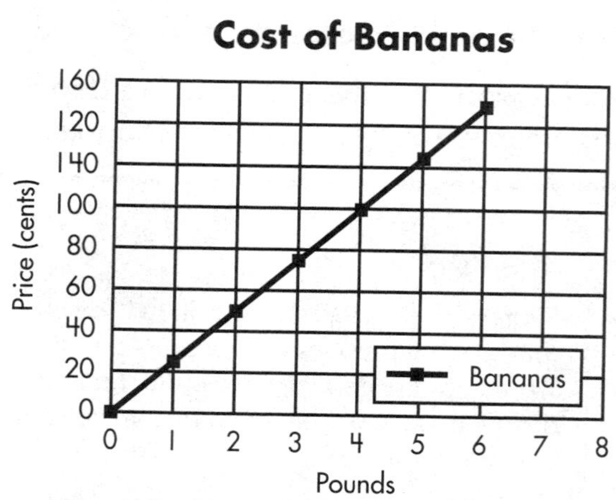

---

1. The price of bananas at another store can be determined by the equation $P = \$0.35n$, where P is the price and n is the number of pounds of bananas. What is the constant of proportionality (unit rate)?

____

2. Jane is making trail mix.

Serving Size	1	2	3	4
cups of nuts (x)	1	2	3	4
cups of fruit (y)	2	4	6	8

Create a graph to determine if the quantities of nuts and fruit are proportional for each serving size. Graph nuts: fruit as ordered pairs.

Fruit (cups)

Nuts (cups)

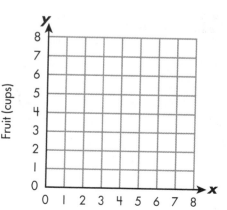

3. Is the relationship proportional? How do you know?

________, ____________________

____

____

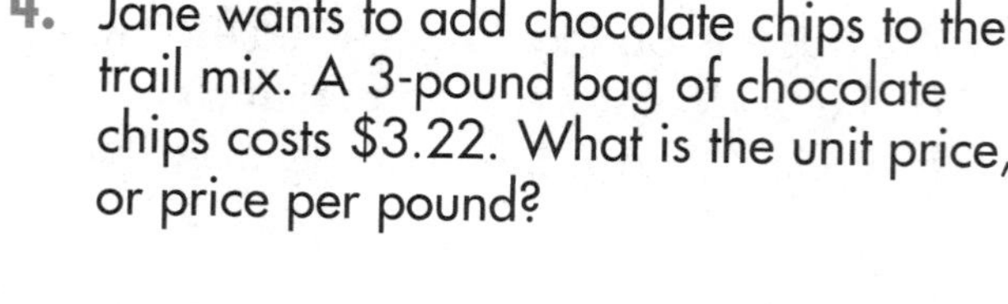

4. Jane wants to add chocolate chips to the trail mix. A 3-pound bag of chocolate chips costs $3.22. What is the unit price, or price per pound?

____

5. Jane made 32 cups of trail mix over 16 nights. How many nights will Jane have to spend making trail mix in order to make 38 cups of trail mix? How many cups will she make in 1 night?

________ nights

________ cups

NAME ______________________

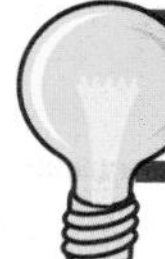

Check What You Learned

Ratio and Proportion

Read the problem carefully and solve. Show your work under each question.

Barry works for an architectural design firm. His latest project involves the construction of a condominium building.

1. Barry designs the layout of the parking garage for the condominium building. For each condo, Barry plans for 2 parking spaces. If there are 125 condo units, how many parking spaces are there?

   ____

2. For every 10 rooms, 4 will have carpeted flooring. If there are 350 total rooms in the building, how many will have carpeted flooring?

   ____

3. Three out of every 5 condominium units will have a balcony. If there are 125 condo units, how many condos will have a balcony?

   ____

4. One floor of the building will have 27 condominium units. If 2 out of every 9 units on this floor are next to a stairwell, how many units will be near a stairwell?

   ____

5. A scale drawing for a bedroom in the building has a ratio of 2 inches = 6 feet. If the width of the bedroom on the drawing is 3 inches, what is the width of the actual bedroom?

   ________ feet

6. A scale drawing for the lobby of the building has a ratio of 8 centimeters = 24 feet. If the width of the lobby on the drawing is 12 centimeters, what is the width of the actual lobby?

   ________ feet

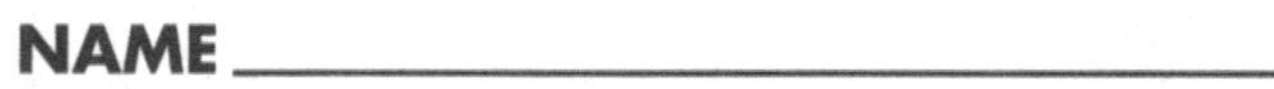

NAME ______________________

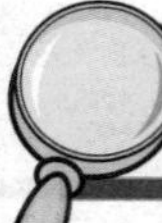

CHAPTER 6 PRETEST

Check What You Know

Customary Measurement

Read the problem carefully and solve. Show your work under each question.

Emma spends 14 days at summer camp. The camp is on a 4.2–mile stretch of a lake. Emma swims every day while at camp.

1. Emma's bag packed with clothing and personal items for camp weighs 26.5 pounds. How many ounces does her bag weigh?

   ________ ounces

2. The camp sits on a 4.2–mile stretch of the lake. What is this distance in yards?

   ________ yards

3. Emma swims for 195 minutes in the first week. How many hours does she swim?

   ________ hours

4. How many seconds did Emma swim during the first week of camp?

   ________ seconds

5. Emma brings a water bottle to camp that holds 2.5 pints of water. How many quarts of water does the bottle hold?

   ________ quarts

6. One day, Emma fills her water bottle with lemonade. How many cups of lemonade are in the bottle?

   ________ cups

NAME ____________________

Lesson 6.1 Units of Length (inches, feet, yards, and miles)

Read the problem carefully and solve. Show your work under each question.

Amira lives 5.3 miles from school. Her house is 45 feet away from the house next door and 243 feet from her cousin's house. She also lives 124 yards from the local market.

Helpful Hint

Use the table and multiply or divide to convert units of measure.
1 foot (ft.) = 12 inches (in.)
1 yard (yd.) = 3 ft. = 36 in.
1 mile (mi.) = 1,760 yd. = 5,280 ft.

1. How many feet does Amira live from school?

   ________ feet

2. What is the distance, in yards, between Amira's house and school?

   ________ yards

3. How many inches does Amira live from the house next door?

   ________ inches

4. How many yards does Amira live from her cousin's house?

   ________ yards

5. How many inches does Amira live from the local market?

   ________ inches

NAME ____________________

Lesson 6.2 Liquid Volume (cups, pints, quarts, gallons)

Read the problem carefully and solve. Show your work under each question.

Chris plans for a brunch. He has a pitcher that holds 2 quarts of liquid. He buys 3 gallons of iced tea. He also buys 0.75 gallon of tomato juice and makes 6 pints of soup.

Helpful Hint

Use the table and multiply or divide to convert units of measure.
1 pint (pt.) = 2 cups (c.)
1 quart (qt.) = 2 pt. = 4 c.
1 gallon (gal.) = 4 qt. = 8 pt. = 16 c.

1. Chris fills the pitcher with orange juice. How many cups of orange juice are in the pitcher?

   ________ cups

2. How many cups of iced tea did Chris buy?

   ________ cups

3. How many quarts of iced tea did Chris buy?

   ________ quarts

4. How many pints of tomato juice did Chris buy?

   ________ pints

5. How many cups of soup did Chris make?

   ________ cups

NAME ______________________

Lesson 6.3 Weight (ounces, pounds, tons)

Read the problem carefully and solve. Show your work under each question.

Carla wants to know the weight of different objects. She finds that her dad's truck weighs 1.13 tons. Her dog weighs 42.6 pounds. Carla's couch weighs 158 pounds and her camera weighs 1.2 pounds.

Helpful Hint

Use the table and multiply or divide to convert units of measure.
1 pound (lb.) = 16 ounces (oz.)
1 ton (T.) = 2,000 lb. = 32,000 oz.

1. How many pounds does the truck weigh?

   ________ pounds

2. How many ounces does Carla's dog weigh?

   ________ ounces

3. Carla wants to convert the weight of her couch into tons. What is the weight of her couch in tons?

   ________ ton

4. How many ounces does the truck weigh?

   ________ ounces

5. How many ounces does Carla's camera weigh?

   ________ ounces

NAME ______________________

Lesson 6.4 Time

Read the problem carefully and solve. Show your work under each question.

Brad records the amount of time it takes to do certain tasks. It takes him 2.3 hours to complete his homework. It takes him 135 seconds to brush his teeth. He usually sleeps 9 hours each night. He spent $13\frac{1}{2}$ days on vacation last year.

Helpful Hint

Use the table and multiply or divide to convert units of measure.

1 minute (min.) = 60 seconds (sec.)
1 hour (hr.) = 60 min. = 3,600 sec.
1 day = 24 hr. = 1,440 min.

1. How many minutes does it take for Brad to do his homework?

   ________ minutes

2. How many minutes does it take for Brad to brush his teeth?

   ________ minutes

3. What is the amount of time, in days and hours, that Brad sleeps in a week?

   ________ days ________ hours

4. How many hours did Brad spend on vacation last year?

   ________ hours

5. How many minutes did Brad spend on vacation last year?

   ________ minutes

NAME ______________________

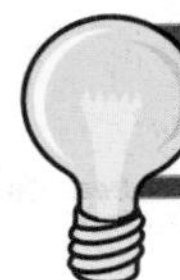

Check What You Learned

Customary Measurement

Read the problem carefully and solve. Show your work under each question.

Harry takes an art class. The class meets for 18 sessions and each session is 75 minutes. The art class is 0.5 mile from Harry's house.

1. In class, Harry makes a sculpture that weighs 73.6 pounds. How many tons does the sculpture weigh?

   ________ ton

2. How many inches is Harry's house from the art class?

   ________ inches

3. How many hours long is each art class?

   ________ hours

4. How many seconds is each art class?

   ________ seconds

5. Harry adds 3 cups of water to his clay to make it softer. What is this amount of water expressed as quarts?

   ________ quart

6. Harry added 4.5 pints of water to another batch of clay. How many cups of water is this?

   ________ cups

CHAPTER 6 POSTTEST

NAME ____________________

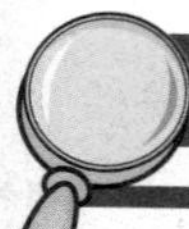

Check What You Know

Metric Measurement

Read the problem carefully and solve. Show your work under each question.

Drew needs containers for storage. He buys a shipping box that has a length of 150 centimeters and a width of 0.55 meter. The box can hold up to 28 kilograms of weight. Drew also buys a large plastic bin that can hold up to 83.2 liters of liquid.

1. Drew wants to find out how many kiloliters the large plastic bin can hold. Convert 83.2 liters to kiloliters.

   ________ kiloliter

2. Drew has 7,050 milliliters of punch that he wants to put in the plastic bin. He converts the amount to liters to see if it will fit in the bin. What is 7,050 milliliters written in liters?

   ________ liters

3. Drew's mother asks him how many grams the box can hold. How many grams does he tell her?

   ________ grams

4. How many metric tons can the shipping box hold?

   ________ metric ton

5. How many kilometers wide is the box?

   ________ kilometer

6. Drew calculates the length of the box in millimeters. How many millimeters in length is the box?

   ________ millimeters

NAME ____________________

Lesson 7.1 Units of Length (millimeters, centimeters, meters, and kilometers)

Read the problem carefully and solve. Show your work under each question.

Addie lives 12 kilometers from her grandmother's house and 266 meters from a gas station. She makes a gift for her grandmother using 450 millimeters of ribbon and 38 centimeters of yarn.

Helpful Hint

1 centimeter (cm) = 10 millimeters (mm)
1 meter (m) = 100 cm = 1,000 mm
1 kilometer (km) = 1,000 m

1 mm = 0.1 cm = 0.001 m
1 cm = 0.01 m
1 m = 0.001 km

1. Addie visits her grandmother on her birthday. How many meters away is her grandmother's house?

________ meters

2. Addie wants to know how many centimeters of ribbon she used to make her grandmother's gift. How many centimeters of ribbon did she use?

________ centimeters

3. Addie decides to calculate the distance from her house to the gas station in millimeters. Find the distance in millimeters.

________ millimeters

4. How many meters of yarn does Addie use to make the gift for her grandmother?

________ meter

5. Addie wants to know how many centimeters she lives from her grandmother's house. Write 12 kilometers as centimeters.

________ centimeters

NAME ________________________

Lesson 7.2 Liquid Volume (milliliters, liters, and kiloliters)

Read the problem carefully and solve. Show your work under each question.

Travis likes chemistry and often sets up his own experiments for fun. During one experiment he has 3.5 liters of orange juice, 55 milliliters of seltzer water, 0.007 kiloliter of cranberry juice, and 22.4 liters of ginger ale.

Helpful Hint

1 liter (L) = 1,000 milliliters (mL)
1 kiloliter (kL) = 1,000 liters

1 mL = 0.001 m
1 liter = 0.001 kL

1. How many liters of cranberry juice does Travis have?

   ________ liters

2. How many liters of orange juice and cranberry juice does he have in all?

   ________ liters

3. Travis's sister asks him how many milliliters of ginger ale he has. Write the volume of ginger ale in milliliters.

   ________ milliliters

4. How many liters of seltzer water does Travis have?

   ________ liter

5. Travis measures the orange juice in milliliters as part of the experiment. How many milliliters of orange juice does he have?

   ________ milliliters

NAME ______________________

Lesson 7.3 Weight (milligrams, grams, kilograms, and metric tons)

Read the problem carefully and solve. Show your work under each question.

Cole completes a project on the weight mass of various items within his community. He researches and records the weight of many types of items for the project.

Helpful Hint

1 gram (g) = 1,000 milligrams (mg)
1 kilogram (kg) = 1,000 g
1 metric ton (MT) = 1,000 kg

1 mg = 0.001 g
1 g = 0.001 kg
1 kg = 0.001 MT

1. A box of crackers at the store weighs 0.84 kilogram. Cole converts the weight to grams. What is the weight of the box of crackers in grams?

   ________ grams

2. The town dump has 42,000,000 kilograms of garbage. What is this weight in metric tons?

   ________ metric tons

3. A meal at the local diner has 2.7 grams of sodium. Cole wants to know this amount in milligrams. Rewrite 2.7 grams in milligrams.

   ________ milligrams

4. A chair at a furniture store weighs 11 kilograms. What is the weight of the chair in metric tons?

   ________ metric ton

5. A frozen entree from the market weighs 326 grams. Cole rewrites this weight in milligrams. How many milligrams does the entree weigh?

   ________ milligrams

NAME ____________________

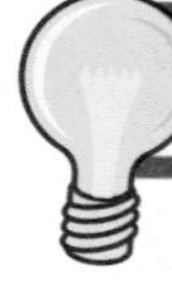

Check What You Learned

Metric Measurement

Read the problem carefully and solve. Show your work under each question.

Fiona works for a delivery service. The delivery truck is 16.4 meters in length. The truck can hold 0.5 metric ton of cargo. There is a separate container in the truck for liquids. This container can hold up to 2,100 liters.

1. Fiona wants the truck to deliver 1.8 kiloliters of a cleaning fluid to a customer. What is 1.8 kiloliters written as liters?

   ________ liters

2. How many milliliters of liquid can the container hold?

   ________ milliliters

3. Fiona wants to know how many kilograms of cargo the truck can hold, so she can notify a customer. How many kilograms of cargo can the truck hold?

   ________ kilograms

4. Fiona has a customer that has a large shipment measured in grams. How many grams can the truck hold?

   ________ grams

5. Fiona calculates the length of the truck in kilometers. How many kilometers in length is the truck?

   ________ kilometer

6. How many millimeters long is the truck?

   ________ millimeters

NAME ____________________

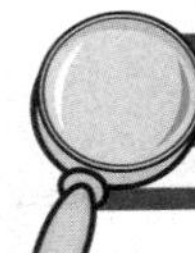

Check What You Know

Probability and Statistics

Read the problem carefully and solve. Show your work under each question.

Carter asks 40 of his friends what their favorite type of music is. He records the data on paper and then makes a circle graph to display the results. The circle graph is shown to the right.

Favorite Type of Music

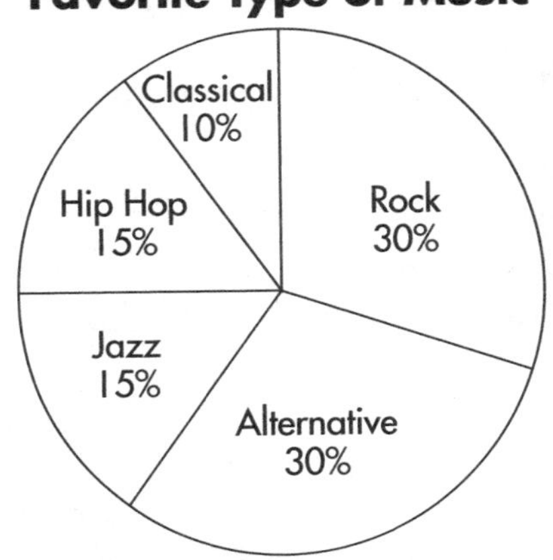

40 people responded

1. How many people said Rock music is their favorite?

   ________ people

2. Carter compares the data for each person he interviewed. Which two types of music account for three-fifths of the people interviewed?

   ____

3. How many people said Hip Hop music is their favorite?

   ________ people

4. How many people from Carter's survey chose Jazz or Classical as their favorite type of music?

   ________ people

5. If the number of people who chose Rock tripled, how many people would have chosen Rock music?

   ________ people

6. When Carter was giving his report in school, he was asked how many people chose Alternative, Jazz, or Classical. How did Carter respond?

   ________ people

CHAPTER 8 PRETEST

NAME ___________________________

Check What You Know

Probability and Statistics

Read the problem carefully and solve. Show your work under each question.

Marisa tracks the rainfall each month for March, April, May, and June. She records the data and then makes a histogram to display the data. The histogram is shown to the right.

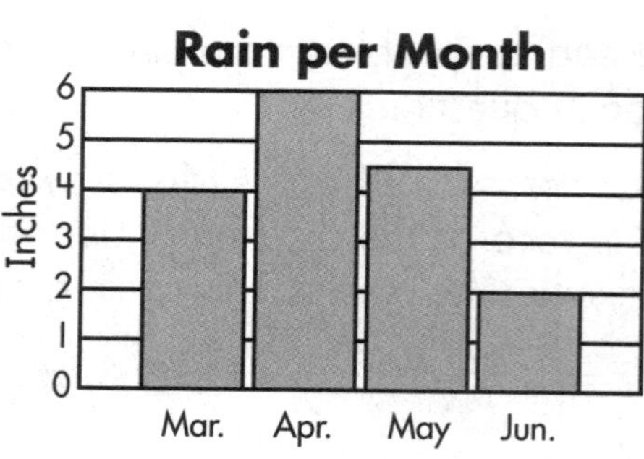

1. Marisa looks to the graph to see how many inches of rain fell in May. How many inches of rain fell in May?

   ________ inches

2. How many more inches did it rain in April than in March?

   ________ inches

3. Marisa shows the histogram to her dad. Her dad wants Marisa to tell him how many inches it rained in all 4 months. How many inches did it rain altogether?

   ________ inches

4. Last year, it rained 4 more inches in June than it rained this year. How many inches did it rain in June last year?

   ________ inches

5. Marisa wants to know how many inches it would have rained in April if two less inches of rain had fallen than she recorded. How many inches of rain would there have been?

   ________ inches

6. Marisa brings her histogram to school. Her teacher asks her how many more inches it rained in April than it did in June. What did she say?

   ________ inches

NAME ______________________

Lesson 8.1 Bar Graphs

Read the problem carefully and solve. Show your work under each question.

Ivan created a survey to find out the favorite sports of the boys and girls in his grade at school. He drew the graph to the right to show the results.

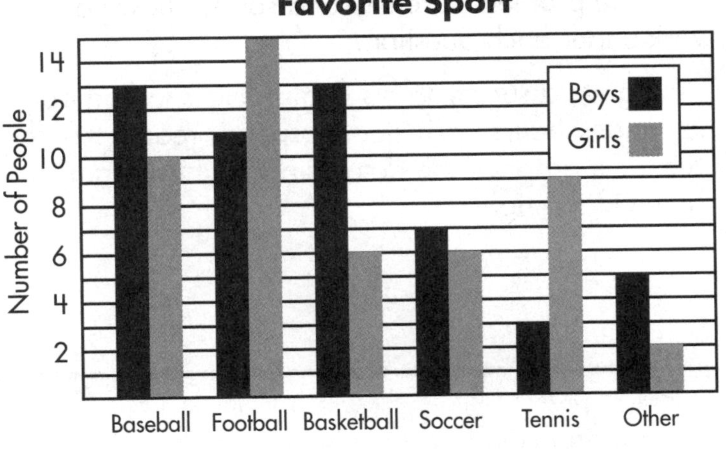

Helpful Hint

Use the key given in a double-bar graph to help you identify the numbers of boys and girls who identified each favorite sport.

1. How many people responded to the survey in all?

   ________ people

2. Ivan compares the number of boys who chose basketball to the number of boys who chose football. How many more boys chose basketball than football?

   ________ boys

3. Ivan calculates how many girls chose either soccer or other as their answer for the survey. How many girls chose either soccer or other?

   ________ girls

4. How many total people chose basketball as their favorite sport?

   ________ people

5. Ivan compares the number of girls who chose football to the number of girls who chose soccer. How many more girls chose football than soccer?

   ________ girls

NAME ______________________

Lesson 8.2 Histograms

Read the problem carefully and solve. Show your work under each question.

Iman gave a survey to his English class to find out how many hours each student spends reading each week. He graphed the data using the histogram shown to the right.

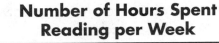

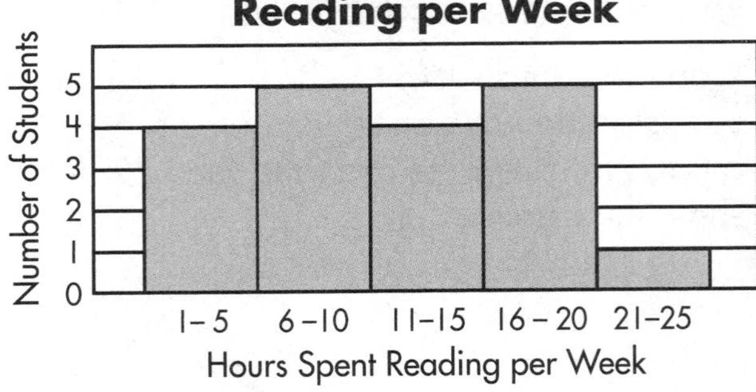

Helpful Hint

Each bar in the histogram represents an interval of 5 hours. The intervals are equal and the bars represent continuous data.

1. Iman wants to know how many students read between 16 and 25 hours per week. How many students read between 16 and 25 hours per week?

   ________ students

2. How many more students read between 16 to 20 hours per week than read between 11 to 15 hours per week?

   ________ student

3. If the survey represents every student in the English class, how many students are there in this class?

   ________ students

4. Iman calculates the number of students that read between 11 and 20 hours per week. How many students read between 11 and 20 hours per week?

   ________ students

5. How many more students read between 11 and 15 hours per week than read between 21 and 25 hours per week?

   ________ students

NAME ______________________

Lesson 8.3 Line Graphs

Read the problem carefully and solve. Show your work under each question.

James plays offense on a hockey team. He keeps track of his performance for the first 10 games of the season. He then graphs the data in the line graph shown to the right.

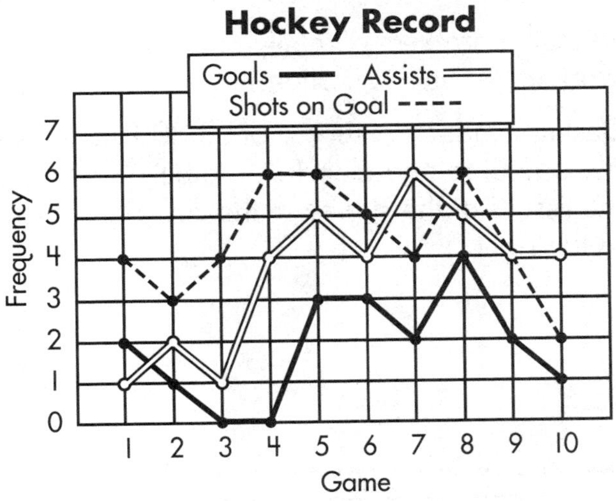

Hockey Record

Goals —— Assists ═══ Shots on Goal - - - -

Frequency: 0 1 2 3 4 5 6 7

Game: 1 2 3 4 5 6 7 8 9 10

Helpful Hint

Use the key shown in the graph to properly read which line represents goals, assists, and shots on goal.

1. During which game did James have the most assists?

game ________

2. James calculates his total shots on goal. How many shots on goal did he have in the 10 games in all?

________ shots on goal

3. During which games did James get 2 goals?

games ________

4. How many more assists did James have in game 7 than in game 2?

________ assists

5. James analyzes his goals for the 10 games. During which games did he have zero goals?

games ________

NAME ____________________

Lesson 8.4 Circle Graphs

Read the problem carefully and solve. Show your work under each question.

Destini conducts a survey of all 800 students in her school to find their favorite berry. She graphs the results of the survey in the circle graph shown to the right.

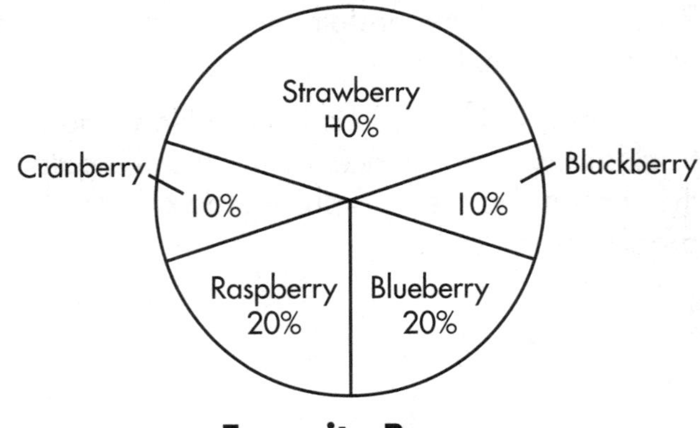

Favorite Berry

Helpful Hint

Each sector shows the percent of people who prefer each berry.

The circle is divided into sectors that add up to 100%. Each sector represents a percentage of the total number of people.

1. Destini says that two berries together account for one-fifth of the people surveyed. Which two berries together total one-fifth of the people in the survey?

   ____________ and ____________

2. Destini calculates how many people prefer blackberries. How many people prefer blackberries?

   ________ people

3. How many people prefer either cranberries or strawberries?

   ________ people

4. How many people prefer blueberries?

   ________ people

NAME ____________________

Lesson 8.5 Scattergrams

Read the problem carefully and solve. Show your work under each question.

Zoe collects data for a charity walk-a-thon relay. She recorded the number of miles some teams walked and the number of hours they walked. She records the results in the scattergram to the right.

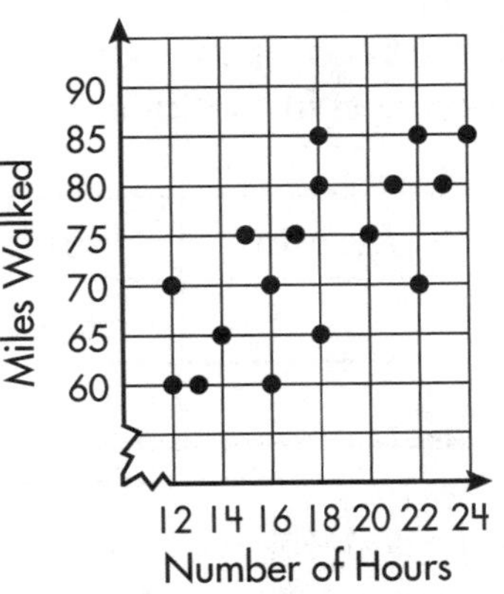

Helpful Hint

A **positive relationship** exists in a scattergram if, as one value increases, the other value increases as well. A **negative relationship** exists in a scattergram if, as one value increases, the other value decreases. If there is no trend to be found in the scattergram, then **no relationship** exists within the data.

1. One team had 20 hours of walking. How many miles did the team walk?

   ________ miles

2. Three teams walked for 18 hours. What were the distances they walked?

   ________________ miles

3. How many teams walked more than 75 miles?

   ____

4. How many teams walked for 20 hours or more?

   ____

5. What type of relationship—positive, negative, or none—was there between the number of hours walked and the number of miles walked?

   ____

NAME ____________________

Lesson 8.6 Measures of Central Tendency

Read the problem carefully and solve. Show your work under each question.

Dave records the outside temperature at noon for seven consecutive days. The temperatures are recorded in the table below.

Monday	Tuesday	Wednesday	Thursday	Friday	Saturday	Sunday
62° F	65° F	75° F	78° F	70° F	77° F	70° F

Helpful Hint

The **mean** is the average of a set of numbers. The **median** is the middle number of a set of numbers that is ordered from least to greatest. The **mode** is the number that appears most often in a set of numbers. The **range** is the difference between the greatest and least numbers in the set.

1. Dave wants to find the median temperature for the week. What is the median temperature for the week?

   ____

2. Dave thought that there were some days that seemed cold and some days that seemed hot. What was the range of the temperatures?

   ____

3. Dave wants to know which temperature occurred the most often during the week, so he finds the mode of the temperatures. What is the mode of the data?

   ____

4. Dave wants to find the mean temperature for the week so he can share it with his classmates. What is the mean temperature for the week?

   ____

5. If the temperature on the 8th day was 55° F, which measure would change the most?

   ____

NAME ______________________

Lesson 8.7 Stem-and-Leaf Plots

Read the problem carefully and solve. Show your work under each question.

Wren collects information on the ages of the houses in his neighborhood. He decides to display these ages in the stem-and-leaf plot shown to the right.

Stems	Leaves
1	1 3 3 6
2	2 4 7
3	0 3 7 9
4	1 4 9

Key: 4|1 = 41

Helpful Hint

The right column of a stem-and-leaf plot shows the **leaves**—the ones digit of each number. The other digits form the **stems** and are shown in the left column. The **key** explains how to read the plot.

1. After he creates the stem-and-leaf plot, Wren wants to determine the oldest house in his neighborhood. What is the age of the oldest house?

   ________ years

2. What is the age of the newest house in his neighborhood?

   ________ years

3. Wren's father asks him how many houses are between 25 and 35 years old. What is Wren's answer?

   ________ houses

4. Wren's teacher takes a look at the graph. She asks Wren to tell her how many houses are less than 30 years old. What is Wren's response?

   ________ houses

5. What is the mean age of houses in Wren's neighborhood?

   ________ years

NAME ___________________________

Lesson 8.8 Frequency Tables

Read the problem carefully and solve. Show your work under each question.

After giving a test to her class, Mrs. Ling decides to make a frequency table to show the number of hours each student studied for the test. The table is shown below. The actual hours studied were: 6, 10, 2, 4, 5, 7, 9, 8, 3, 6, 8, 11, 7, 1.

Test Scores			
Hours Studied	Frequency	Cumulative Frequency	Relative Frequency
0–1.9	1	1	7.1%
2–3.9	2	3	14.3%
4–5.9	2	5	14.3%
6–7.9	4		28.6%
8–9.9	3	12	
10–11.9	2	14	14.3%

Helpful Hint

A **frequency table** shows how often a range of numbers occurs. **Cumulative frequency** is the total of a frequency and all of the frequencies below it. **Relative frequency** is the percent of a specific category compared to all of the categories.

1. Mrs. Ling wants to know how many of the students studied in the 2–3.9 hours range. How many students were in that range?

   ________ students

2. What was the cumulative frequency for 6–7.9 hours?

   ________ students

3. How many students studied for more than 5.9 hours?

   ________ students

4. What is the total number of students who took the test?

   ________ students

5. What was the relative frequency of students who studied 8–9.9 hours? Round your answer to the nearest tenth of a percent.

   ________ number of hours studied

NAME ____________________

Lesson 8.9 Line Plots

Read the problem carefully and solve. Show your work under each question.

Antonio conducts a survey to find the number of soccer balls each member of his soccer team owns so players can practice in their neighborhoods on a weeknight. After the survey, he graphs the results using a line plot. The line plot is shown to the right.

Number of Soccer Balls

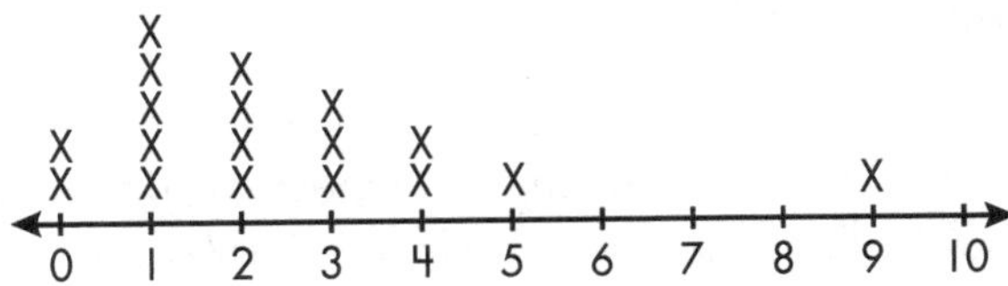

Helpful Hint

A **line plot** is a graph that shows the frequency of data on a number line. Line plots make it easy to identify the mode, range, and any outliers in a data set. **Outliers** are data points that are much larger or smaller than other values.

1. How many team members do not own any soccer balls?

________ members

2. The coach of the soccer team wants to know how many members of the team have at least 4 soccer balls. How many members is this?

________ members

3. How many soccer balls are there in all?

________ soccer balls

4. Antonio compares the members of the team that have only 1 soccer ball with the members of the team that have exactly 5 soccer balls. How many more members have only 1 soccer ball?

________ members

5. When Antonio shows the line plot he made based on the survey to his coach, the coach asks him what the outlier is for the data. How many soccer balls represent the outlier for the data?

________ soccer balls

NAME ____________________

Lesson 8.10 Box-and-Whisker Plots

Read the problem carefully and solve. Show your work under each question.

Ginny interviews 24 of her friends to find the number of movies each friend watched over the summer. After she collects the data, Ginny graphs the results using a box-and-whisker plot. This plot is shown to the right.

Movies Watched Over the Summer

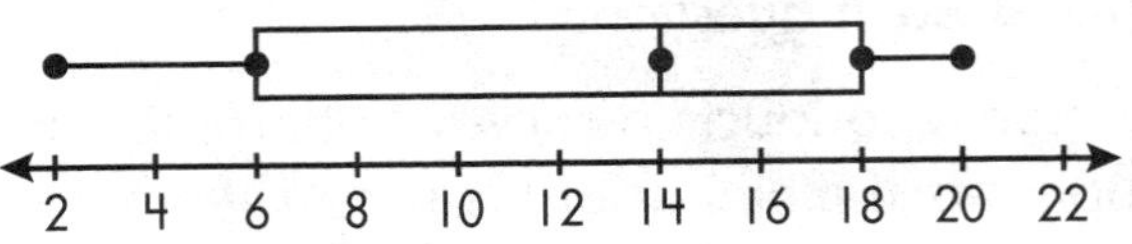

> **Helpful Hint**
>
> A **box-and-whisker plot** displays data along a number line. Quartiles are used to divide the data into four equal parts.

1. What is the median number of movies watched?

   ________ movies watched

2. What is most number of movies watched by a student?

   ________ movies watched

3. How many of Ginny's friends watched between 14 and 18 movies?

   ________ friends

4. What percent of Ginny's friends watched between 6 and 18 movies?

   ________ percent

5. What is the lower quartile for the data?

   ________ movies watched

NAME ______________________

Lesson 8.11 Tree Diagrams

Read the problem carefully and solve. Show your work under each question.

Cody is doing an experiment with a penny and a cube with sides numbered from 1–6. He wants to draw a tree diagram to show the sample space for all the possible outcomes (possible results) for tossing a penny and rolling the number cube at the same time.

Helpful Hint

A **sample space** is a set of all possible outcomes for an activity or experiment. To determine the sample space, it is helpful to organize the possibilities using a list, chart, picture, or tree diagram.

1. Make a tree diagram to show all of the possible outcomes.

2. How many possible outcomes are there?

   ________ possible outcomes

3. In how many possible outcomes does the penny land on heads?

   ________ outcomes

4. How many possible outcomes involve rolling a number less than 5?

   ________ outcomes

5. Cody found a spinner with 3 equal sections. How many possible outcomes are there for flipping the coin, rolling the number cube, and spinning the spinner all at the same time?

   ________ outcomes

NAME ______________________

Lesson 8.12 Data Sets

Read the problem carefully and solve. Show your work under each question.

The mean absolute deviation (MAD) is the degree of variability of a data set. The greater the MAD value, the more variability.

Liam compared the average height some of the players on his favorite cricket and volleyball teams.

Cricket Team – Height of players in inches: 60, 55, 59, 52, 76, 72, 65

Volleyball Team – Height of players in inches: 55, 72, 70, 71, 68, 50, 65

The shortest player is 50 inches and the tallest player is 76 inches. Which team's average player is taller?

First, find the average. Cricket team = 62.71 inches; Volleyball team = 64.42 inches

The mean height of the cricket players is 62.71 inches, and the mean height of the volleyball players is 64.42 inches. The average volleyball player is taller.

Helpful Hint

The MAD for any set can be calculated by:

1. Finding the mean of each set.
2. Determining the deviation of each variable from the mean by using subtraction.
3. Averaging all the values.

1. Jill compares the mean age of the tennis team members to the mean age of the soccer team members.

Tennis team ages:
2, 3, 8, 6, 7, 6, 9, 10, 4

Soccer team ages:
5, 6, 9, 2, 11, 10, 11, 3, 4

Which team is older, on average?

____

2. What is the average age difference?

________ years

3. Melinda compares the mean of how much Caroline and Jessi raised for a fundraiser over 8 days (amounts in $).

Caroline: 54, 68, 21, 47, 23, 96, 25, 32

Jessi: 62, 94, 15, 72, 63, 48, 75, 16

Which person's average amount raised was higher?

____

4. On the average day, what is the difference between their fundraising levels?

$________

5. Pablo compares the mean number of sales in a week between a hat shop and a scarf shop (sales in $).

Hat shop: 48, 42, 18, 32, 39, 41, 30

Scarf shop: 97, 84, 93, 15, 63, 22, 44

Which shop averages higher sales? What is the average?

________________, $________

NAME ____________________

Lesson 8.13 Calculating Probability

Read the problem carefully and solve. Show your work under each question.

Luis has a box of different colored markers. The box contains 4 red markers, 6 blue markers, 3 purple markers, 2 green markers, and 1 black marker.

Helpful Hint

An **outcome** is any of the possible results of an activity or experiment. **Probability** is the likelihood that a specific outcome or set of outcomes will occur. Probability is the ratio of desired outcome(s) to the sample space. It can be expressed as a ratio, fraction, decimal, or percent.

1. What is the probability that a red marker is randomly chosen from the box? Write your answer as a fraction in simplest form.

   ____

2. What is the probability of randomly choosing a purple marker from the box? Write your answer as a ratio.

   ____

3. What is the probability of randomly choosing a green marker out of the box? Write your answer as a decimal.

   ____

4. What is the probability of randomly choosing a yellow marker? Write your answer as a percent.

   ____

5. What is the probability of randomly choosing either a blue or green marker from the box? Write your answer as a percent.

   ____

NAME ________________

Lesson 8.14 Calculating Probability

Read the problem carefully and solve. Show your work under each question.

A two-sided coin is tossed 3 times. What is the probability that the coin will land on "heads" twice and "tails" once (in any order)? The possible outcomes of 3 coin tosses:

TTT	**HTT**
TTH	**(HTH)**
THT	**(HHT)**
(THH)	**HHH**

There are 3 different ways to get 2 heads and 1 tails.

The probability is $\frac{3}{8} = 0.375 = 37.5\%$

1. A two-sided coin is tossed 50 times. What is the probability that it will land on tails twice and heads once (in any order)?

   ____

2. How many different ways can you arrange the letters in the word TOY?

   ____

3. A two-sided coin is tossed 2 times. What is the probability that it will land on heads once and tails once (in any order)?

   ____

4. How many different ways can you arrange the letters in the word BEST?

   ____

5. Aiden, Nick, and Jade take a test. Make a diagram to show how many different possible ways they can place on the test. Assume there are no ties.

   How many different ways can they place on the test?

   ____

NAME ____________________

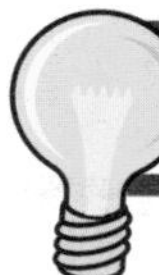

Check What You Learned

Probability and Statistics

Read the problem carefully and solve. Show your work under each question.

Nathan takes a survey to find out how many hours per week the 20 people in his guitar class practice playing guitar. He displays the results in a circle graph shown to the right.

Hours of Guitar Practice Per Week

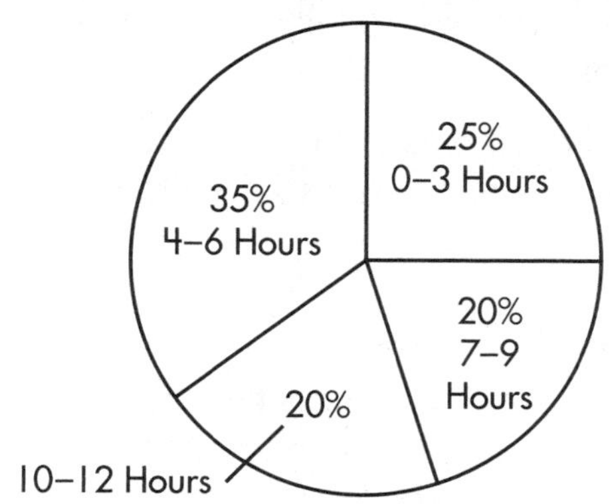

20 people responded.

CHAPTER 8 POSTTEST

1. Nathan writes down how many people practice guitar 4–6 hours per week. How many people does he write down?

   ________ people

2. Nathan is asked how many more people practice 0–3 hours per week than practice 7–9 hours per week. What is his answer?

   ____

3. How many people practice guitar either 4–6 hours per week or 7–9 hours per week?

   ________ people

4. Nathan's cousin is one of the people surveyed who practice 0–3 hours per week. How many other people practice 0–3 hours per week?

   ________ people

5. How many more people practice 4–6 hours per week than 7–9 hours per week?

   ________ people

6. If the number of people who practice 10–12 hours per week doubles, how many people would then practice 10–12 hours per week?

   ________ people

NAME ______________________

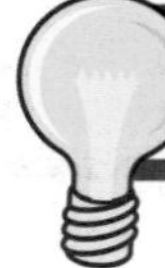

Check What You Learned

Probability and Statistics

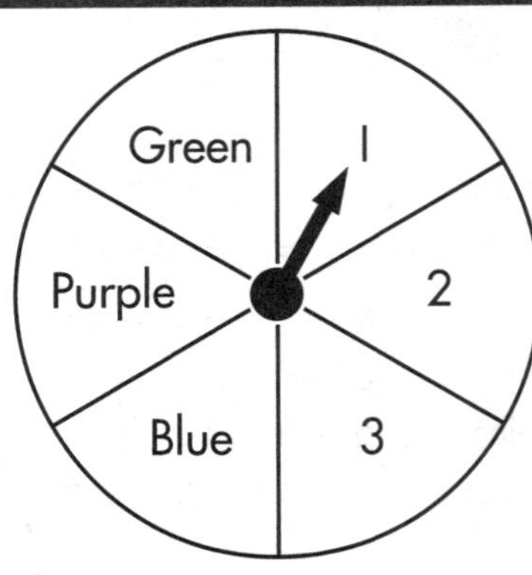

Read the problem carefully and solve. Show your work under each question.

Callista likes to make her own probability experiments. She decides to make the spinner shown to the right for an experiment.

CHAPTER 8 POSTTEST

1. Callista wants to know the probability that the spinner will land on a color. What is the probability that the spinner will land on a color? Write your answer as a decimal.

   ____

2. Callista hopes that the spinner will land on an odd number. What is the probability that the spinner will land on an odd number? Write your answer as a ratio in simplest form.

   ____

3. Callista has a friend that wants to know the probability that the spinner will land on either an even number or a color. What is the probability? Show your answer as a fraction in simplest form.

   ____

4. Callista hopes that the spinner will land on the number 2. What is the probability that the spinner will land on the number 2? Write your answer as a fraction.

   ____

5. Callista wants to know the probability that the spinner will land on any section except the color green. Write your answer as a percent rounded to the nearest tenth.

   ____

6. What is the probability that the spinner will land on any number or the color blue? Write your answer as a decimal rounded to the nearest tenth.

   ____

NAME ____________________

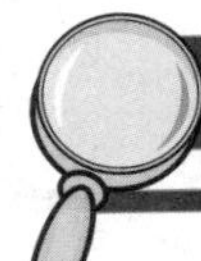

Check What You Know

Geometry

Read the problem carefully and solve. Show your work under each question.

Dawn drew the figure to the right for an art class. In the class, she is studying various angles that can be used when she draws or paints. She also learns about various geometric figures in the art class.

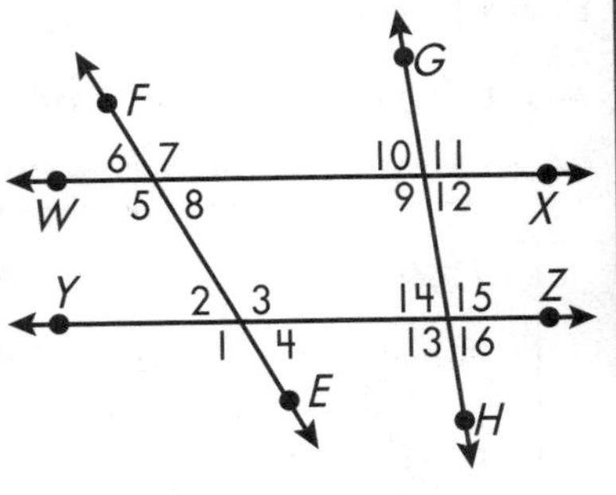

1. Dawn measures angle 8. What is the measure of angle 8?

______

2. How would Dawn identify the ray that starts at point *Z* and passes through point *Y*?

______

3. Dawn looks at the drawing to classify the angle represented by the number 4. Is angle 4 obtuse, right, or acute?

______

4. In Dawn's drawing, $\overleftrightarrow{WX}$ and $\overleftrightarrow{YZ}$ are parallel. If the measure of angle 11 is 110°, what is the measure of angle 10?

______

5. In the art class, Dawn learns to identify several different figures. What is the name of the figure below?

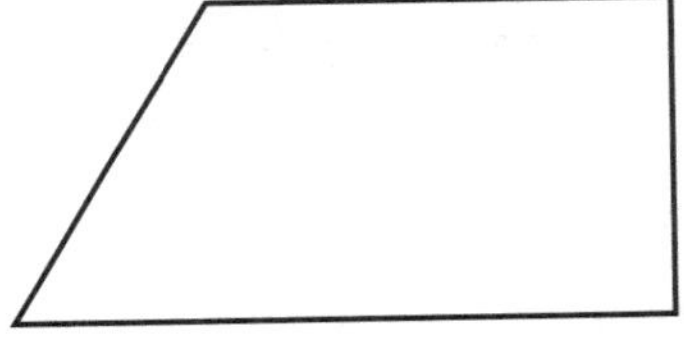

______

6. Dawn drew the following shape to represent her backyard. What is the name of the shape?

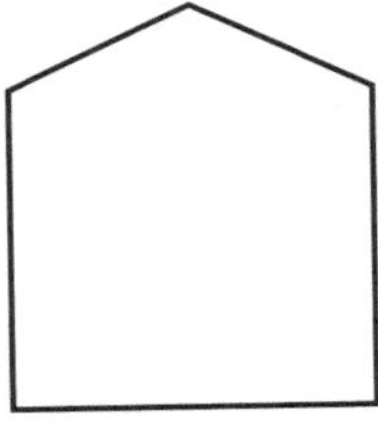

______

NAME ______________________

Lesson 9.1 Points and Lines

Read the problem carefully and solve. Show your work under each question.

April draws a design. She likes to label points and lines to help plan the design.

Helpful Hint

A line and a line segment use different symbols. A line continuously extends in two directions.

1. April included the following line in her design. How would you name the line, using geometric notation?

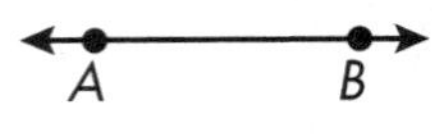

_______ or _______

2. She plans to add line *GH* to her design. Draw the line *GH* below.

3. In the middle of the design, she decided to add the following line segment. How would she name this line segment?

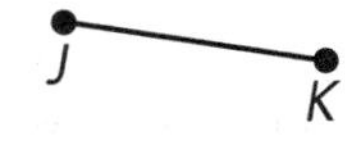

_______ or _______

4. Next to line segment *JK*, April draws line segment *WX* into the design. Identify line segment *WX* using geometric notation.

_______ or _______

5. April decides to change line segment *WX* to line *WX*. Identify line *WX* using geometric notation.

_______ or _______

NAME ___________________________

Lesson 9.2 Rays and Angles

Read the problem carefully and solve. Show your work under each question.

Alvin is helping to plan a playground for the neighborhood. The playground plan has many rays and angles.

Helpful Hint

An angle is the union of two rays. The middle of the angle is where the two rays meet.

1. One corner of the playground is represented using the angle shown below. Use geometric notation to name the angle in two ways.

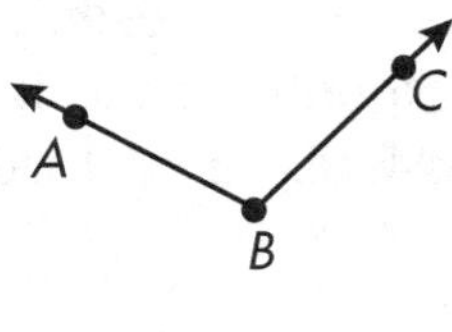

_______ or _______

2. Alvin draws a ray on the plan that shows the direction people will enter the playground. How would he label ray *MN* on the plans?

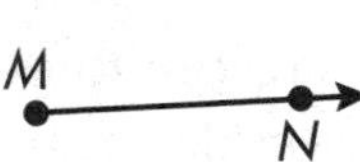

____

3. Alvin combined two rays, $\overrightarrow{BA}$ and $\overrightarrow{BC}$, to make an angle at the edge of the playground plan. Draw and label this angle.

4. Alvin was asked to draw angle *RQS* to represent the relationship of the slide to the ground. He drew the angle shown below. Did Alvin draw the angle correctly?

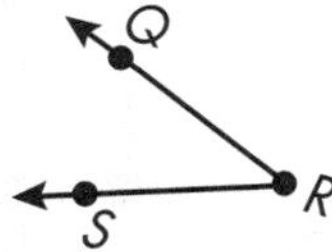

____

5. The gate and the fence on the playground form the angle shown below. Name two geometric figures that are combined to make this angle.

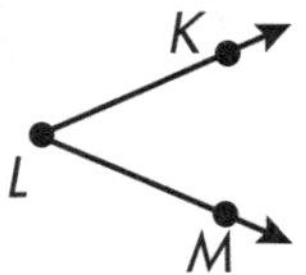

____

NAME ______________________________

Lesson 9.3 Measuring Angles

Read the problem carefully and solve. Show your work under each question.

Alexis works in a mall. She notices all sorts of angles in the mall.

Helpful Hint

Use a protractor to measure an angle. Angles can be classified as **acute**, **obtuse**, or **right**. An acute angle measures less than 90°. An obtuse angle measures more than 90°. A right angle measures 90°.

1. A display in the mall contains the angle shown below. What type of angle is this?

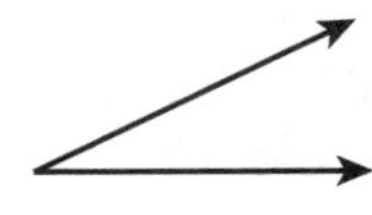

______

2. Alexis uses a protractor to find the actual measurement of the angle shown in question 1. What is the measure of the angle?

______

3. The edge of the counter where Alexis works forms the angle shown below. Use a protractor to determine the measure of this angle. Then, classify the angle.

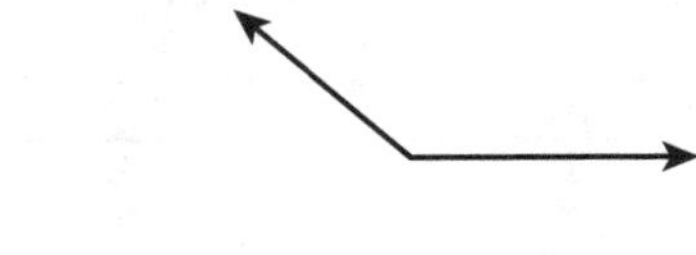

______ ______

4. The angle below represents Alexis's walk from the mall entrance to the store where she works. Measure and classify the angle.

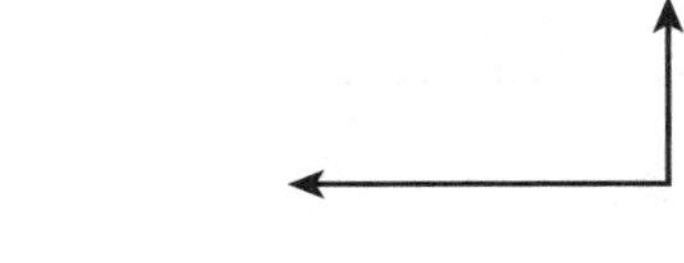

______

5. Alexis told her mom that she can get to the mall office by walking straight from the entrance, then making an 85° turn and walking straight to get to the office. What kind of angle represents Alexis's route?

______

NAME ______________________

Lesson 9.4 Vertical, Supplementary, and Complementary Angles

Read the problem carefully and solve. Show your work under each question.

Chang uses lines and angles to create a map of the streets near his home. The map is represented by the drawing to the right.

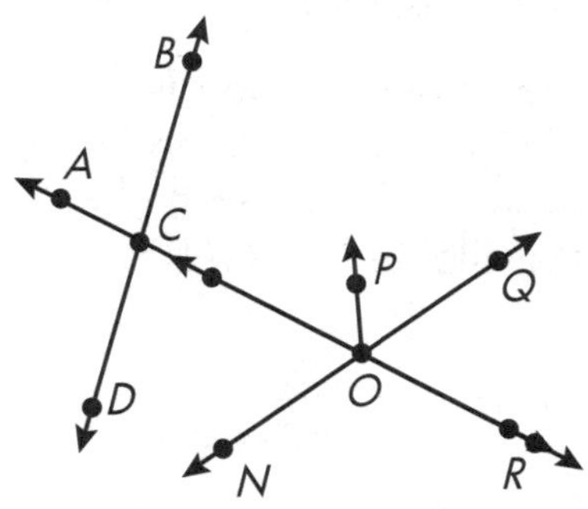

Helpful Hint

Vertical angles are opposite angles that have the same measure. **Supplementary** angles are two angles whose measures have a sum of 180°. **Complementary** angles are two angles whose measures have a sum of 90°. A **bisector** divides an angle into angles of equal measure.

1. Chang has a friend that lives at the corner represented by $\angle BCO$. Name the angle that is vertical to this angle.

________ ________

2. Chang notices that there appears to be two angle bisectors on the map. Which parts of the map appear to be a bisector?

____

3. Chang lives at the corner of $\angle ACD$. Name an angle that is supplementary to $\angle ACD$.

________ or ________

4. Chang's cousin lives along angle $\angle DCA$. What is the relationship of angle $\angle DCA$ and $\angle BCA$?

____

5. Which angle must have the same measure as $\angle ACB$?

____

NAME ____________________

Lesson 9.5 Transversals

Read the problem carefully and solve. Show your work under each question.

Ivy likes to make pieces of art by putting together pieces of colored paper. Her father is helping her by cutting the pieces of colored paper. The figure to the right shows the initial plan for Ivy's art. In the figure, line *EF* is parallel to line *GH*.

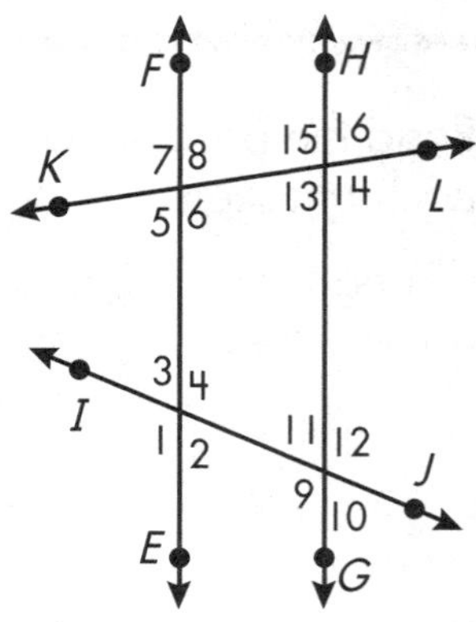

Helpful Hint

If the two lines being crossed are parallel, then:

- **Alternate interior angles** have the same measure.
- **Alternate exterior angles** have the same measure.
- **Corresponding angles** have the same measure.

1. Ivy notices that some of the angle pairs for the design are equal. She identifies $\angle 15$ and another angle as alternate interior angles. What is the other angle?

   ____

2. Ivy tells her dad that $\angle 10$ and $\angle 3$ are equivalent. What term describes the relationship between these two angles?

   ____

3. Ivy tells her dad that she knows the measure of $\angle 5$, and therefore knows three other angles that have the same measure. One is a vertical angle, one is a corresponding angle, and one is an alternate exterior angle. Which three angles does she mean?

   ________ ________ ________

4. Ivy names the angle that is an alternate interior angle with $\angle 2$.Which angle does she name?

   ____

5. Ivy knows about angle relationships because she has studied transversals. Name the transversals in her plan.

   ____

NAME ______________________________

Lesson 9.6 Triangles (by angles) and Triangles (by side)

Read the problem carefully and solve. Show your work under each question.

Zeb is building a triangular sandbox for his younger sister. He isn't sure what type of triangle he wants to use for the shape of the sandbox, so he experiments by drawing plans with several different triangles.

Helpful Hint

Triangles can be named by their angles and side lengths. **Equilateral triangles** have three equal sides and 60° angles. **Isosceles triangles** have two equal sides and angles. **Scalene triangles** have no equal sides and angles.

1. Zeb draws a triangle for his sister, shown below. Based on its angles, what type of triangle is this?

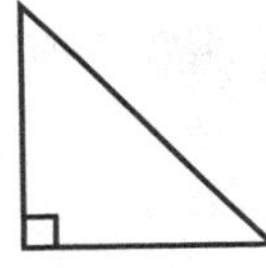

____

2. Zeb's sister draws a different triangle, shown below. Based on its sides, what type of triangle is this?

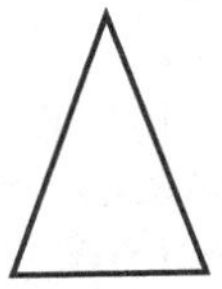

____

3. Zeb tells his sister that they could use 3 pieces of wood they already have to make the edges of the sandbox. The 3 pieces of wood are all different lengths. Based on the lengths of the pieces, what type of triangle would these pieces of wood make?

____

4. Zeb's sister likes the idea of having 2 of the sandbox edges the same length, so she drew the triangle shown below. Based on its side lengths and angles, name the type of triangle that Zeb's sister drew.

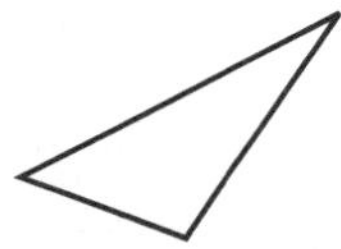

____

5. After considering all the possibilities, Zeb and his sister decide that they will build an equilateral triangle for the sandbox. Describe the side lengths and angles of this triangle.

____

____

____

NAME ______________________________

Lesson 9.7 Quadrilaterals

Read the problem carefully and solve. Show your work under each question.

Erin is studying quadrilaterals. She learns that small changes in a quadrilateral can give it a new name. She practices the definitions of quadrilaterals by drawing figures on index cards and then writing the definitions on the back of the cards.

Helpful Hint

A **quadrilateral** is a closed figure with 4 sides. A **parallelogram** is a quadrilateral whose opposite sides are parallel and congruent. A **rectangle** is a parallelogram with four right angles. A **rhombus** is a parallelogram with four congruent sides. A **square** has four right angles and four congruent sides. A **trapezoid** is a quadrilateral with only one pair of parallel sides.

1. The definition on the back of one card reads, "a parallelogram with 4 congruent sides." Draw and label two different figures that fit this description.

2. Erin's sister asks her if all squares are also rectangles. How does Erin respond?

____

____

3. The shape below is on the front of one card. Which 2 terms will Erin use to name the shape?

____________________ and __________

4. Erin sees the figure shown below on another card as she reviews for a quiz. What terms can be used to name this figure?

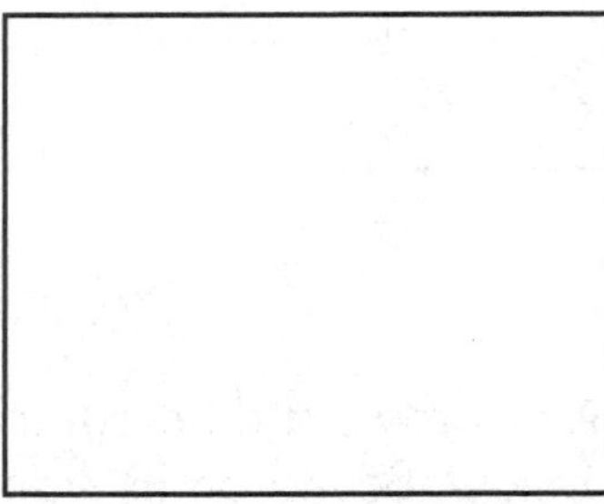

____

5. Erin's sister asks if any square can also be called a rhombus. How should Erin answer the question?

____

____

NAME ______________________

Lesson 9.8 Polygons

Read the problem carefully and solve. Show your work under each question.

Jerry draws different polygons in the sand at the beach. He plays a game where he asks each family member to identify the polygons he draws.

Helpful Hint

A **polygon** is a closed figure whose sides are all line segments. Polygons can be classified by the number of sides they have. For example, a 5-sided polygon is called a **pentagon** and a 6-sided polygon is called a **hexagon**. Some other prefixes are: **hepta-** (7), **octa-** (8), **nona-** (9), and **deca-** (10).

1. Jerry draws a 10-sided figure. What is the name of the polygon?

   ____

2. Jerry drew the figure below. What is the name of this figure?

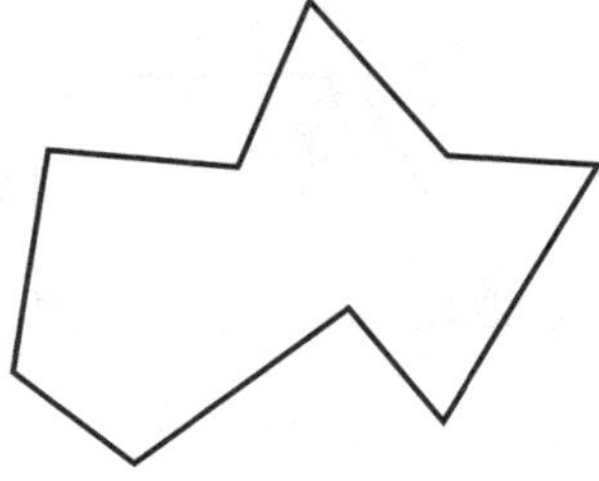

   ____

3. Jerry drew a heptagon. Draw a heptagon below.

4. If Jerry looks at this object from the top, draw what he will see.

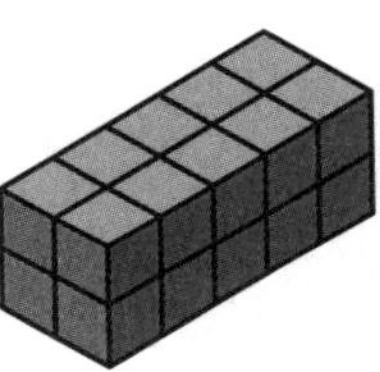

5. Draw three different cross sections from the square pyramid.

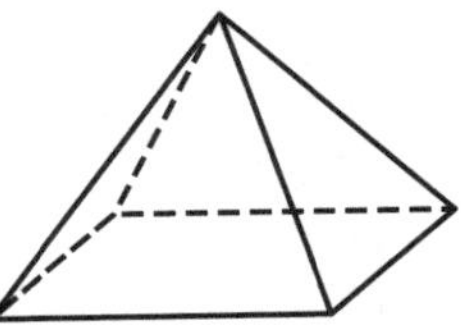

NAME ______________________

Lesson 9.9 Similar Figures

Read the problem carefully and solve. Show your work under each question.

Ella draws pairs of figures and writes the ratio of their sides in order to determine if the figures are similar.

Helpful Hint

Two figures are **similar** if their corresponding angles are congruent and the lengths of their corresponding sides are proportional. Write a ratio to determine if the sides are proportional.

1. Ella draws the figures below. What would the missing measure have to be for the triangles to be similar?

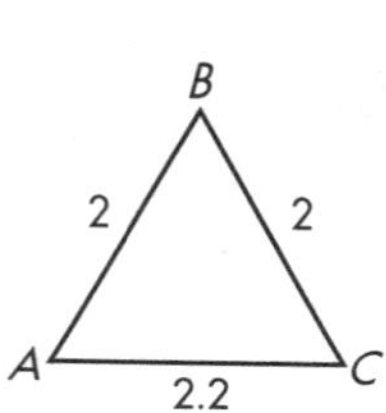

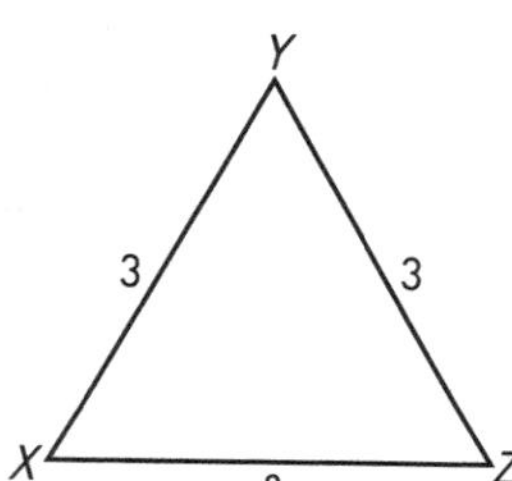

______

2. Ella draws the figures below to model drawings for her new kitchen. How can you tell that the figures are not similar without calculating the ratios?

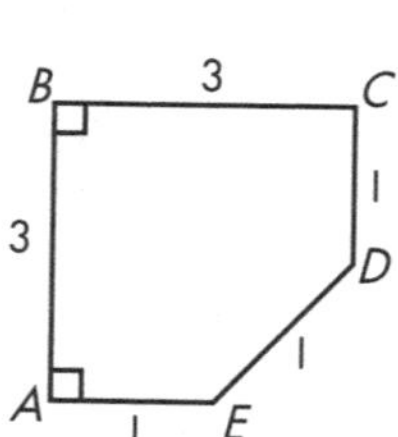

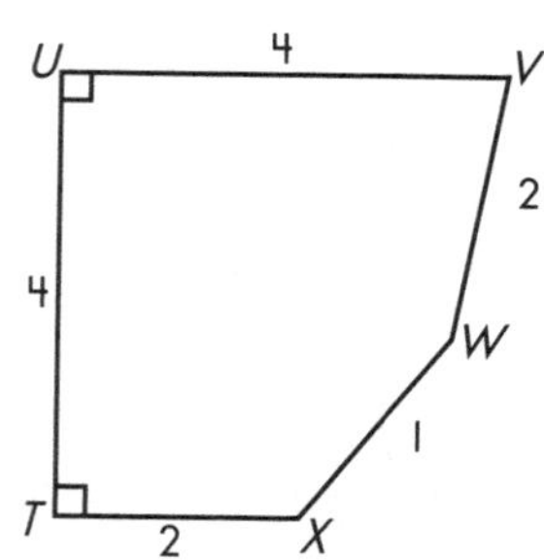

____

3. Ella draws two pictures of kites below. Are the kites similar?

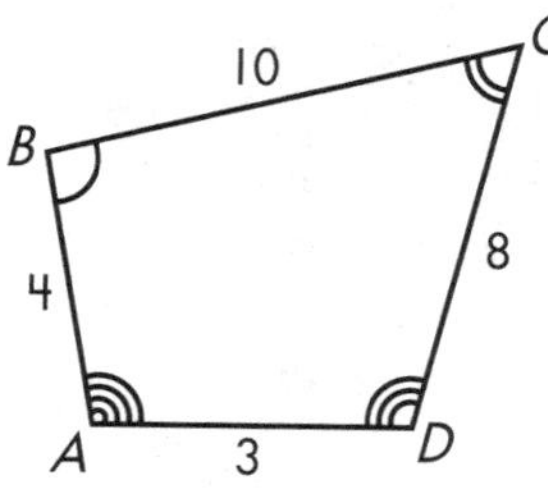

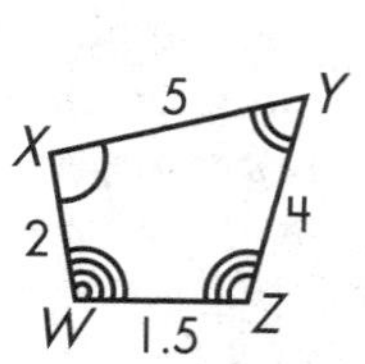

______

4. Ella draws the figures below to model drawings for her patio. Using ratios of the side lengths, show if the figures are similar or not similar.

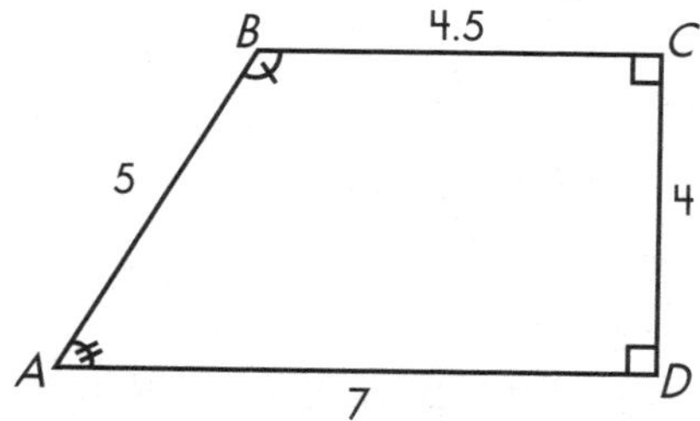

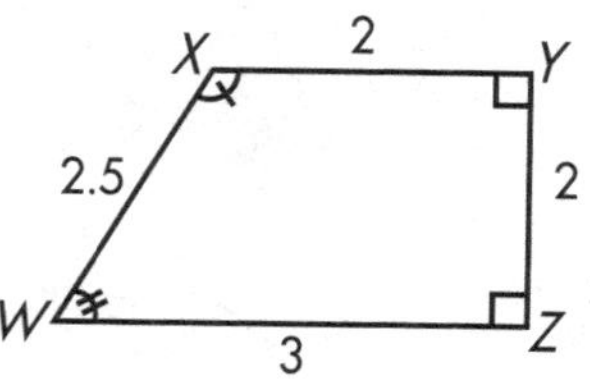

______

NAME ______________________

Lesson 9.10 Plotting Ordered Pairs

Read the problem carefully and solve. Show your work under each question.

Irene draws a coordinate plane and plots points to help her decide where to paint flowers on her bedroom wall. The grid is shown to the right.

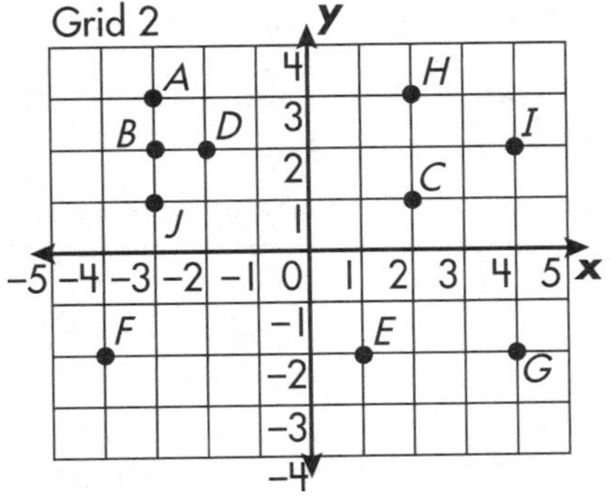

Helpful Hint

In a **coordinate plane**, the axes are labeled x and y. The coordinates of a point are represented by the ordered pair (x, y). The plane is divided into four quadrants. The x-value of the ordered pair tells you how to move along the horizontal axis and the y-value tells you how to move along the vertical axis.

1. Irene plans to paint a lilac flower at point (4, 2) on the grid. Which letter represents this point?

______

2. If Irene moves point H two units to the right, what will be the coordinate location of the new point on the grid?

______

3. Irene plans to paint a rose at point (−3, 3) on the grid. Which letter represents this point?

______

4. Irene is trying to decide what type of flower to paint at point (−3, 2). She thinks that she will paint a lily at this point. Which letter represents point (−3, 2)?

______

5. Irene plans to paint a daisy on the grid at a spot that is marked with the letter G. Which ordered pair represents point G?

______

NAME ______________________________

Lesson 9.11 Transformations

Read the problem carefully and solve. Show your work under each question.

Felipe uses transformations to make designs on T-shirts. He then paints the transformed shapes different colors.

Helpful Hint

A **transformation** is a change of the position or size of an image. In a **translation**, an image slides in any direction. In a **reflection**, an image is flipped over a line. In a **rotation**, an image is turned around on a point. In a **dilation**, an image is enlarged or reduced.

1. Felipe uses the transformation below to make his most popular T-shirt. What type of transformation is represented on the T-shirt?

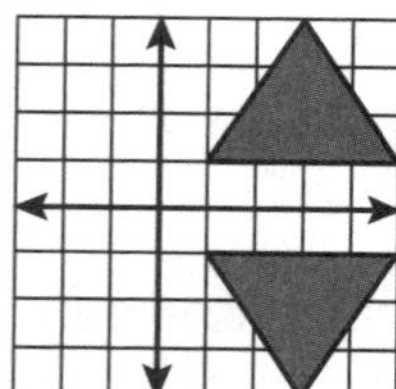

____

2. One customer requested the figures below as the image on a T-shirt. What type of transformation do these shapes represent?

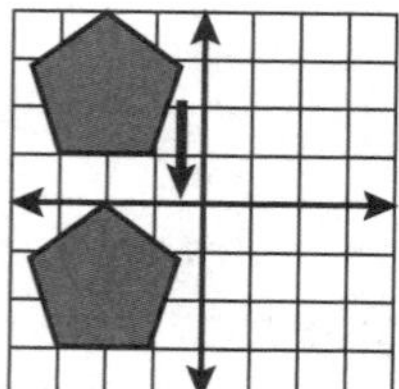

____

3. The figure below was requested on a T-shirt by Felipe's neighbor. What type of transformation is represented on the T-shirt?

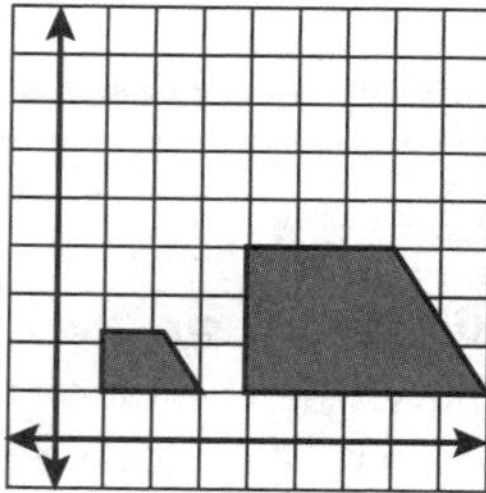

____

4. The design shown below is the first image that Felipe ever put on a T-shirt. Which type of transformation is represented by this image?

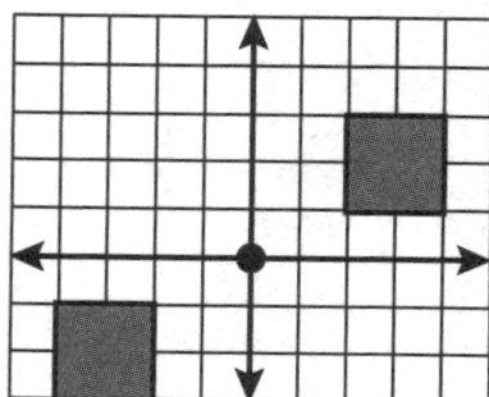

____

5. Felipe is making a new design for T-shirts. The design is represented by the figure below. What type of transformation is shown?

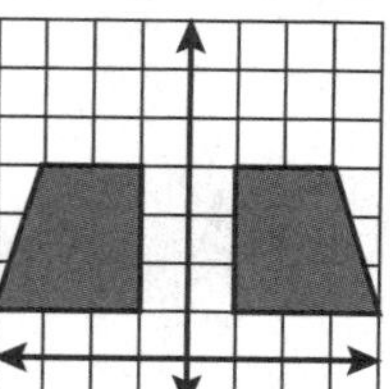

____

NAME ______________________

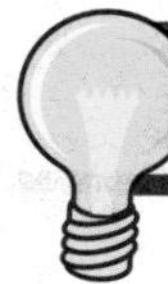

Check What You Learned

Geometry

Read the problem carefully and solve. Show your work under each question.

Wyatt reviews figures that he has learned in class. He practices what he has learned by sketching shapes.

1. Wyatt draws the following triangle. Then, he asks his brother to name the triangle based on its sides and angles. How does he name the triangle?

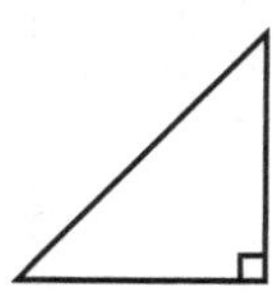

____

2. Wyatt draws the following two rectangles. Are the rectangles similar or not similar?

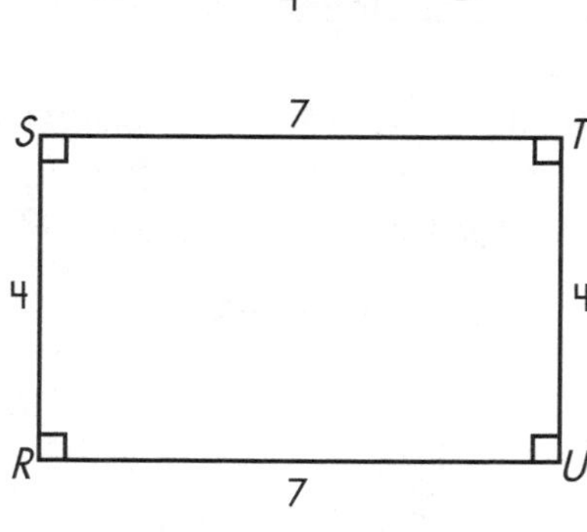

____

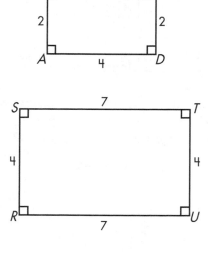

3. Wyatt draws the transformation shown below to practice identifying transformations and points on a coordinate grid. What transformation does the drawing represent? What ordered pair is represented by point *A*?

________ and ________

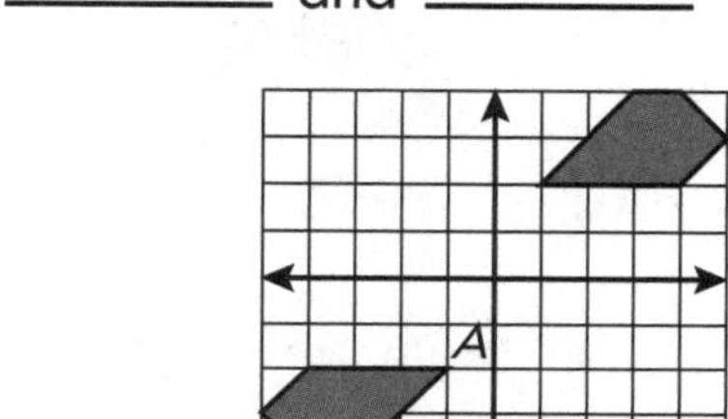

4. Wyatt draws the angle shown below. He wants to draw an angle that is complementary to this angle. Draw an angle that is complementary to this angle.

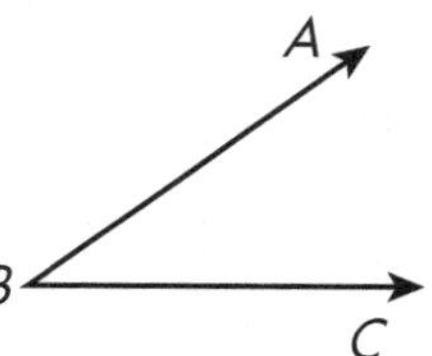

CHAPTER 9 POSTTEST

NAME ____________________

Check What You Know

Perimeter, Area, and Volume

Read the problem carefully and solve. Show your work under each question.

Greg spends a week over the summer at an overnight camp. He records many things about his environment while at camp.

1. The layout of the camp is represented by the drawing shown below. There is a fence around the property. How long is the fence?

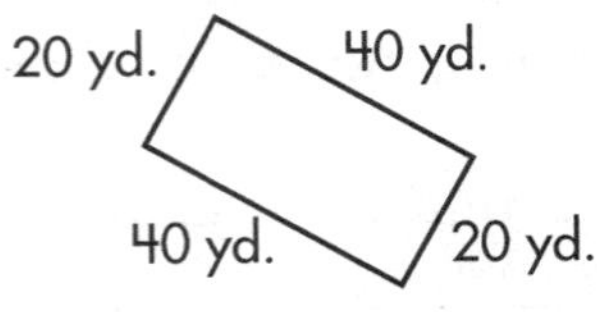

_______ yards

2. The camp has a pool that is in the shape of a circle, shown below. There is a tile trim around the edge of the pool. How long is the tile trim?

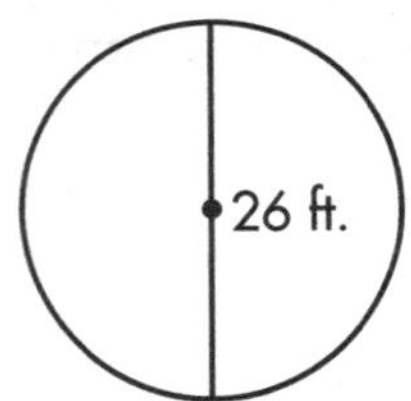

_______ feet

3. The pool has a depth of 5 feet. How much water can the pool hold?

_______ cubic feet

4. Greg makes a clay slate in one of his activities at camp. The picture below shows the slate. What is the area of the slate?

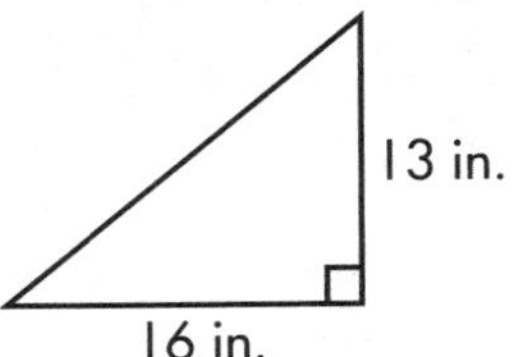

_______ square inches

5. The figure below is a wood storage box that Greg makes at camp. What is the volume of the box?

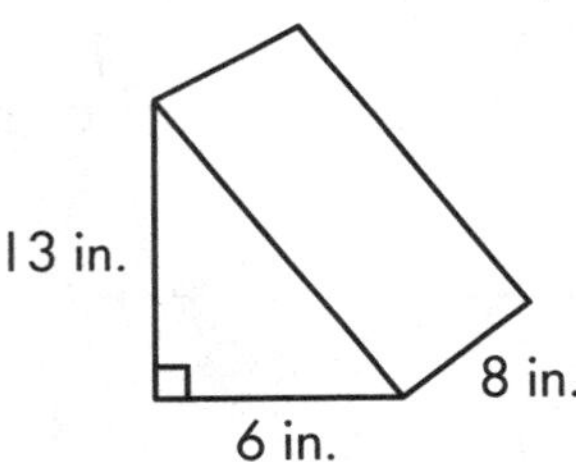

_______ cubic inches

6. Greg makes the following object while at camp and wants to paint its sides. What is the surface area of the object?

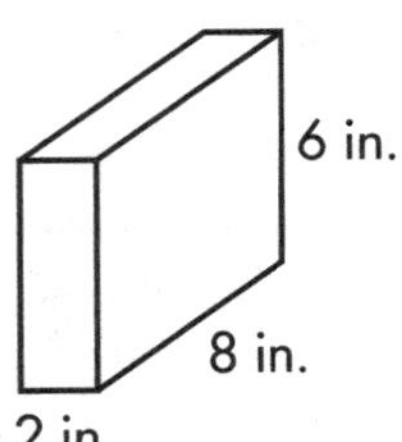

_______ square inches

NAME ____________________

Lesson 10.1 Perimeter

Read the problem carefully and solve. Show your work under each question.

Joanna works for a fencing company. Her job is to determine the amount of fencing needed for various clients.

Helpful Hint

The **perimeter** of a figure is the sum of the lengths of its sides. If two or more sides are equal, the formula can be simplified with multiplication.

1. Joanna needs to determine the perimeter of an animal pen. How many yards is the perimeter of the pen?

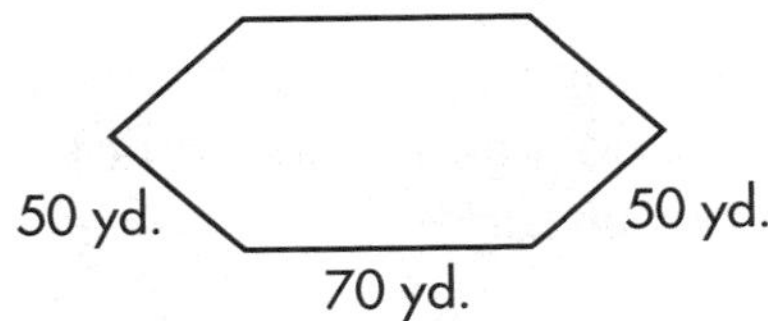

_______ yards

2. The figure below represents a city park in the shape of a regular pentagon. The city puts a fence around the park. How many yards of fencing is needed?

30 yd. 30 yd. 30 yd.

_______ yards

3. A parking lot is represented by the rectangle below. Joanna's company is hired to put a fence around the lot. How many yards of fencing will be needed?

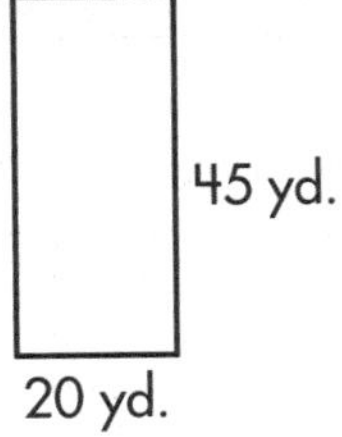

_______ yards

4. A dog park is in the shape of the square below. Joanna's company is going to put a fence around this park. How many meters of fencing will be needed?

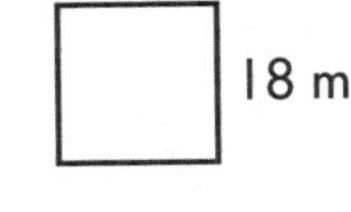

_______ meters

5. The lot for a school is shown below. Joanna was called in to figure out how much fencing is needed. How many feet of fencing is needed to enclose the lot?

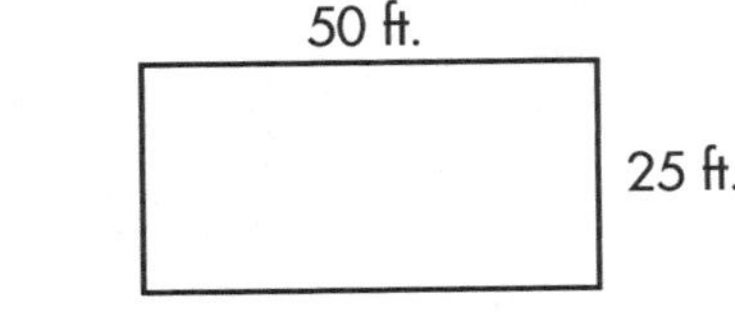

_______ feet

NAME ______________________

Lesson 10.2 Area of Rectangles

Read the problem carefully and solve. Show your work under each question.

Ivan sells rugs that are either square or rectangular in shape. He prices the rugs based on their square footage.

Helpful Hint

Area is the number of square units it takes to cover a figure. To find the area of a rectangle, multiply the length by the width.

1. Ivan sells the rug below to a new customer. What is the area of this rug?

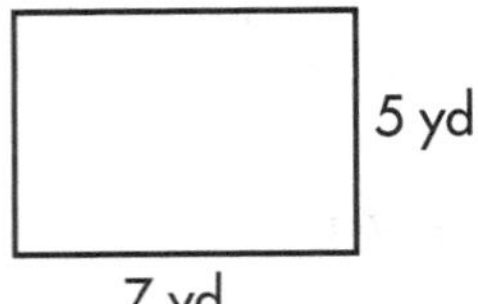

_______ square yards

2. The most popular rug that Ivan sells is represented by the figure below. A customer at the store wants to know the area of this rug. Write the area below.

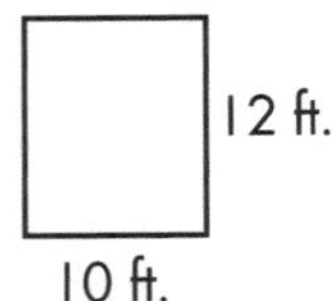

_______ square feet

3. On Saturday, Ivan sells a large rug to a restaurant. The rug measures 24 feet by 18 feet. What is the area of the rug?

_______ square feet

4. Ivan sells the rug shown below with an area of 308 square feet. What is the width of this rug?

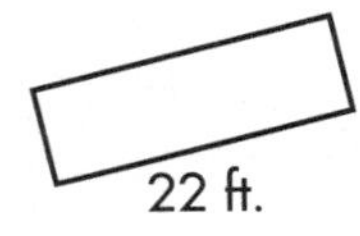

_______ feet

5. A hotel buys the square rug below for the lobby. What is the area of this rug?

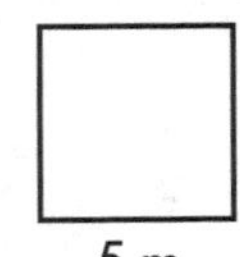

_______ square meters

NAME ______________________________

Lesson 10.3 Area of Triangles

Read the problem carefully and solve. Show your work under each question.

Hugo makes ceramic tiles that are triangular in shape. He sells his tiles to friends and businesses in the town where he lives.

Helpful Hint

The area of a triangle is the product of $\frac{1}{2}$ the base times the height.

1. One type of tile Hugo makes that is often purchased for kitchen counters is shown below. Find the area of the tile.

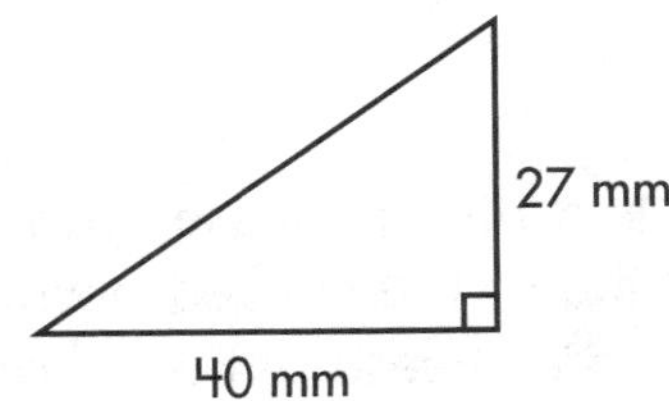

________ square millimeters

2. Hugo makes tiles for his mother in the shape shown below. She plans to use them in her living room. What is the area of each tile?

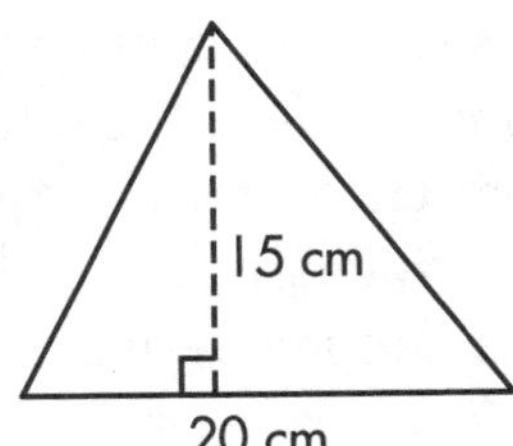

________ square centimeters

3. Hugo makes a pattern using only tiles like the one shown below. He wants to know how many tiles can fit on the counter where he is building out the pattern. Find the area of each tile.

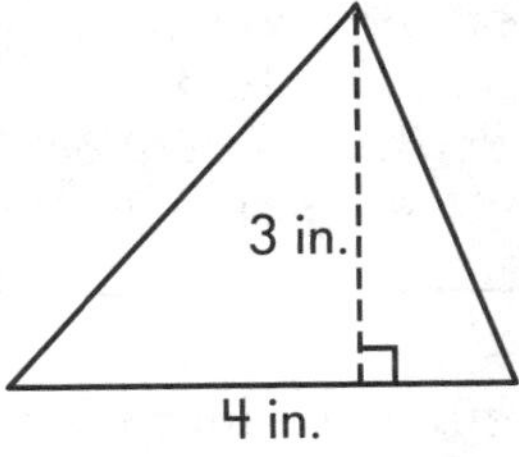

________ square inches

4. Hugo makes the tile below for a storefront sign. The area of the tile is 552 square inches. What is the height?

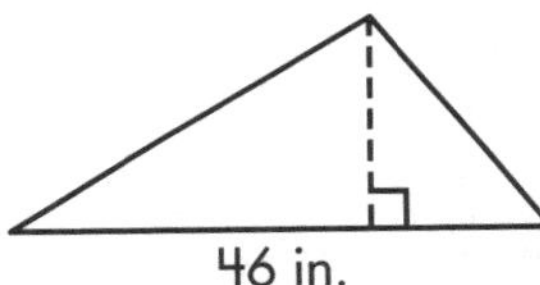

________ inches

5. A set of tiles like the one below is made for a project. Hugo needs to find the area of each tile used. What is the area of each tile?

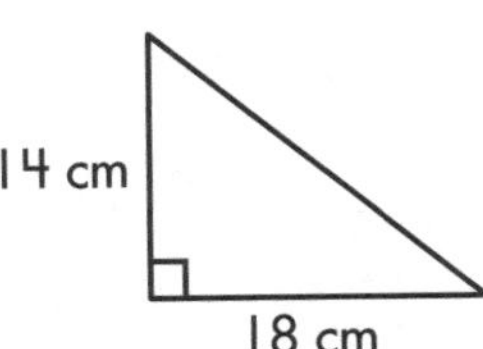

________ square centimeters

NAME ____________________

Lesson 10.4 Circumference of Circles

Read the problem carefully and solve. Show your work under each question.

Essie works at a pizza shop. She helps with all aspects of the pizza shop. For the items below, use 3.14 for π.

Helpful Hint

A **circle** is a set of points that are all the same distance from a given point, called a **center**. The **perimeter** of a circle is called the **circumference**. The **diameter** is a segment that passes through the center of the circle and has both endpoints on the circle. The **radius** is a segment that has the circle and its center as its endpoints.

1. The main circular dining section in the pizza shop has a diameter of 40 feet. What is the circumference of the dining section?

________ feet

2. Each table was protected with a plastic strip around the outside edge. Each table has a diameter of 3 feet. What is the length of each plastic strip?

________ feet

3. An individual-sized pizza has a radius of 4 inches. What is the circumference?

________ inches

4. Essie puts a rim of cheese around the edge of the medium-sized pizza. The length of the cheese rim is 37.68 inches long. Find the radius of the pizza.

________ inches

5. The pizza shop sells a large pizza that has an 8-inch radius. Essie needs to know the circumference of the large pizza to order the correct size boxes for delivery. What is the circumference of this pizza?

________ inches

NAME ______________________

Lesson 10.5 Area of Circles

Read the problem carefully and solve. Show your work under each question.

Javon works for a company that makes kitchenware. Javon is in charge of determining the amount of materials they will need to make circular plates, vases, and platters.

Helpful Hint

The *area* of a circle is found by using the formula $A = \pi r^2$. Remember, π can be expressed as 3.14.

1. The circle below represents one of the plates the company makes. What is the area of this plate?

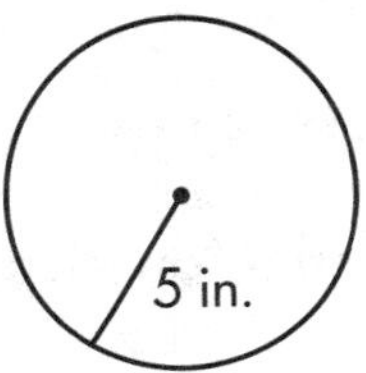

_______ square inches

2. The bottom of a vase is in the shape of a circle. Javon measures the diameter of the bottom and it is 18 cm. What is the area of the bottom of the vase?

_______ square centimeters

3. A large ceramic wheel that the company sells is shown below. What is the area of the wheel?

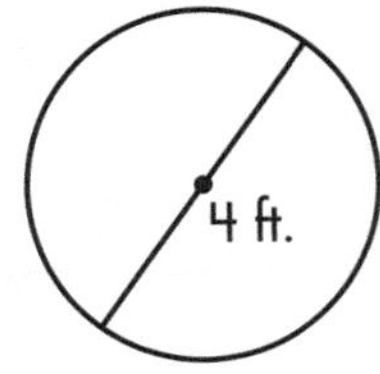

_______ square feet

4. A platter made at Javon's company is in the shape of a circle with a radius of 8 inches. What is the area of the platter?

_______ square inches

5. Javon packages plates that are 24 cm in diameter. He wants to know the area of each plate. What is the area of each plate?

_______ square centimeters

NAME ______________________

Lesson 10.6 Area of Irregular Shapes

Read the problem carefully and solve. Show your work under each question.

Olivia learns about irregular shapes in school. Then, she begins to notice all sorts of irregular shapes in the world around her.

Helpful Hint

To find the area of irregular shapes, separate the shapes into figures for which you can find the area, like triangles, squares, and rectangles. Then, add those areas together.

1. Olivia looks at a drawing of her parents' property and then draws the shape below to represent it. What is the area of the property?

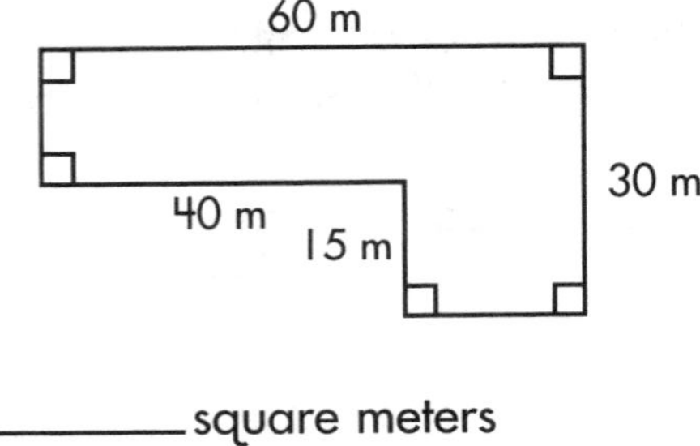

_________ square meters

2. Olivia's family has a cottage by a lake. The picture below shows the layout of the cottage. What is the area?

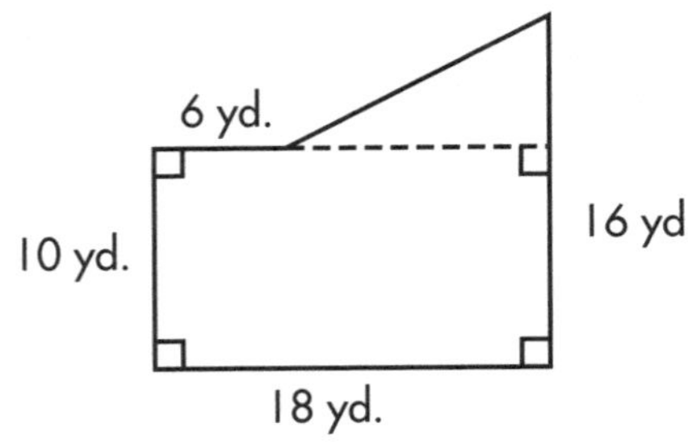

_________ square yards

3. Olivia finds a plastic shape in her house that has the dimensions shown below. What is the area of the shape?

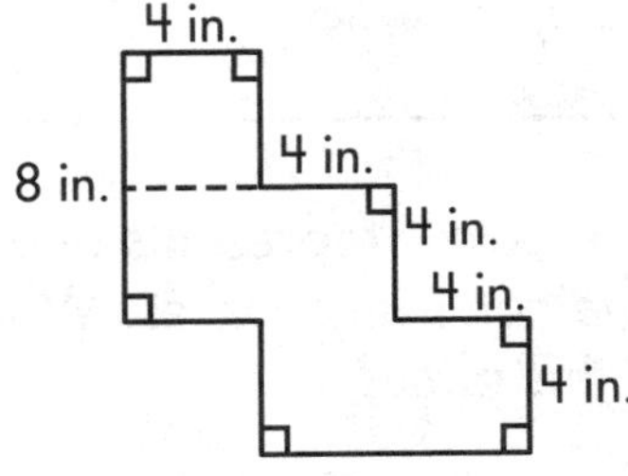

_________ square inches

4. To help her father order paint for the front of the house, Olivia calculates the area using the drawing shown below. What is the area?

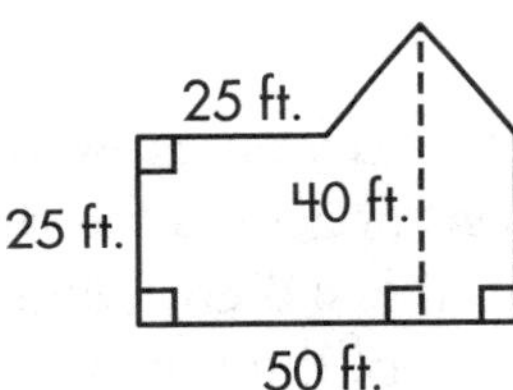

_________ square feet

5. Olivia makes a card to give to her father for Father's Day. The shape of the card is shown below. The area of the card is 75 square inches. What is the height?

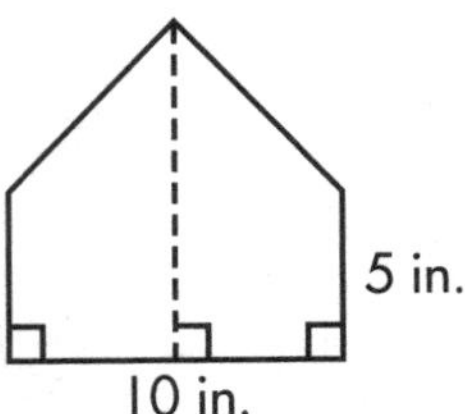

_________ inches

NAME ____________________

Lesson 10.7 Surface Area (Rectangular Solids)

Read the problem carefully and solve. Show your work under each question.

Mr. Benson sells packaging boxes. The boxes come in a variety of sizes.

Helpful Hint

The **surface area** of a solid is the sum of the areas of all the faces (or surfaces of the solid). The surface area of a rectangular solid can be found by the formula $SA = 2lw + 2lh + 2wh$.

1. The most popular box Mr. Benson sells has the dimensions of 32 cm by 12 cm by 26 cm. What is the surface area of this box?

_______ square centimeters

2. Mr. Benson has a customer who wants to know the surface area of the box below so she can buy enough gift wrap for the box. What is the surface area of the box?

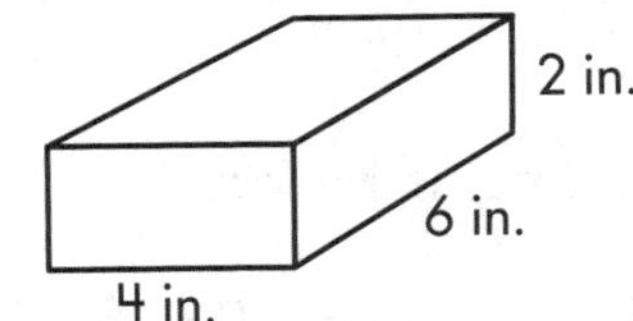

_______ square inches

3. One of Mr. Benson's customers buys the box below to send some books through the mail. What is the surface area of the box?

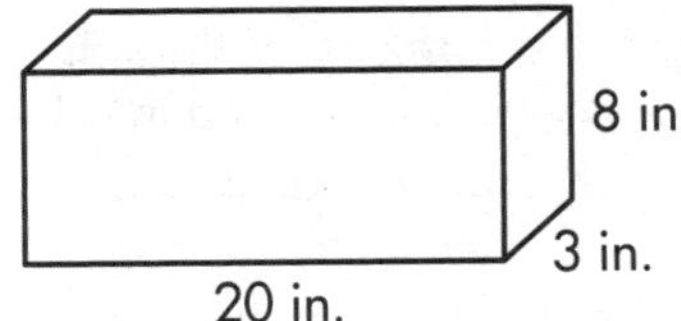

_______ square inches

4. The picture below represents the building that Mr. Benson works in. The surface area of the building is 416 square yards. What is the height of the building?

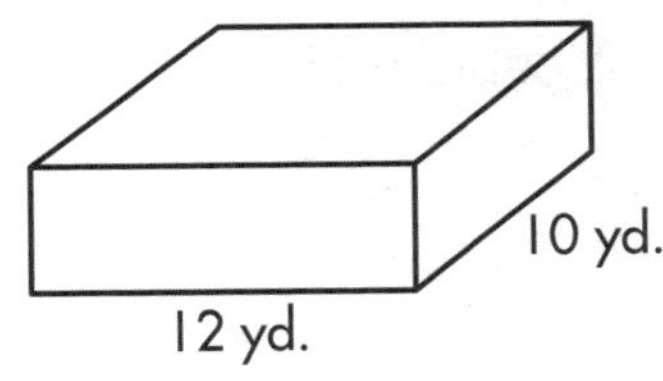

_______ yards

5. Mr. Benson buys a jewelry box for his daughter. The box measures 7 inches by 5 inches by 3 inches. What is the surface area of the box?

_______ square inches

NAME ______________________

Lesson 10.8 Volume of Rectangular Solids

Read the problem carefully and solve. Show your work under each question.

Daysha works on a container ship that carries cargo. Daysha records the volume of each container that is loaded onto the ship.

Helpful Hint

The **volume** of a rectangular solid is the product of the length times the width times the height. The formula for the volume is $V = lwh$. Volume is expressed in cubic units.

1. One of the containers on the ship contains cameras. The dimensions of this container are shown below. Find the volume of the container.

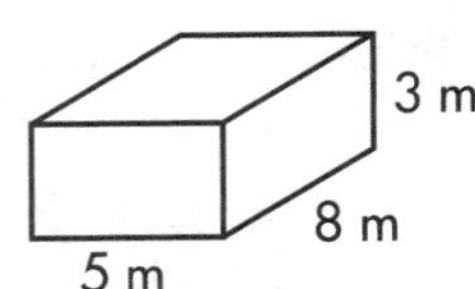

________ cubic meters

2. The container shown below is filled with office supplies and loaded onto the ship by Daysha. The volume of the container is 225 cubic feet. What is the width?

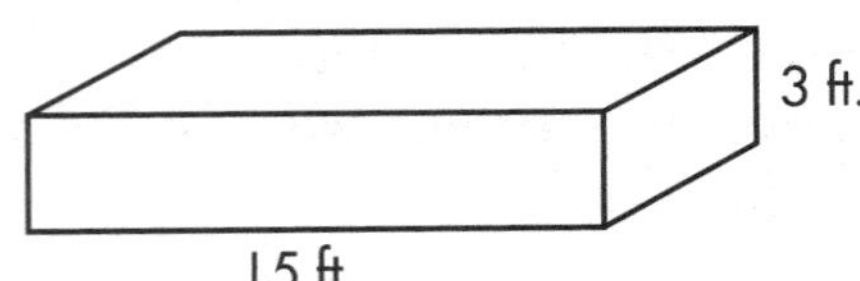

________ feet

3. Daysha loads a container onto the ship that is packed with furniture. The drawing below shows the dimensions of this container. What is its volume?

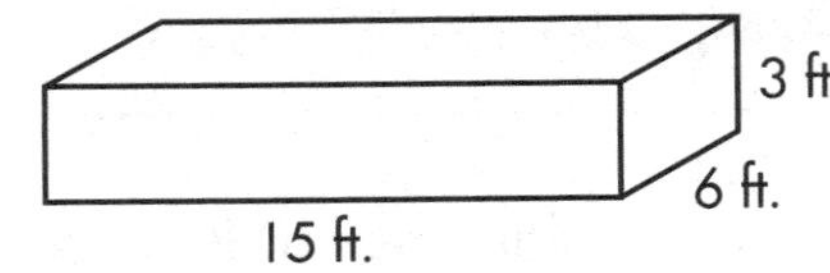

________ cubic feet

4. One of the heavier containers Daysha loads onto the ship is shown below. What is the volume of this container?

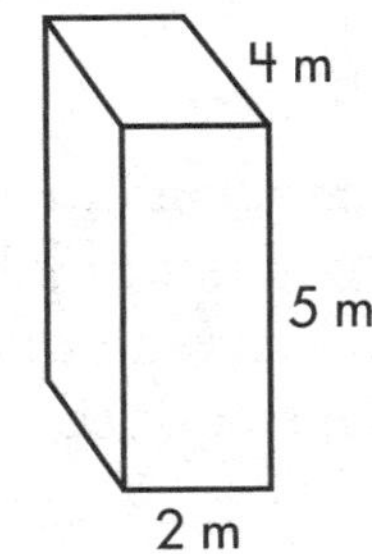

________ cubic meters

5. One of the containers Daysha loads onto the ship is shown below. The volume of the container is 1,200 cubic feet. What is the length of the container?

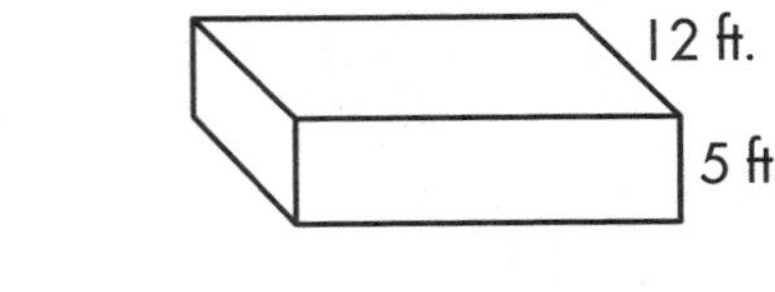

________ feet

NAME ______________________

Lesson 10.9 Volume of Triangular Solids

Read the problem carefully and solve. Show your work under each question.

Ashton makes models and doorstops using blocks of wood. When he is planning what to make, he calculates the volume of each piece so he knows how much wood to purchase.

Helpful Hint

The bases of a triangular solid are triangles. To find the volume, multiply the area of one base times the height.

1. The first piece of wood that Ashton uses in his model is the block shown below. What is the volume of the block?

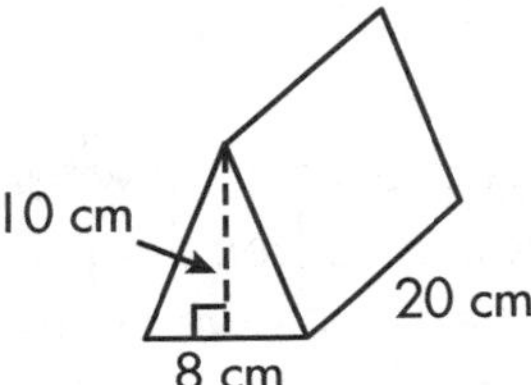

_________ cubic centimeters

2. The second block Ashton makes for the model is shown below. What is the volume of this block?

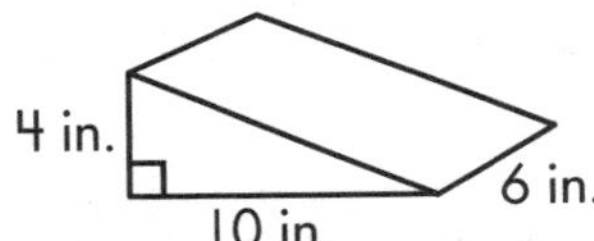

_________ cubic inches

3. The piece of wood shown below will be used as a decorative doorstop. What is its volume?

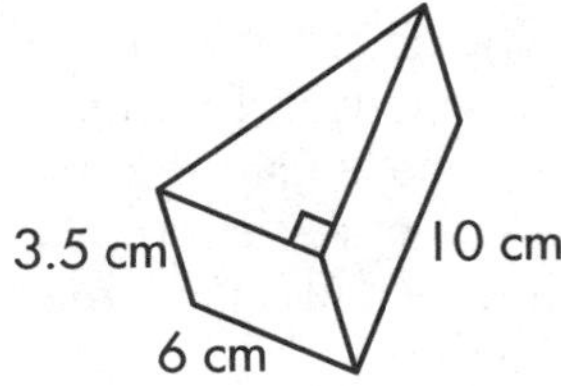

_________ cubic centimeters

4. Ashton packs his blocks onto a container shown below. What is the volume of the container?

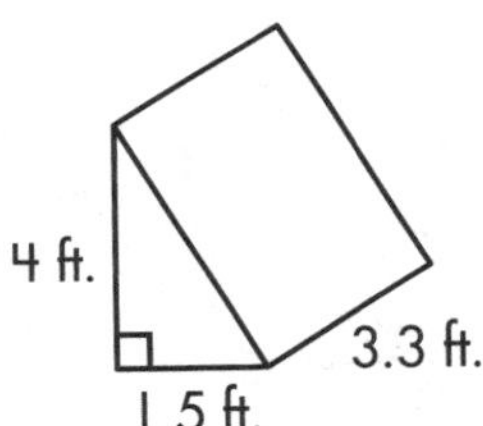

_________ cubic feet

5. Ashton adds the final block, shown below, to his model. What is the volume of this block?

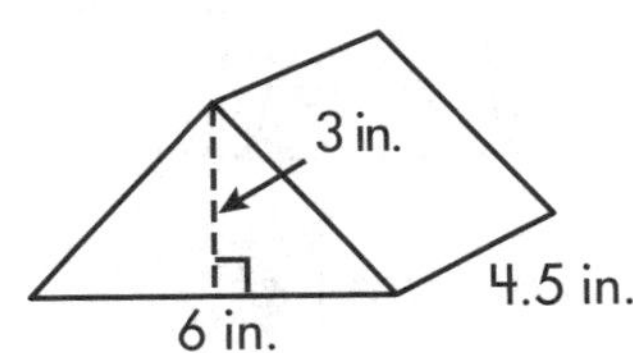

_________ cubic inches

NAME ____________________

Lesson 10.10 Surface Area (Cylinders)

Read the problem carefully and solve. Show your work under each question.

Cheryl has just learned about cylinders in geometry. She collects all the cylinders she can find to practice finding the surface area of a cylinder. Use 3.14 for π.

Helpful Hint

A **cylinder** can be represented on a flat surface as two circles for the bases and a rectangle. The height of the cylinder is the width of the rectangle. The circumference of the base is the length. The surface area is the sum of the area of these three surfaces. It is found by the formula $2\pi r^2 + 2\pi rh$.

1. Cheryl finds that she has a cooler for ice in the shape of a cylinder. A diagram of the cooler is shown below. What is the surface area of the cooler?

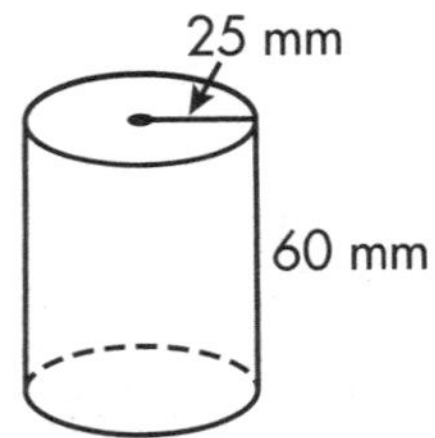

________ square millimeters

2. An old container, shown below, was used to ship a rug to Cheryl's house. What is the surface area of the container?

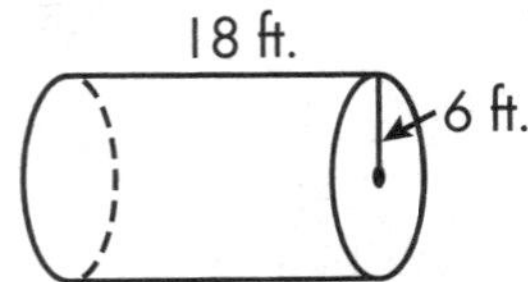

________ square feet

3. A container used to store sea salt is shown below. The surface area of the container is 439.6 square inches. What is the height?

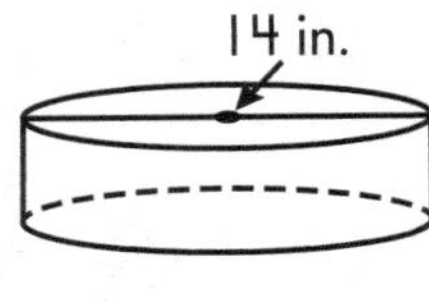

________ inches

4. Cheryl has a container where she stores old blankets and bedding. A picture of the container is shown below. What is the surface area of the cylinder?

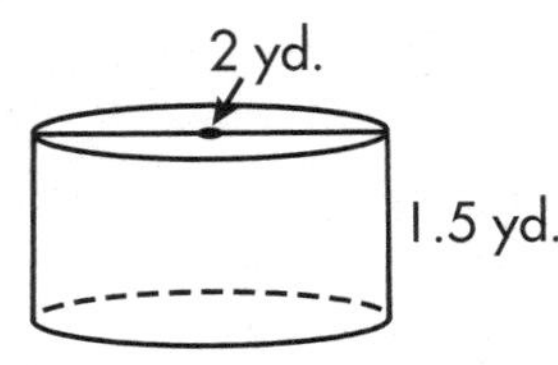

________ square yards

5. There is a hatbox in Cheryl's garage like the one shown below. What is the surface area of the box?

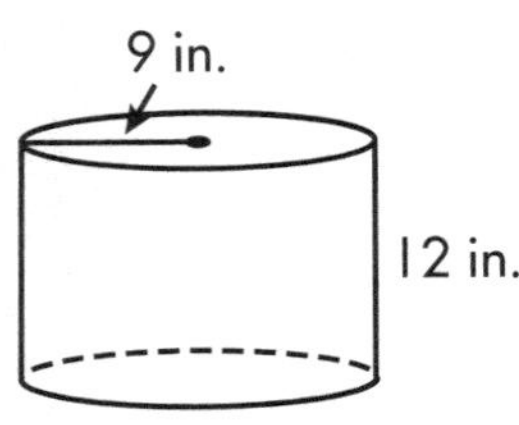

________ square inches

NAME ______________________________

Lesson 10.11 Volume of Cylinders

Read the problem carefully and solve. Show your work under each question.

Bill has a set of plastic storage containers. He calculates the volume of each container.

Helpful Hint

The volume of a cylinder is the product of the area of the base (B) times the height. The formula for the volume of a cylinder is $V = Bh$.

1. Bill stores rice in the container below. How much rice will the container hold?

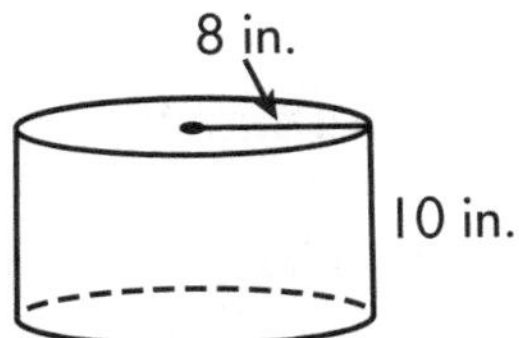

_______ cubic inches

2. Bill usually stores homemade salad dressing in the container below. How many cubic centimeters of dressing can the container hold?

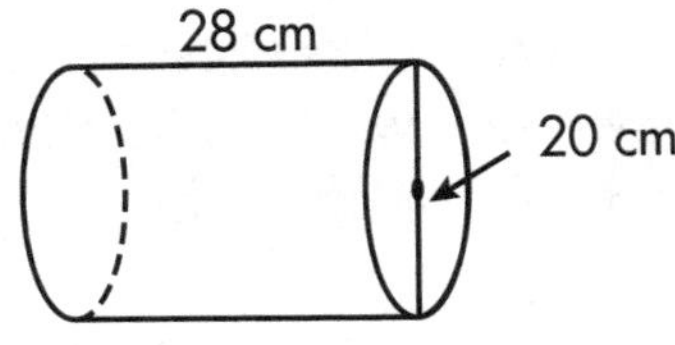

_______ cubic centimeters

3. The container below is used by Bill to store dried herbs. Find the volume of the container.

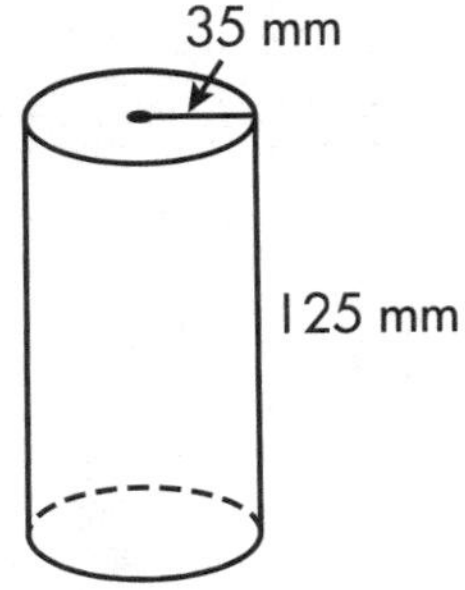

_______ cubic millimeters

4. The container below can hold 530.66 cubic inches of coffee. What is its height?

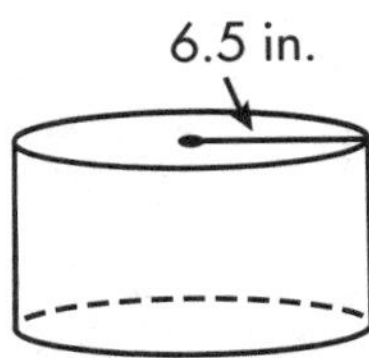

_______ inches

5. Bill uses the container shown below to store pasta. How much pasta can the container hold?

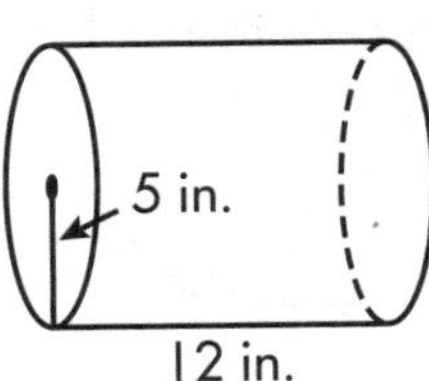

_______ cubic inches

NAME ____________________

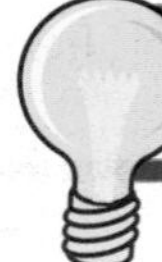

Check What You Learned

Perimeter, Area, and Volume

Read the problem carefully and solve. Show your work under each question.

Delia works in the maintenance department for a local business.

CHAPTER 10 POSTTEST

1. Delia has an office space, shown below, that is in the shape of a square. She needs to run an electric cord around the edge of the space. How long will the cord be?

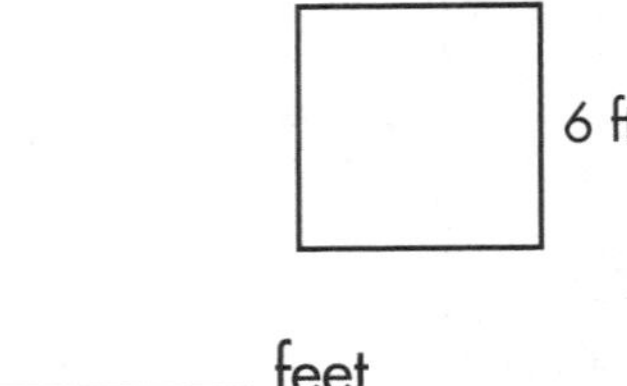

_________ feet

2. On her wall, Delia has a small clock, shown below. What is the circumference of the clock?

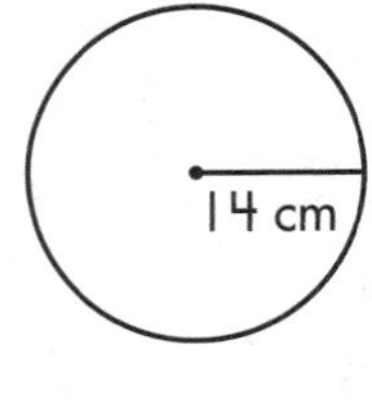

_________ centimeters

3. The diagram below represents Delia's office building. The maintenance crew needs to calculate the total volume of the building for the new air-conditioning system. What is the volume of the building?

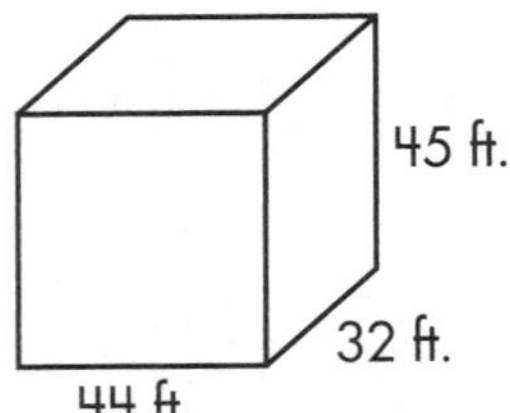

_________ cubic feet

4. The company that Delia works for has a lunchroom. The picture below shows the room. What is its area?

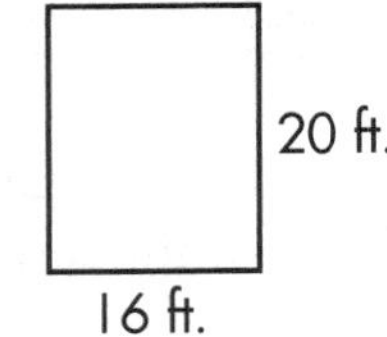

_________ square feet

5. Delia has a novelty coffee mug that is in the shape shown below. What is the volume of this mug?

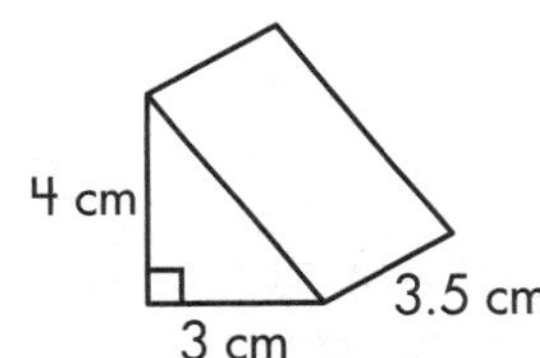

_________ cubic centimeters

6. The bin Delia has to store her paper clips in is shown below. What are the surface area and volume of the bin?

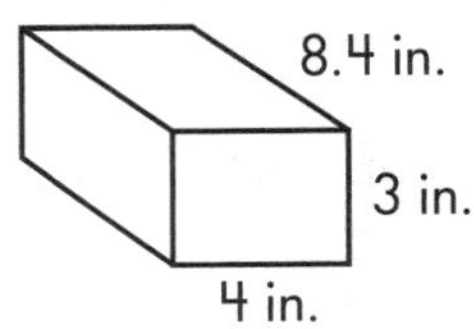

_________ square inches

_________ cubic inches

NAME ______________________

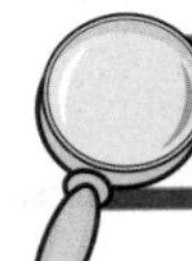

Check What You Know

Variables, Expressions, and Equations

CHAPTER 11 PRETEST

Read the problem carefully and solve. Show your work under each question.

Dylan likes to work with numbers. He likes to make everyday situations into puzzles that he can then solve. The problems below show some examples of how he does this.

1. Dylan has two books by the same author. Book A was published five years earlier than the other book. If book A is represented by the letter x, what statement can Dylan write to represent the age of the other book?

   ____

2. Dylan ordered a box of pencils. The box contains y pencils. Dylan divides the pencils evenly among 4 friends. What expression does Dylan write to find how many pencils each friend gets?

   ____

3. Dylan adds a number, n, to 8 and gets a total of 26. What equation could Dylan write to represent this situation?

   ____

4. Dylan buys 3 orange drinks on Tuesday and 5 orange drinks on Wednesday. The drinks cost $2 each. Write an equation using the Distributive Property to represent this situation.

   ____

5. Dylan plays a game with cards. The following expression shows how many points he got. How many points did Dylan get?

   $-5 + (-3) \div (2 - 1)$

   ____

6. In one of Dylan's puzzles, he has the expression 2^{-2}. How is this written as a fraction?

   ____

NAME ____________________

Lesson 11.1 Variables, Expressions, and Equations

Read the problem carefully and solve. Show your work under each question.

Drew is researching his family history for a class project. He compares the ages of many of his family members. He uses variables, expressions, and equations to represent the ages of his family members.

Helpful Hint

An **expression** is a way of naming a number. A **numerical expression** contains only numbers. A **variable expression** contains numbers and variables. An **equation** is a mathematical sentence that states that two expressions are equal. An **inequality** is a mathematical sentence that states that two expressions are not equal.

1. Drew starts his project with his immediate family members. Drew is 4 years older than his sister, Carol. If Carol is represented by the letter *c*, what expression represents Drew's age in relation to his sister's age?

   ____

2. Drew's father is 5 years younger than his mother. If *m* represents his mother's age, what expression represents Drew's father's age?

   ____

3. Drew's grandmother is 72 years old. Drew's mother is *y* years younger than Drew's grandmother, and she is 45 years old. Write an equation using subtraction that represents this situation.

   ____

4. Drew is three times the age of his cousin, Steve. Write an equation to represent this relationship. Use division, *d* for Drew, and *s* for Steve.

   ____

5. Drew's sister Carol is more than twice the age of their youngest sibling, Abe. Write an inequality to represent this situation using *c* for Carol's age and *a* for Abe's age.

   ____

NAME ___________________

Lesson 11.2 Number Properties

Read the problem carefully and solve. Show your work under each question.

Zaina and Hunter often work on their homework together. They are writing problems for each other where they have to name the property used in the problem.

Helpful Hint

Associative property:
$a + (b + c) = (a + b) + c$

Commutative property: $a + b = b + a$

Identity property: $a \times 1 = a$ and $a + 0 = a$

Multiplication property of zero: $a \times 0 = 0$

1. Zaina writes the following equation and Hunter is asked to identify the number property. What is Hunter's answer?

   $25 + p = p + 25$

   ____

2. Hunter asks Zaina to write a difficult equation. Zaina writes the equation below. Hunter says he can solve it immediately without making any calculations. Which number property did Hunter use?

   $41 \times 115 \times 0 \times 52 \times 1{,}273 = ?$

   ____

3. Hunter says that the expression $4 \times (t \times 5)$ has the same value as $(4 \times t) \times 5$. Which number property helps Hunter make this statement?

   ____

4. Zaina says: "Adding zero to any number does not change its value." Which property is represented by Zaina's statement?

   ____

5. Hunter writes the following equation. Which number property is represented by this equation?

   $9{,}456{,}845 \times 1 = 9{,}456{,}845$

   ____

NAME ___________________________

Lesson 11.3 The Distributive Property

Read the problem carefully and solve. Show your work under each question.

Irene studies the distributive property and finds ways to use it in her everyday life. The situations shown below demonstrate this concept.

Helpful Hint

The **distributive property** combines multiplication with addition or subtraction. The property states:
$a \times (b + c) = (a \times b) + (a \times c)$
$a \times (b - c) = (a \times b) - (a \times c)$

1. Irene rents a canoe for 2 hours in the morning and for 3 more hours in the afternoon. The rental company charges $15 per hour for the rental. Write an expression using the distributive property to represent this situation.

   ____

2. Irene orders 4 boxes of notepads one week and 7 boxes of notepads the next week. Each box costs *a* dollars. She writes the following expression: $(a \times 4) + (a \times 7)$

   Rewrite the expression using the distributive property.

   ____

3. Irene buys 5 pairs of shirts. The shirts cost $22 each. Use the distributive property to write an expression that will make it easier for Irene to determine the total cost of the shirts.

   ____

4. Irene and four friends each had coupons for $2 off admission to a water park. If admission is $11, write an expression using the distributive property to represent the total cost of admission for all 5 people.

   ____

5. Irene has to paint 8 mugs. It takes *v* minutes to paint a mug and *m* minutes to dry. Write an equation relating two expressions that will help Irene calculate the total amount of time it will take to finish the mugs. Use the distributive property.

   ____

NAME ______________________

Lesson 11.4 Order of Operations

Read the problem carefully and solve. Show your work under each question.

Ahmed likes to represent everyday situations in his life using expressions.

Helpful Hint

Order of operations

1. All operations within parentheses
2. All exponents
3. All multiplication and division, from left to right
4. All addition and subtraction, from left to right

1. Ahmed buys cans of seltzer water in packs of six cans. One day, he buys 4 packs of six cans and then another 3 individual cans of seltzer. He uses the expression below to represent the purchase. How many cans in total did he buy?

   $3 + 4 \times 4$

   ____

2. Ahmed writes the expression below to show how players were divided into teams for a game and how extra players were added. What is the value of the expression?

   $18 \div (2 + 1) + 2$

   ____

3. Ahmed played a game using the expression below. If he answered correctly, he gets to write the next expression. What is the value of the expression?

   $42 \div 6 + 8$

   ____

4. Ahmed tosses 5 pennies into a wishing well. He then tosses 2 more pennies in the pool. He did this 2 days in a row. Use the expression below to find the total number of pennies Ahmed tossed into the well.

   $2 \times (2 + 5)$

   ____

5. Ahmed writes the expression below to represent the number of games he has acquired or lost over the past few years. How many games does he have?

   $(8 - 4) \times (4 + 2) + 2$

   ____

NAME ______________________

Lesson 11.5 Solving Addition and Subtraction Equations

Read the problem carefully and solve. Show your work under each question.

Lin sells cars for a living. She keeps track of her sales data each week.

Helpful Hint

Subtraction Property of Equality: When two expressions are equal, if you subtract the same number from both expressions, the difference will also be equal.

Addition Property of Equality: When two expressions are equal, if you add the same number to both expressions, the sums will also be equal.

1. Lin sells 7 more cars this week than she did in week *a*. She sold 16 cars this week. How many cars did she sell in week *a*?

   $7 + a = 16$

   ____

2. Lin writes the following equation to represent the total number of cars she expects to sell this week, *b*, minus the number of cars she has already sold. How many cars does she expect to sell?

   $b - 17 = 3$

   ____

3. Lin writes the following equation to represent the number of cars she sells in one day, *d*, plus another day. How many cars does she sell on day *d*?

   $9 = d + 4$

   ____

4. Lin writes the following equation to represent the selling price of a car minus the cost for the dealership to get the car. What was the cost, *c*, of the car?

   $\$4,000 - c = \$350$

   ____

5. Lin writes the following equation to represent the number of cars she needs to sell in week *g*. How many cars does she need to sell in week *g*?

   $15 = g + 12$

   ____

NAME ___________________________

Lesson 11.6 Solving Multiplication and Division Equations

Read the problem carefully and solve. Show your work under each question.

Mrs. Ross orders supplies for her classroom and then distributes them to the students in her classroom.

Helpful Hint

Division Property of Equality: When two expressions are equal, if they are divided by the same number, the quotients will also be equal.

Multiplication Property of Equality: When two expressions are equal, if they are multiplied by the same number, the products will also be equal.

1. Mrs. Ross orders pencils that come in packs of 16. The equation below represents the pencils she ordered. How many packs did she order?

   $n \times 16 = 32$

   ____

2. Mrs. Ross orders notepads that come in packs of 4. The equation below represents the notepads she ordered. How many notepads did she order in total?

   $m \times 4 = 24$

   ____

3. Mrs. Ross orders binders. She divides them evenly among the 24 students. Each student gets 3 binders. Use the equation below to find the total number of binders.

   $a \div 24 = 3$

   ____

4. Mrs. Ross orders highlighters for her students. She divides them evenly among the students. Each student gets 6 highlighters. Use the equation below to find the number of students.

   $144 \div s = 6$

   ____

5. Mrs. Ross orders pens that come in packs of 12. The equation below represents the pens she ordered. How many pens did she order in total?

   $z \times 12 = 48$

   ____

NAME ______________________

Lesson 11.7 Writing Expressions

Read the problem carefully and solve. Show your work under each question.

All varieties of muffins are $3.50 a box. Jake buys blueberry muffins and chocolate muffins. There are two ways to write an expression that represents the total cost, T, of the muffins if b represents the number of blueberry muffins and c represents the number of chocolate muffins.

Find the cost of each variety of muffin and then add to find the total:

$$T = \$3.50b + \$3.50c$$

or

Multiply $3.50 by the number of boxes (regardless of variety).

$$T = \$3.50\ (b + c)$$

1. Janet and Toby both get paid $9 per hour. This week, Toby makes an additional $27 in overtime. Write an expression that represents the total weekly wages of both if J = the number of hours that Janet worked and T = the number of hours that Toby worked.

   ____

2. What is another way to write the expression in question 1?

   ____

3. Patricia, Hugo, and Sun work at a music store. Each week, Patricia works three more than twice the number of hours that Hugo works. Sun works two less hours than Hugo. Let x represent the number of hours Hugo works each week. Write an expression that represents how many hours Patricia works.

   ____

4. Write an expression that represents how many hours Sun works.

   ____

NAME ______________________

Lesson 11.8 Adding, Subtracting, Multiplying, and Dividing Integers

Read the problem carefully and solve. Show your work under each question.

Owen is the manager for the high school football team. He keeps track of team statistics.

Helpful Hint

The sum of two positive integers is positive. The sum of two negative integers is negative. The product or quotient of two integers with the same sign is positive. The product or quotient of two integers with different signs is negative.

1. Owen writes the expression below to represent the yards gained in the last three plays of a game. Find the sum.

   $14 + (-7) + (-3)$

   ____

2. The expression below is used by Owen to find the difference in yards gained by two different players. What is the difference?

   $15 - (-10)$

   ____

3. Each time the team loses, they lose 7 points in the standings. Use the expression below to show the total number of points lost from their 5 losses.

   $5 \times (-7)$

   ____

4. Owen writes the expression below to represent the average yards lost in the team's worst 8 plays last week. What was the average loss per play?

   $-32 \div 8$

   ____

5. Owen uses the expression below when calculating one of the team's statistics at the end of the year. What is the product?

   $-7 \times (-3)$

   ____

NAME ________________

Lesson 11.9 Integers and Inverses

Read the problem carefully and solve. Show your work under each question.

The highest elevation in North America is Mt. McKinley, which is 20,320 feet above sea level. The lowest elevation is Death Valley, which is 282 feet below sea level. The distance from the top of Mt. McKinley to the bottom of Death Valley is the same as the distance from +20,320 to −282 on a number line. Add +20,320 to 0, and 0 to −282 for a total of 20,602 feet.

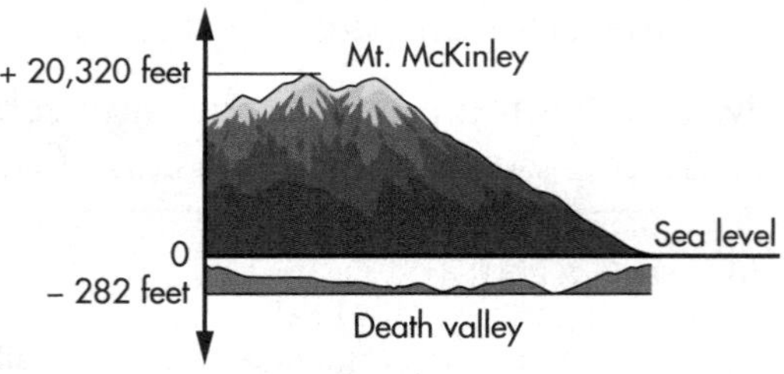

Helpful Hint

This situation uses opposites. Above sea level is the opposite of below sea level. Some more examples of opposites are increase, decrease; forward, backward; and positive, negative.

1. Paul had $26. He owed $26 to his friend Jess. How much money did Paul have after he paid Jess?

   ____

2. Mt. Everest, the highest elevation in Asia, is 29,028 feet above sea level. The Dead Sea, the lowest elevation, is 1,312 feet below sea level. What is the difference between these two elevations?

   ____

3. In Minneapolis, Minnesota, the temperature was −14°F in the morning. If the temperature dropped 7°F, what is the temperature now?

   ____

4. A submarine is 800 feet below sea level. If it ascends 250 feet, what is its new position?

   ____

5. In the Sahara Desert one day, it was 136°F. In the Gobi Desert, a temperature of −50°F was recorded. What is the difference between these two temperatures?

   ____

6. Metal mercury at room temperature is a liquid. Its freezing point is −39°C. The freezing point of alcohol is −114°C. How much warmer is the freezing point of mercury than the freezing point of alcohol?

   ____

NAME ____________________

Lesson 11.10 Multiplying and Dividing Powers

Read the problem carefully and solve. Show your work under each question.

Yuri keeps track of various data in New Evansville. He uses exponents to represent large numbers.

Helpful Hint

A **power** is a number that is expressed using an **exponent**. The **base** is the number that is multiplied, and the exponent tells how many times the base is used as a factor.

1. Yuri writes the expression 6^3 to represent the number of seventh-grade students in the school district. How many seventh-grade students are in the district?

   ________ students

2. Yuri uses the expression 4^4 to represent the number of clients for an accounting firm in town. How many clients does the firm have?

   ____

3. The expression $5^2 \times 5^3$ represents the number of buildings times the number of occupants in the local college dormitories. What is the simplified form of this expression using one exponent?

   ____

4. There are 64 stoplights in town. How can this number be written using an exponent with a base of 2?

   ____

5. Yuri wants to rewrite 2^6 as the product of two expressions, both with exponents using 2 as the base. What does Yuri write?

   ________ $\times$ ________

NAME ______________________________

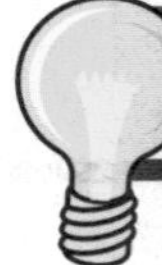

Check What You Learned

Variables, Expressions, and Equations

Read the problem carefully and solve. Show your work under each question.

Hector writes variables, expressions, and equations to help him study for a test.

1. Hector brings x pairs of shorts on a 5-day vacation. He plans to wear 2 pairs per day. How many pairs of shorts did Hector bring on vacation?

   ________ pairs of shorts

2. Hector runs a total of 12 miles. If he runs c miles each hour, write an expression to show the number of miles he runs each hour.

   ____

3. Hector has 2^3 cans of peanuts, and each can contains 2^8 peanuts. How many peanuts does Hector have in all? Write your answer as a number with one exponent.

   ________ peanuts

4. Hector has 48 paperclips, and he gives h paper clips to a friend. If he is left with 32 paperclips, write an equation that shows this situation.

   ____

5. Hector gains 9 points in a game. Then in the next round, he loses 12 points. He writes the expression below to show this. How many points does he have in total?

   $9 + (-12) =$ ________

CHAPTER 11 POSTTEST

NAME ____________________

Final Test Chapters 1–11

Read the problem carefully and solve. Show your work under each question.

Evan is attending a picnic. Among the things he packs are 4 quarts of lemonade, a 34-inch loaf of french bread, and 57 ounces of potato salad.

1. Each quart of lemonade costs $4.29. How much money does Evan spend on lemonade for the picnic?

   ____

2. Another person brings 3 quarts of lemonade. How many gallons of lemonade are there in all?

   ________ gallons

3. How many feet of bread does Evan bring to the picnic? Show your answer as a mixed numeral.

   ________ feet

4. How many pounds of potato salad does Evan bring to the picnic?

   ________ pounds

5. The cost of the potato salad is $27.96. If 12 people each eat the same amount of potato salad and there is none left over, how much is the cost per person?

   ____

6. The picnic lasted 126 minutes. How many hours is this?

   ________ hours

NAME ______________________________

Final Test Chapters 1–11

Read the problem carefully and solve. Show your work under each question.

Daysha buys a business making smoothies. She has chosen to purchase a smoothie machine because it is light enough to transport. The weight of the machine is 4.2 kilograms. The machine can hold up to 5 liters of liquid.

1. Daysha wants to know how many metric tons the machine weighs. Write the weight of the machine in metric tons.

________ metric tons

2. Daysha makes a batch of smoothies and fills the machine $\frac{6}{20}$ full with strawberries. What percent of the smoothie machine is full?

____

3. What is the total number of milliliters that the smoothie machine can hold?

________ milliliters

4. The smoothie machine cord measures 58 centimeters in length. How many millimeters long is the cord?

________ millimeters

5. Daysha writes the simple interest rate from her account, 3%, as a decimal. How do you write 3% as a decimal?

____

6. Daysha deposits $500 she made over the weekend in her bank account. The account earns 3% simple interest. How much will the $500 yield after 5 years?

____

NAME ______________________

Final Test Chapters 1–11

Read the problem carefully and solve. Show your work under each question.

India is surveying people from her booth at the mall. One survey asks 20 people their favorite color of car. The results are shown in the circle graph to the right.

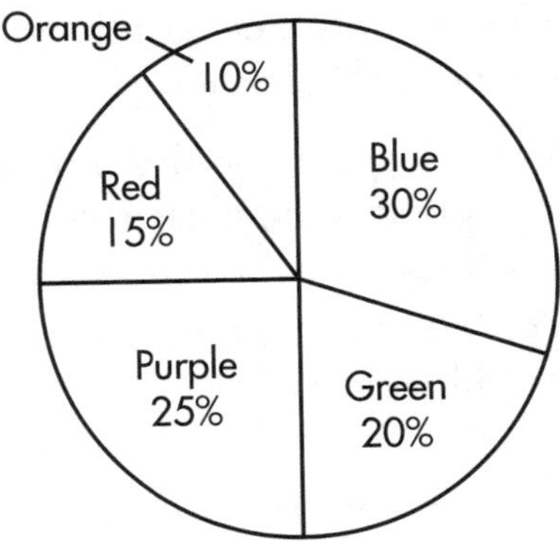

Favorite Color of Car

1. How many people said that green or red was their favorite color?

   ________ people

2. India surveys 20 people to find the number of hours each week that they exercise. The results in hours are: 2, 0, 4, 7, 1, 4, 3, 1, 3, 9, 1, 5, 3, 5, 2, 1, 3, 4, 2, 1. Make a line plot to show these results.

3. In her booth, India has a jar with different flavors of tea bags. The jar contains 12 tea bags, and 3 of them are green tea. Write the percentage of the tea bags that are green tea as a decimal and as a fraction.

   ________ and ________

4. The figure below is a drawing from one of India's surveys about car hood ornaments. Determine if the two shapes are similar, and what type of transformation was used to make the larger figure.

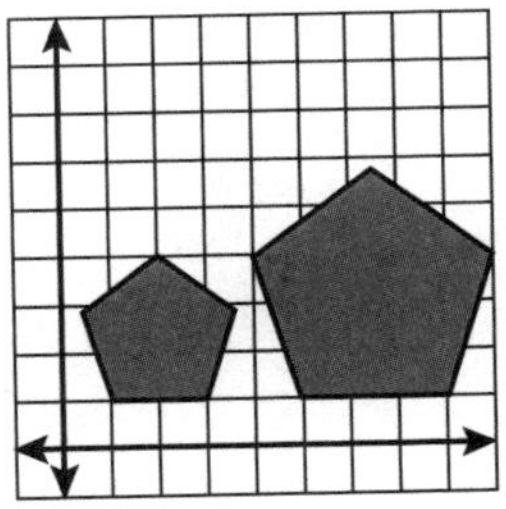

   ________ and ________

5. India uses the circle below to represent the clock in her booth. She wants to buy a decorative frame and a piece of glass to cover it. What is the circumference and area of the clock? Use 3.14 for π.

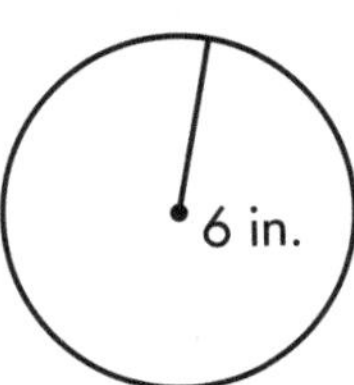

   ________ inches

   ________ square inches

NAME ____________________

Final Test Chapters 1–11

Read the problem carefully and solve. Show your work under each question.

Mrs. Jung created the box-and-whisker plot to the right to represent the class scores on a recent history test.

Test Scores on History Test

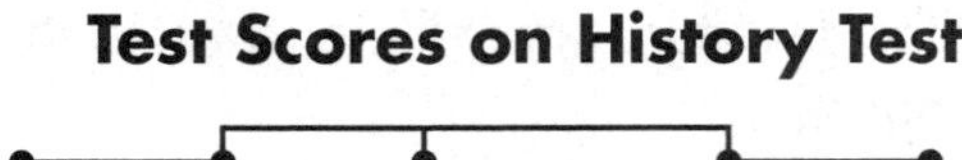

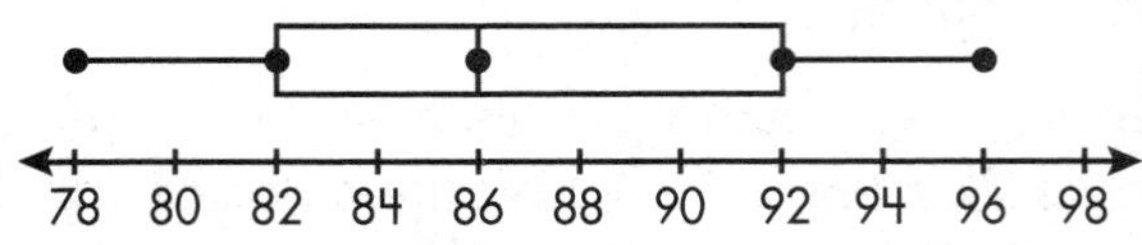

1. What is the median score of the history test?

____

2. The actual scores for the test are: 86, 92, 83, 79, 80, 81, 92, 83, 84, 87, 89, 92, 94, 78, 95, 96, and 85. What is the mean test score, rounded to the nearest whole number?

____

3. Mrs. Jung makes a stem-and-leaf plot using the list of actual scores from the test. Make a stem-and-leaf plot.

4. Mrs. Jung tells her students the range of the data for the test scores. What is the range?

____

5. To help decide who gets form A of the test, Mrs. Jung rolls a 12-sided number cube. It is numbered on each side with a number from 1–12. What is the probability that she will roll either a 2 or a 5? Write your answer as a percent rounded to the nearest whole percent.

____

6. Mrs. Jung has a container, shown below, to hold pencils and erasers. She wants to cover it with decorative fabric. What is the surface area and the volume of the container?

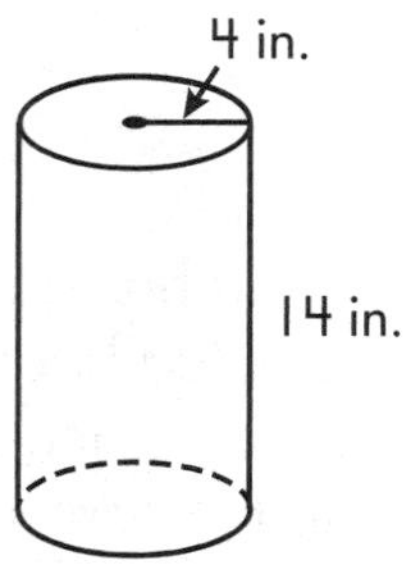

_______ square inches

_______ cubic inches

NAME ____________________

Final Test Chapters 1–11

Read the problem carefully and solve. Show your work under each question.

Jayla is getting her home ready for sale. She drew a floorplan and sketches of her house to include with the sale announcement.

1. Jayla draws the angle shown below to represent the angle of a wall in her closet. How would you name the angle using a symbol and letters?

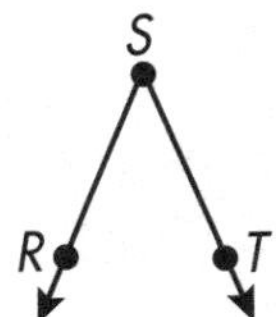

_______ or _______

2. Jayla draws the triangle below to represent a window in her house. How would you name the triangle based on its sides and angles?

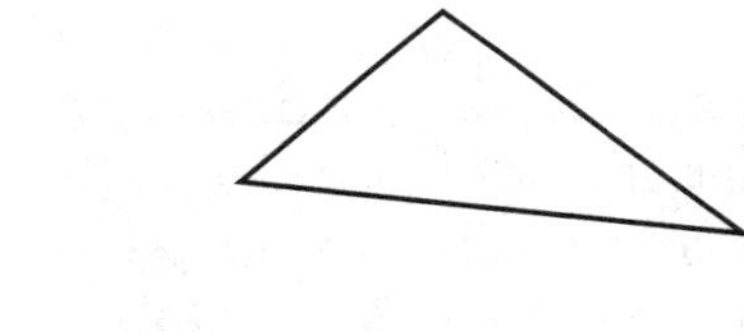

____

Use the drawing below of Jayla's garden layout for numbers 3–5.

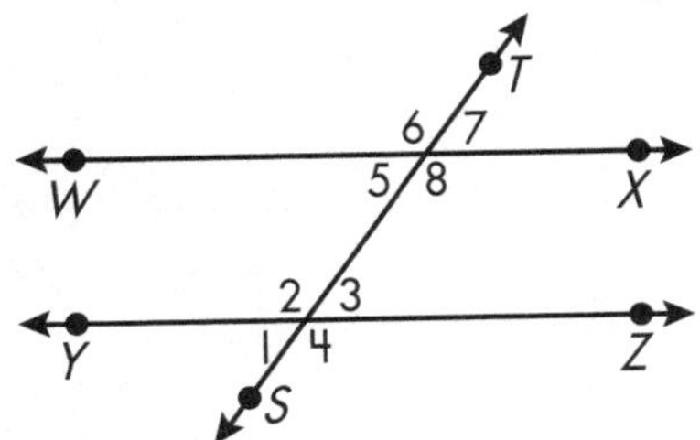

3. Which angle is vertical to ∠7?

∠ _______

4. Which angle along with ∠2 makes a pair of alternate interior angles?

∠ _______

5. Jayla wants to know which angle is a corresponding angle to ∠1. Which angle corresponds to ∠1?

∠ _______

6. Jayla buys p paint cans at $18.22 each. She spends a total of $91.10. Jayla writes the equation below to represent the situation. How many cans of paint does she buy?

$\$18.22 \times p = \$91.10$

_______ cans of paint

NAME ____________________

Final Test Chapters 1–11

Read the problem carefully and solve. Show your work under each question.

Grace works in a bank. The dimensions of the bank are shown on the right.

32 ft.

12 ft.

1. Grace calculates the perimeter and area of the bank building. What is the perimeter? What is the area?

________ feet ________ square feet

2. The expression below represents 2 deposits of \$17 and 2 deposits of \$85 into Grace's savings account. Use the distributive property to rewrite the expression.

2(\$17) + 2(\$85)

____

3. Grace writes the following equation to represent the amount of money that she has in her bank account after buying groceries that total \$45. How much money did she start with in her account?
$x - \$45 = \$378$

____

4. The following expression represents the calculations Grace made with a savings account. What is the value of the expression?
$2 + 4 \times 4 - 5$

____

5. Grace has a box on her desk where she keeps her personal belongings. The box measures 6 inches by 14 inches by 5 inches. What is the volume of the box?

________ cubic inches

NAME ______________________ DATE ____________

Scoring Record for Posttests, Mid-Test, and Final Test

		Performance			
Chapter Posttest	Your Score	Excellent	Very Good	Fair	Needs Improvement
1	____ of 6	6	5	3–4	2 or fewer
2	____ of 6	6	5	3–4	2 or fewer
3	____ of 6	6	5	3–4	2 or fewer
4	____ of 6	6	5	3–4	2 or fewer
5	____ of 6	6	5	3–4	2 or fewer
6	____ of 6	6	5	3–4	2 or fewer
7	____ of 6	6	5	3–4	2 or fewer
8	____ of 12	11–12	9–10	7–8	6 or fewer
9	____ of 4	4	3	2	1 or fewer
10	____ of 6	6	5	3–4	2 or fewer
11	____ of 5	5	4	3	2 or fewer
Mid-Test	____ of 24	22–24	20–21	16–19	15 or fewer
Final Test	____ of 34	31–34	27–30	19–26	18 or fewer

Record your test score in the Your Score column. See where your score falls in the Performance columns. Your score is based on the total number of required responses. If your score is fair or needs improvement, review the chapter material.

Grade 7 Answers

Chapter 1

Pretest, page 1

1. 24,368
2. 399,028
3. 40,620
4. 2,707
5. 2,031
6. 42,561

Lesson 1.1, page 2

1. 201,587
2. 56,647
3. 334,361
4. 132,774
5. 41,523

Lesson 1.2, page 3

1. 1,472
2. 63,612
3. 23,718
4. 39,648
5. 147,250

Lesson 1.3, page 4

1. 615; 2
2. 65
3. 732
4. 61; 22
5. 1,464

Posttest, page 5

1. 122,800
2. 8,174
3. 194,814
4. 27,174
5. 1,130
6. 4,529

Chapter 2

Pretest, page 6

1. 12
2. $\frac{8}{12} < \frac{9}{12}, \frac{3}{4}$
3. $1\frac{5}{12}$
4. $4\frac{3}{4}$
5. $86\frac{5}{8}$
6. $\frac{5}{12}$

Lesson 2.1, page 7

1. $\frac{11}{30}$
2. $\frac{2}{15}$
3. The probability of the event occurring is a fraction between 0 and 1.
4. $\frac{4}{15}$
5. $\frac{1}{12}$

Lesson 2.2, page 8

1. Marlene: $\frac{10}{12}$, Bianca: $\frac{5}{12}$
2. Kareem
3. $\frac{20}{24} > \frac{15}{24}$
4. 24
5. Paul

Lesson 2.3, page 9

1. $3\frac{4}{7}$
2. $3\frac{3}{4}$
3. $\frac{37}{8}$
4. $\frac{20}{9}$
5. $\frac{33}{5}$

Lesson 2.4, page 10

1. $1\frac{27}{56}$
2. $\frac{1}{8}$
3. $1\frac{4}{15}$
4. $3\frac{9}{35}$
5. $\frac{5}{12}$

Lesson 2.5, page 11

1. $3\frac{3}{8}$
2. 4
3. $7\frac{1}{3}$
4. $\frac{1}{4}$
5. $\frac{2}{9}$

Lesson 2.6, page 12

1. $\frac{19}{15}$
2. $\frac{1}{45}$
3. $\frac{7}{33}$
4. $\frac{9}{4}$
5. $\frac{9}{29}$

Lesson 2.7, page 13

1. $2\frac{2}{7}$
2. $1\frac{5}{6}$
3. $8\frac{2}{3}$
4. $\frac{7}{8}$
5. $1\frac{1}{4}$

Posttest, page 14

1. 10
2. $\frac{7}{10} < \frac{4}{5}$
3. $1\frac{1}{2}$
4. $1\frac{1}{8}$
5. $153\frac{1}{32}$
6. $3\frac{1}{12}$

Grade 7 Answers

Chapter 3

Pretest, page 15

1. $4,874.85
2. 3.375
3. $4,318.35
4. $676.38
5. 13
6. $1,947.60

Lesson 3.1, page 16

1. 0.125
2. 1.75
3. 0.285
4. $\frac{7}{50}$
5. $3\frac{3}{8}$

Lesson 3.2, page 17

1. 32.548
2. 13.315
3. 14.03
4. 21.435
5. 38.748

Lesson 3.3, page 18

1. 19.27
2. 18.14
3. 8.575
4. 21.06
5. 2.92

Lesson 3.4, page 19

1. 14.175
2. 18.275
3. 47.5
4. 1.875
5. 24.65

Lesson 3.5, page 20

1. $14.15
2. $32.99
3. $1.98
4. $26.78
5. 1.1784

Lesson 3.6, page 21

1. 40
2. 48
3. 60
4. 170
5. 1.1342

Lesson 3.7, page 22

1. 30
2. 42
3. 17
4. 30
5. 264.12; 264

Posttest, page 23

1. $2,755.08
2. $12.35
3. $694.30
4. $533.28
5. 12
6. $2\frac{14}{25}$

Chapter 4

Pretest, page 24

1. 0.25
2. $1\frac{3}{4} > 1.7$
3. $\frac{3}{10}$
4. $\frac{1}{3}$, 34%, 0.35
5. 12%
6. 6

Lesson 4.1, page 25

1. $\frac{39}{50}$; 0.78
2. $\frac{4}{5}$; 0.8
3. $\frac{13}{20}$; 0.65
4. $\frac{47}{50}$; 0.94
5. $\frac{22}{25}$; 0.88

Lesson 4.2, page 26

1. $40\% > \frac{1}{4}$
2. $3.68 < 3\frac{4}{5}$
3. $\frac{1}{4} > 0.15$
4. 40%, 3.68, $3\frac{4}{5}$
5. 105%, $\frac{11}{10}$, 1.111, $1\frac{1}{4}$

Lesson 4.3, page 27

1. $\frac{2}{25}$
2. 35%
3. $\frac{11}{50}$
4. 50%
5. $1\frac{1}{4}$

Lesson 4.4, page 28

1. 0.12
2. 58%
3. 6%
4. 0.02
5. 0.62

Lesson 4.5, page 29

1. 9
2. 12
3. 6
4. 18
5. 51

Grade 7 Answers

Lesson 4.6, page 30

1. $16.50
2. $1,511.25
3. $8.36; $463.98
4. $33.02
5. $68.40; $1,1413.60

Posttest, page 31

1. 0.14
2. $0.62 < \frac{5}{8}$
3. $1\frac{7}{20}$
4. 4%, 0.44, $\frac{3}{4}$
5. $13\frac{1}{2}$%, $1\frac{1}{4}$, 1.3, $\frac{11}{8}$
6. 42

Mid-Test Chapters 1–4

Mid-Test, page 32

1. 1,555,700
2. 188,900
3. 2,733,600
4. 227,800
5. 11
6. 8

Mid-Test, page 33

1. 38
2. 6.8
3. 52
4. $\frac{112}{5}$
5. 57.12
6. 542

Mid-Test, page 34

1. $382.50
2. $438.75
3. $1,245
4. $2\frac{1}{2}$%
5. $1,580
6. $9,200

Mid-Test, page 35

1. 12
2. 12
3. 63
4. 27
5. 9
6. 30

Chapter 5

Pretest, page 36

1. 49
2. 22
3. 100
4. 12
5. 20
6. 6

Lesson 5.1, page 37

1. yes
2. no
3. yes
4. yes
5. 5

Lesson 5.2, page 38

1. 128
2. 24
3. 128
4. 12
5. 98

Lesson 5.3, page 39

1. 6
2. 4
3. 27
4. 126
5. 15

Lesson 5.4, page 40

1. 0.35
2. 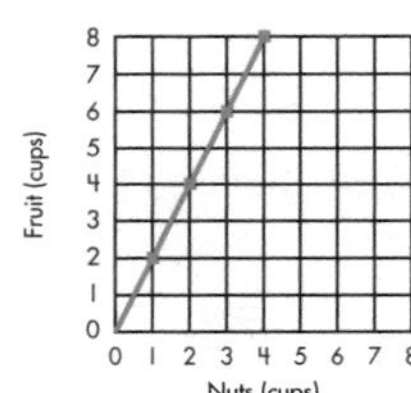

3. yes; For each of the other serving sizes, there are 2 cups of fruit for every 1 cup of nuts (2:1).
4. $1.07
5. 19; 2

Posttest, page 41

1. 250
2. 140
3. 75
4. 6
5. 9
6. 36

Grade 7 Answers

Chapter 6

Pretest, page 42

1. 424
2. 7,392
3. 3.25
4. 11,700
5. 1.25
6. 5

Lesson 6.1, page 43

1. 27,984
2. 9,328
3. 540
4. 81
5. 4,464

Lesson 6.2, page 44

1. 8
2. 48
3. 12
4. 6
5. 12

Lesson 6.3, page 45

1. 2,260
2. 681.6
3. 0.079
4. 36,160
5. 19.2

Lesson 6.4, page 46

1. 138
2. 2.25
3. 2 days 15 hours
4. 324
5. 19,440

Posttest, page 47

1. 0.0368
2. 31,680
3. 1.25
4. 4,500
5. 0.75
6. 9

Chapter 7

Pretest, page 48

1. 0.0832
2. 7.05
3. 28,000
4. 0.028
5. 0.00055
6. 1,500

Lesson 7.1, page 49

1. 12,000
2. 45
3. 266,000
4. 0.38
5. 1,200,000

Lesson 7.2, page 50

1. 7
2. 10.5
3. 22,400
4. 0.055
5. 3,500

Lesson 7.3, page 51

1. 840
2. 42,000
3. 2,700
4. 0.011
5. 326,000

Posttest, page 52

1. 1,800
2. 2,100,000
3. 500
4. 500,000
5. 0.0164
6. 16,400

Chapter 8

Pretest, page 53

1. 12
2. Rock and Alternative
3. 6
4. 10
5. 36
6. 22

Pretest, page 54

1. $4\frac{1}{2}$
2. 2
3. $16\frac{1}{2}$
4. 6
5. 4
6. 4

Lesson 8.1, page 55

1. 100
2. 2
3. 8
4. 19
5. 9

Grade 7 Answers

Lesson 8.2, page 56
1. 6
2. 1
3. 19
4. 9
5. 3

Lesson 8.3, page 57
1. 7
2. 40
3. 1, 7, 9
4. 4
5. 3 and 4

Lesson 8.4, page 58
1. cranberry, blackberry
2. 80
3. 400
4. 160 people

Lesson 8.5, page 59
1. 75
2. 65, 80, 85
3. 6
4. 6
5. positive

Lesson 8.6, page 60
1. 70° F
2. 16° F
3. 70° F
4. 71° F
5. range

Lesson 8.7, page 61
1. 49
2. 11
3. 3
4. 7
5. 28.5

Lesson 8.8, page 62
1. 2
2. 9
3. 9
4. 14
5. 21.4%

Lesson 8.9, page 63
1. 2
2. 4
3. 44
4. 4
5. 9

Lesson 8.10, page 64
1. 14
2. 20
3. 6
4. 50%
5. 6

Lesson 8.11, page 65
1.

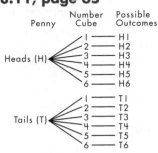

Penny	Number Cube	Possible Outcomes
Heads (H)	1	H1
	2	H2
	3	H3
	4	H4
	5	H5
	6	H6
Tails (T)	1	T1
	2	T2
	3	T3
	4	T4
	5	T5
	6	T6

2. 12
3. 6
4. 8
5. 36

Lesson 8.12, page 66
1. soccer team
2. 0.66 years
3. Jessi
4. $9.87
5. scarf shop = $57.71

Lesson 8.13, page 67
1. $\frac{1}{4}$
2. 3:16
3. 0.125
4. 0%
5. 50%

Lesson 8.14, page 68
1. $\frac{50}{8}$
2. 6
3. $\frac{2}{4}$
4. 24
5. 6; ANJ, AJN, JNA, JAN, NJA, NAJ

Posttest, page 69
1. 7
2. 1 person
3. 11
4. 4
5. 3
6. 8

Posttest, page 70
1. 0.5
2. 1:3
3. $\frac{2}{3}$
4. $\frac{1}{6}$
5. 83.3%
6. 0.7

Grade 7 Answers

Chapter 9

Pretest, page 71

1. 60°
2. $\overrightarrow{ZY}$
3. acute
4. 70°
5. trapezoid
6. pentagon

Lesson 9.1, page 72

1. $\overleftrightarrow{AB}$ $\overleftrightarrow{BA}$
2. $\overleftrightarrow{G \quad H}$
3. $\overline{JK}$, $\overline{KJ}$
4. $\overline{WX}$, $\overline{XW}$
5. $\overleftrightarrow{WX}$, $\overleftrightarrow{XW}$

Lesson 9.2, page 73

1. ∠ABC, ∠CBA
2. $\overrightarrow{MN}$
3. ∠ABC
4. no
5. $\overrightarrow{LK}$, $\overrightarrow{LM}$

Lesson 9.3, page 74

1. acute angle
2. 25°
3. 140°, obtuse angle
4. 90°, right angle
5. acute

Lesson 9.4, page 75

1. ∠DCA or ∠ACD
2. $\overrightarrow{OQ}$ and $\overrightarrow{OP}$
3. ∠ACB or ∠DCR
4. supplementary
5. ∠DCR or ∠RCD

Lesson 9.5, page 76

1. ∠6
2. alternate exterior angles
3. ∠8, ∠13, ∠16
4. ∠11
5. $\overleftrightarrow{IJ}$ and $\overleftrightarrow{KL}$

Lesson 9.6, page 77

1. right
2. isosceles
3. scalene
4. obtuse scalene
5. All three sides will be congruent, and all three angles will be congruent.

Lesson 9.7, page 78

1. 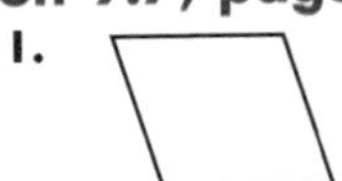 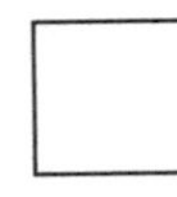

   rhombus square

2. Yes. A square is also a parallelogram with four right angles.
3. trapezoid, quadrilateral
4. quadrilateral, rectangle, parallelogram
5. Yes. A square is also a rhombus because a square has four congruent sides.

Lesson 9.8, page 79

1. decagon
2. nonagon
3. 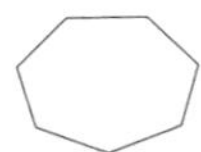
4. 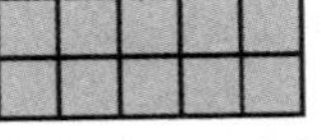
5. 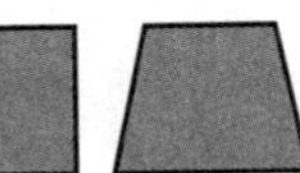 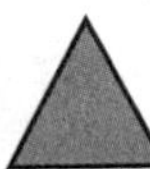

Lesson 9.9, page 80

1. 3.3
2. The corresponding angles are not all congruent, and corresponding sides are not all proportional.
3. similar
4. not similar

Lesson 9.10, page 81

1. *l*
2. (4, 3)
3. *A*
4. *B*
5. (4, −2)

Lesson 9.11, page 82

1. reflection
2. translation
3. dilation
4. rotation
5. reflection

Posttest, page 83

1. right, isosceles triangle
2. not similar
3. rotation, (−1, −2)
4. D A B C

Grade 7 Answers

Chapter 10

Pretest, page 84

1. 120
2. 81.64
3. 2,653.3
4. 104
5. 312
6. 152

Lesson 10.1, page 85

1. 340
2. 150
3. 130
4. 72
5. 150

Lesson 10.2, page 86

1. 35
2. 120
3. 432
4. 14
5. 25

Lesson 10.3, page 87

1. 540
2. 150
3. 6
4. 24
5. 126

Lesson 10.4, page 88

1. 125.6
2. 9.42
3. 25.12
4. 6
5. 50.24

Lesson 10.5, page 89

1. 78.5
2. 254.34
3. 12.56
4. 200.96
5. 452.16

Lesson 10.6, page 90

1. 1,200
2. 216
3. 80
4. 1,437.5
5. 10

Lesson 10.7, page 91

1. 3,056
2. 88
3. 488
4. 4
5. 142

Lesson 10.8, page 92

1. 120
2. 5
3. 270
4. 40
5. 20

Lesson 10.9, page 93

1. 800
2. 120
3. 105
4. 9.9
5. 40.5

Lesson 10.10, page 94

1. 13,345
2. 904.32
3. 3
4. 15.7
5. 1,186.92

Lesson 10.11, page 95

1. 2,009.6
2. 8,792
3. 480,812.5
4. 4
5. 942

Posttest, page 96

1. 24
2. 87.92
3. 63,360
4. 320
5. 21
6. 141.6; 100.8

Chapter 11

Pretest, page 97

1. $x - 5$
2. $y \div 4$
3. $n + 8 = 26$
4. $2(3) + 2(5) = 2(3 + 5)$
5. -8
6. $\frac{1}{4}$

Lesson 11.1, page 98

1. $c + 4$
2. $m - 5$
3. $72 - y = 45$
4. $d \div 3 = s$
5. $c > 2a$

Lesson 11.2, page 99

1. commutative property
2. multiplication property of zero
3. associative property
4. identity property
5. identity property

Grade 7 Answers

Lesson 11.3, page 100

1. $15(2 + 3)$
2. $a(4 + 7)$
3. $(5 \times 20) + (5 \times 2)$
4. $5(11 - 2)$
5. $8(v \times m) = (8 \times v) + (8 \times m)$

Lesson 11.4, page 101

1. 19
2. 8
3. 15
4. 14
5. 26

Lesson 11.5, page 102

1. 9
2. 20
3. 5
4. $3,650
5. 3

Lesson 11.6, page 103

1. 2
2. 6
3. 72
4. 6
5. 4

Lesson 11.7, page 104

1. $9J + 9T + 27$
2. $9(J + T) + 27$ or $(9J) + (9T + 27)$
3. $2x + 3$
4. $x - 2$

Lesson 11.8, page 105

1. 4
2. 25
3. −35
4. −4
5. 21

Lesson 11.9, page 106

1. $0
2. 30,340
3. −21°F
4. −550
5. 186°F
6. 75°C

Lesson 11.10, page 107

1. 216
2. 256
3. 5^5
4. 2^6
5. $2^2 \times 2^3$

Posttest, page 108

1. 10
2. $12 \div c$
3. 2^{11}
4. $48 - h = 32$
5. −3

Final Test Grade 7

Final Test, page 109

1. $17.16
2. 1.75
3. $2\frac{5}{6}$
4. $3\frac{9}{16}$
5. $2.33
6. 2.1

Final Test, page 110

1. 0.0042
2. 30%
3. 5,000
4. 580
5. 0.03
6. $575

Final Test, page 111

1. 7
2. **Hours of Exercise**

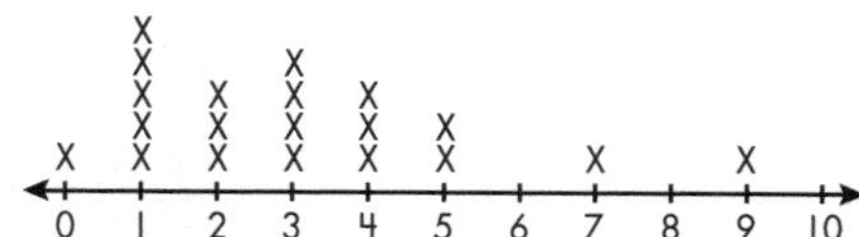

3. 0.25; $\frac{1}{4}$
4. similar, dilation
5. 37.68; 113.04

Final Test, page 112

1. 86
2. 87
3. Stem-and-leaf plot:

Stems	Leaves
7	8 9
8	0 1 3 3 4 5 6 7 9
9	2 2 2 4 5 6

Key: 7|8 = 78

4. 18
5. 17%
6. 452.16; 703.36

Final Test, page 113

1. ∠*RST* or ∠*TSR*
2. obtuse, scalene triangle
3. 5
4. 8
5. 5
6. 5

Final Test, page 114

1. 88; 384
2. 2($17 + $85)
3. $423
4. 13
5. 420

Notes